Critical Care Paramedicine
A Case-Based Approach

Critical Care Paramedicine
A Case-Based Approach

Edited by

David Anderson, Ben Meadley
and
Alexander Olaussen

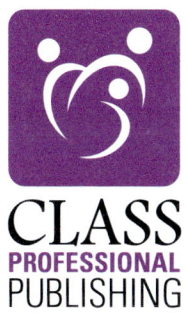

CLASS
PROFESSIONAL
PUBLISHING

Class Professional Publishing have made every effort to ensure that the information, tables, drawings and diagrams contained in this book are accurate at the time of publication. The book cannot always contain all the information necessary for determining appropriate care and cannot address all individual situations; therefore, individuals using the book must ensure they have the appropriate knowledge and skills to enable suitable interpretation. Class Professional Publishing does not guarantee, and accepts no legal liability of whatever nature arising from or connected to, the accuracy, reliability, currency or completeness of the content of *Critical Care Paramedicine*. Users must always be aware that such innovations or alterations after the date of publication may not be incorporated in the content. Please note, however, that Class Professional Publishing assumes no responsibility whatsoever for the content of external resources in the text or accompanying online materials.

Text © David Anderson, Ben Meadley and Alexander Olaussen, 2025

All rights reserved. Without limiting the rights under copyright reserved above, no part of this publication may be reproduced, stored in or introduced into a retrieval system, or transmitted, in any form or by any means (electronic, mechanical, photocopying, recording or otherwise) without the prior written permission of the publisher of this book.

The information presented in this book is accurate and current to the best of the authors' knowledge.

The authors and publisher, however, make no guarantee as to, and assume no responsibility for, the correctness, sufficiency or completeness of such information or recommendation.

Printing history
This edition first published in 2025.
The authors and publisher welcome feedback from the users of this book.

Please contact the publisher:

Class Professional Publishing,
The Exchange, Express Park, Bristol Road, Bridgwater TA6 4RR
Telephone: 01278 472 800
Email: info@class.co.uk
Website: www.classprofessional.co.uk
Class Professional Publishing is an imprint of Class Publishing Ltd

A CIP catalogue record for this book is available from the British Library

ISBN 9781801610377 (paperback)
ISBN 9781801610483 (ePDF)
ISBN 9781801610384 (ePub)

Cover design by Class Professional Publishing
Designed and typeset by PHi Business Solutions
Printed in the UK by Hobbs

This book is printed on paper from responsible sources. Refer to local recycling guidance on disposal of this book.

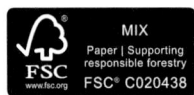

WORLD
LAND
TRUST™

www.carbonbalancedprint.com
CBP2250

Contents

Acknowledgements ix
Preface xi
About the Editors and Contributors xiii

Section 1 Airway 1
Chapter 1 Paramedic-Led Prehospital Rapid Sequence Intubation (RSI) 3
David Anderson, Ben Meadley and Alexander Olaussen

Chapter 2 The Physiologically Difficult Airway 13
Jonathan Begley and Ben Meadley

Chapter 3 The Anatomically Difficult Airway 24
Jason Bendall and Matt Humar

Section 2 Breathing 37
Chapter 4 Mechanical Ventilation 39
Tim Byrne and Nick Roder

Chapter 5 Respiratory Failure 49
Daniel Cudini and Segun Olusanya

Chapter 6 Severe and Life-Threatening Asthma 60
David Anderson and Tatsu Kuwasaki

Section 3 Circulation 69
Chapter 7 Undifferentiated Shock 71
Andy Celestia and Todd Wollum

Chapter 8 Myocardial Infarction (STEMI) 82
Luke Dawson, Ross Salathiel and Dion Stub

Chapter 9 The Management of Unstable Bradycardia 92
Alan Cowley and Mark Durell

Chapter 10 Palpitations and Chest Pain: Paramedic Management of Narrow Complex Tachycardias 100
Andrew Bishop

Chapter 11 Broad Complex Tachycardia 108
Tim Edwards and Kieren Pugh

Contents

Chapter 12	Acute Chest Pain and Shortness of Breath: Cardiogenic Shock Complicating Acute Myocardial Infarction *Jason Bloom and Dave Hawkins*	116
Chapter 13	Massive Upper Gastrointestinal Bleed (UGIB) *Sarah Yong and Michelle Murphy*	124
Chapter 14	Acute Pulmonary Oedema *Nick Trestrail and Luke Hamilton*	133

Section 4   Disability — 145
Chapter 15	Approach to an Altered Level of Consciousness *Luke De La Rue and Natalie Lavergne*	147
Chapter 16	Severe Traumatic Brain Injury *James Manktelow and Virginia Newcombe*	157
Chapter 17	Assessment and Management of Acute Ischaemic Stroke *Skye Coote and Henry Zhao*	168
Chapter 18	Severe/Uncontrolled Pain *Todd Blackburn*	182

Section 5   Exposure — 193
Chapter 19	Hypothermia and Hyperthermia *Eystein Grusd and Justin Hensley*	195
Chapter 20	Prehospital Sepsis Management *Daniel Cudini and Judit Orosz*	200

Section 6   Cardiac Arrest — 209
Chapter 21	High-Performance CPR *Belinda Delardes, Jack Howard and Ziad Nehme*	211
Chapter 22	Refractory Cardiac Arrest and Salvage Extracorporeal Cardiopulmonary Resuscitation (ECPR) *Matthew Thornton, Julia Coull and Sacha Richardson*	218
Chapter 23	Traumatic Cardiac Arrest *Zainab Alqudah and Brian Burns*	228
Chapter 24	Cardiac Arrest in Special Circumstances *Casey Lewis and Claire Bertenshaw*	239
Chapter 25	Termination of Resuscitation *Natalie Anderson*	247

Section 7   Trauma — 255
Chapter 26	The Trapped Patient *Tash Adams*	257

Chapter 27	Shocked Blunt Trauma *Michael Noonan, Ben Meadley and Alexander Olaussen*	266
Chapter 28	Penetrating Trauma *Kat Baird, Peter Sherren and Scott Wallman*	275
Chapter 29	Severe Chest Injury: Tension Pneumothorax *Mark Fitzgerald and Toby St Clair*	284

Section 8 Toxicology 295

Chapter 30	Tricyclic Antidepressant Toxicity *Ben Fitzgerald and Michael Mann*	297
Chapter 31	Acute Behavioural Disturbance: Emergency Pharmacological Sedation *Claire Bertenshaw and Lachlan Parker*	307
Chapter 32	Severe Metabolic Acidosis *Tash Adams and John Glasheen*	317

Section 9 Paediatrics, Obstetrics and Gynaecology 325

Chapter 33	Croup and Epiglottitis *Brad Gander and Claire Wilkin*	327
Chapter 34	Care of the Newborn: Assisting Transition, Stabilisation and Transport *Rosemarie Boland and James Yates*	342
Chapter 35	Maternal Bleeding: Postpartum Haemorrhage and Active Management of the Third Stage of Labour *Mark Durham and Dawn Kerslake*	353

Section 10 Special Circumstances 367

Chapter 36	The Older Patient *David Anderson and Tegwyn McManamny*	369
Chapter 37	Providing Paramedic Care in Resource-Limited Settings *Matt Cannon and Felix Ho*	382

Index **395**

Acknowledgements

We would like to take a moment to express our heartfelt gratitude to the many individuals and organisations who have contributed to the creation of this critical care book for paramedics. Without their invaluable support, expertise and collaboration, this project would not have been possible.

First and foremost, we extend our deepest appreciation to the paramedics, healthcare professionals and colleagues who work tirelessly on the frontlines of patient care. Your dedication, compassion and unwavering commitment to improving the lives of others inspire us every day. It is your collective expertise and real-world experiences that have shaped the practicality and relevance of the content within these pages.

We are immensely grateful to our esteemed collaborators, including researchers, educators and clinicians, who have generously shared their knowledge and insights. Your contributions have enriched the book with evidence-based information, diverse perspectives and invaluable expertise. Your passion for advancing the field of critical care has been instrumental in ensuring the accuracy and relevance of the content.

To the patients and their families, we extend our deepest appreciation. Your trust, resilience and willingness to participate in the healing process have taught us invaluable lessons. You serve as a constant reminder of the profound impact that our work as paramedics can have on individuals and communities. It is your stories and experiences that drive us continually to improve and strive for excellence.

We would also like to express our gratitude to Class Professional Publishing for their unwavering support and belief in the importance of this book. Their expertise in publishing and their dedication to providing educational resources for healthcare professionals have been instrumental in bringing this project to fruition.

Last, we would like to acknowledge you, the reader. Your commitment to enhancing your knowledge and skills as a paramedic is commendable. By engaging with the material in this book and putting it into practice, you play a crucial role in elevating the standard of critical care and making a meaningful impact on patient outcomes. Your dedication and passion for learning inspire us to continue our work in supporting paramedics worldwide.

In conclusion, we are deeply grateful for the collaborative effort and support from all those who have contributed to this critical care book. Together, we can make a difference in the lives of patients, their families and the communities we serve.

Thank you.

DA, BM and AO
Editors

Preface

It is with enormous pleasure that we introduce our case-based critical care paramedicine textbook. As the editors, we aim to capitalise on the expertise of our specialist collaborators from all over the world to empower you to provide exceptional care to critically ill patients, regardless of degree of illness or geography.

Paramedicine is a young, rapidly advancing profession, and the importance of up-to-date, evidence-based practice cannot be overstated. Paramedics are tasked with making critical decisions in time-sensitive situations, where every action may significantly impact outcomes. We have endeavoured to use an evidence-based approach whenever there is existing literature to support the decision. In the absence of such evidence, we have relied on the practical expertise of our contributors, who are all specialist critical care clinicians. This approach ensures that you will learn the most effective and efficient interventions available.

This is a case-based book. It is our experience – as clinicians, educators and students ourselves – that such texts are extremely popular, as they are both exam focused and also well suited to casual reading and 'just in time' learning.

Each chapter is based on a realistic case, which leads into a question and answer based dialogue that lends itself to study for both written exams and vivas, as well as providing an easily digestible format for those not actively studying. Each chapter is written by two or three experts in critical care and paramedicine. We have used our large international network of professional colleagues across Australasia, the UK, Europe, Asia and North America to ensure that the context reflects international best practice.

You will notice some overlap between chapters, and maybe even some repetition of concepts. This is deliberate. We want to give our subject-matter experts the opportunity to share their knowledge and experience, while you as the adult learner can benefit from ideas being presented from different points of view.

We would like to express our sincere gratitude to the researchers, clinicians and educators who have dedicated their efforts to generating and disseminating high-quality evidence. Their commitment to improving patient care has been the cornerstone of this book, and we owe a debt of gratitude to their tireless pursuit of scientific excellence.

We have strived to engage a diverse group of collaborators, but must acknowledge that there are still not as many women among the authors as we would have liked. Despite paramedicine rapidly advancing in terms of diversity and equality, critical care paramedicine remains a male-dominated specialty. We are immensely grateful to the women who have contributed and also to those who considered our offer but had to prioritise other activities. We hope that we have created enough diversity among the expert voices in our book to help inspire female paramedics to consider a career in critical care, and we very much hope that a future edition of this book will have a more diverse authorship, reflective of the evolving workforce.

Preface

Finally, we extend our deepest appreciation to you, the reader. Your dedication to evidence-based practice is a testament to your commitment to delivering the best possible care to your patients. We hope that this book will serve as a trusted companion in your journey as a critical care paramedic, guiding you through the complexities of patient management with a solid foundation in evidence-based principles. We have all been where you are now, and wish we had had a book like this to help us along the way.

David Anderson, Ben Meadley, and Alexander Olaussen
Editors

About the Editors and Contributors

About the Editors

David Anderson
MStJ BSc MBChB MBioeth DipPallMed FCICM
David is the Medical Director of Ambulance Victoria, an intensive care physician at The Alfred Hospital, Melbourne and an Adjunct Associate Professor in the Department of Paramedicine at Monash University. David worked as a paramedic in Auckland, New Zealand before completing medical training at the University of Auckland and then undertaking postgraduate training in intensive care medicine, anaesthesia, palliative medicine and prehospital and retrieval medicine in Auckland, Sydney and Toronto before settling in Melbourne. His clinical interests are prehospital and retrieval medicine, trauma critical care, ECMO, palliative care and bioethics.

Ben Meadley
ASM, BAppSci, DipSci, GradDip ICP, GradCert Aeromed, PhD, FACPara
Ben is an Adjunct Associate Professor at Monash University in the Department of Paramedicine. Ben has more than 25 years experience, gaining expertise in prehospital critical care, paramedic education, paramedic health research, search and rescue, human performance, systems improvement and clinical guideline development. The majority of Ben's experience is working as an Intensive Care Flight Paramedic (MICA) at Ambulance Victoria. He divides his time between clinical, systems improvement and research roles.

Alexander Olaussen
BEH, BMedSc(Hons), MBBS(Hons), FHEA, MACPara
Alex is a paramedic, doctor and a senior lecturer at Monash University in the Department of Paramedicine. Alex has years of clinical and research experience, with expertise in bridging the pre-hospital and in-hospital environments in critical care. The majority of Alex' experience is working as a rural emergency doctor and conducting research related to paramedicine. Alex holds a Fellowship of the Higher Education Academy and divides his time between clinical care, mentoring and fostering novice researchers and optimising educational strategies.

About the Contributors

Natasha (Tash) Adams is a Senior Critical Care Paramedic (CCP) with the Queensland Ambulance Service, working on the Woodridge CCP POD and with the High Acuity Response Unit. Tash has a Graduate Diploma in Intensive Care Paramedic Practice, a Master in Health Care Leadership and a Master in Traumatology. Tash uses her knowledge and experience to contribute to clinical education, professional development, and leadership development

About the Editors and Contributors

within the ambulance sector. Tash also has a passion for progressive trauma care, and is currently contributing to research on blood product administration led by the Gold Coast University Hospital Trauma Service, as well as being actively involved in quality assurance and data collection in her HARU role. Tash has most recently led the Queensland Ambulance Service graduate paramedic program renewal project and continues to value the development of the newest staff to paramedic practice as a priority focus.

Zainab Alqudah is an accomplished professional from Jordan with a diverse background in academia and research in paramedicine. She currently serves as an Assistant Professor in the Faculty of Applied Medical Sciences at Jordan University of Science & Technology (JUST), Jordan, and an Adjunct Lecturer in the Department of Paramedicine at Monash University, Australia. She was a graduate paramedic from JUST in 2011 and completed her MSc in Emergency Health Services at University of Maryland, Baltimore County, US, in 2015. She also holds a PhD in Paramedicine from Monash University. She is an active researcher with prehospital emergency care and resuscitation research expertise. She was recognised with several awards for her contributions and published several research in Q1 journals. She is an active reviewer and a board member of both the Scientific and Community committees at the Arab Resuscitation Council."

Natalie Anderson is a senior lecturer and currently practising nurse with over 25 years of clinical experience in emergency, intensive care, and prehospital settings. Informed by a dual-discipline academic background in nursing (BHSc, PhD) and health psychology (BA, MSc), her research seeks to understand and improve acute care in the context of death, dying and bereavement. Natalie's PhD explored paramedic decisions to commence, continue, withhold or terminate resuscitation, and she continues to undertake, supervise, publish, and present thought-leading research in this important area.

Kat Baird is an Emergency Medicine Consultant at The Royal London Hospital (A Major Trauma Centre) and a Flight Doctor for Essex and Hertfordshire Air Ambulance Trust. She is a Senior Lecturer at Queen Mary's University, London, lecturing on a BSc in Pre-Hospital Medicine. She has previously completed a 14-month secondment to the Physician Response Unit in London, a pre-hospital emergency medicine service.

Jonathan Begley is an anaesthetist and intensive care physician in the Australian Regular Army. His work and volunteer pursuits included prehospital and event medicine for over ten years, and he completed a fellowship in aeromedical retrieval medicine with LifeFlight in Queensland, Australia. Jonathan has published several papers on airway management, one of which earned him recognition as an *Anaesthesia* Top-10 author and the Felicity Hawker Medal. He is an author of the 11th Edition ATLS airway management section, and teaches on the Critically Ill Airway course, among others. Jonathan holds Honours degrees in Medicine/Surgery and Medical Science, a Master of Public Health degree, and a Graduate Diploma in Adult Education. He is an adjunct senior lecturer at Monash University.

Jason Bendall is the Clinical Dean at the Manning Clinical School within the Department of Rural Health. Jason completed his undergraduate studies in 1991 completing an

About the Editors and Contributors

honours degree in medical science before becoming a paramedic. Jason graduated with a medical degree and (MBBS) and a PhD in medicine in 2004 subsequently specialising in anaesthesia. Jason has undertaken further postgraduate studies in clinical epidemiology and biostatistics.

Claire Bertenshaw is an Emergency Medicine Specialist who is the Deputy Medical Director at the Queensland Ambulance Service. She works on road with the High Acuity Response Unit and in the Clinical Hub. She is also employed at the Emergency and Trauma Centre at the Royal Brisbane and Women's Hospital and at LifeFlight Retrieval Medicine as a Pre-Hospital and Retrieval Consultant. Her current interests include point of care ultrasound, recognition of the deteriorating patient, and the clinical assessment of risk.

Andrew Bishop is a MICA Flight Paramedic at Ambulance Victoria and a Teaching Associate at Monash University. Holding a Bachelor of Health Science and postgraduate degrees in Prehospital Intensive Care and Aeromedical Retrieval, he is passionate about ECG interpretation, particularly in recognising Occlusion Myocardial Infarction and the pre-hospital application of Artificial Intelligence in ECG interpretation. His educational focus is on simplifying and making ECG interpretation accessible and practical for pre-hospital care providers of all experience levels.

Todd Blackburn is a Mobile Intensive Care Paramedic with Ambulance Victoria. He has worked extensively throughout Victoria and is extremely passionate about prehospital education. He is also a teaching associate and works closely with Monash University in the postgraduate paramedicine department. His main areas of interest are airway management and pharmacology. He has previously published in *Emergency Medicine Australasia*.

Jason Bloom graduated from the University of Melbourne Medical school in 2013. After completing cardiology training at The Alfred Hospital in Melbourne, Jason undertook a Ph.D., which focused the management of cardiogenic shock. His doctoral research, supported by the National Health and Medical Research Council (NHMRC) and the National Heart Foundation (NHF), explored the epidemiology of cardiogenic shock and the application of vasoactive medications in this clinical setting.

Rosemarie Boland is an Associate Professor in the Department of Obstetrics and Gynaecology at the University of Melbourne, and a statewide perinatal educator with the Paediatric Infant Perinatal Emergency Retrieval (PIPER) service in Victoria- a role she has held since 2000. She completed her PhD in 2014, investigating risk factors for very preterm birth in non-tertiary hospitals and in the pre-hospital environment (paramedic practice). Her postdoctoral research has focused on developing a suite of strategies aimed at improving outcomes of babies born preterm in non-tertiary hospitals and in paramedic practice. Rose has collaborated with Ambulance Victoria for more than a decade to develop clinical practice guidelines and training resources for paramedics in Victoria and provides advice on equipment purchase for care of newborn babies for Ambulance Victoria. She is also the educational developer for the *NeoResus* program, a multidisciplinary neonatal resuscitation training program, taught in 5 states in Australia.

About the Editors and Contributors

Brian Burns is a Prehospital and Retrieval Medicine Physician with NSW Ambulance, an Emergency Physician at Northern Beaches Hospital, Sydney, a clinical professor at the University of Sydney and Macquarie University and an Honorary Senior Lecturer at Queen Mary University London.

Tim Byrne is an Intensivist and Anaesthetist practicing at The Alfred hospital in Melbourne, Australia. He is also a clinical educator with an interest in simulation and educational device design and is a Senior Adjunct Lecturer at Monash University as well as a Research Fellow at Createlab.

Matt Cannon is an accomplished leader in emergency medical services. Currently the CEO of Papua New Guinea St John Ambulance, he has significantly expanded emergency services in the region. Matt's is a registered nurse and paramedic. His extensive background includes serving as a paramedic for NSW Ambulance, as well as working for the NSW Department of Health and the NSW Minister for Health between 2014 and 2015. He is a Board Director with the Council of Ambulance Authorities and contributes academically at the University of Sydney and lectured in paramedicine at Charles Sturt University, Sydney. Matt was honoured as an Officer of the Most Venerable Order of St John by Queen Elizabeth II in 2018, highlighting his commitment to healthcare and emergency medical services. Matt was admitted as a Fellow of the College of Paramedicine in 2023 for his contribution to paramedicine in the Pacific Region.

Andy Celestia is an emergency medicine physician who is completing an emergency medical services (EMS) fellowship at the University of Washington in Seattle, Washington, USA. They work with the medical directors for Seattle and King County Medic One and with the associated Paramedic Training Institute. Clinically, Dr. Celestia works at a University of Washington emergency department in Seattle and as a flight physician for the University's air medical transport service, Airlift Northwest. They were inspired to pursue emergency medicine after taking an EMT-basic course in Los Angeles, California. They received their Doctor of Medicine degree at the University of Michigan Medical School and completed a residency in emergency medicine at the Henry Ford Hospital in Detroit, Michigan, USA. They have a unique background, with a Bachelor of Music from the Berklee College of Music and a Master of Science in Civil and Environmental Engineering from the University of California, Berkeley, with working experience in both fields prior to making the shift into emergency medicine.

Skye Coote is a Stroke Nurse Practitioner and is the Nursing Lead of the Melbourne Mobile Stroke Unit project, based at the Royal Melbourne Hospital. She has an extensive critical care background in both Intensive Care and Emergency Departments. She has a post-graduate diploma in Critical Care Nursing. Since 2010 she has specialised in stroke. During this time, she has completed a Master's Degree in Nursing and stroke fellowship training. She was the first certified Advanced Neurovascular Practitioner in Australia. She is also certified as a Neurovascular Registered Nurse and an Advanced Stroke Coordinator. She currently sits on the Board of Directors of the Association of Neurovascular Clinicians and has previously been a Director and Chair of the Acute Stroke Nurses Education Network. She has won numerous awards for her work in stroke, including clinical excellence and leadership awards.

About the Editors and Contributors

She is frequently invited to present at both national and international conferences and is internationally published.

Julia Coull is an Intensive Care Specialist from Melbourne, Australia and has completed an ECMO fellowship at the Alfred Hospital. She is an Education Lead for the Victorian ECMO Service focusing on curriculum development, minimum education standards and credentialing for ECMO practice and a co-convener of the Foundation ECMO course. She is a key member of the prehospital ECMO for refractory cardiac arrest service based out of the Alfred Hospital. She is also the Clinical Human Factors lead for Alfred Health and used these skills in the prehospital space, designing equipment and organisational workflow for prehospital ECMO application.

Alan Cowley is an Advanced Paramedic in Critical Care with South East Coast Ambulance Service NHS Foundation Trust in the UK. He gained his MSc in in Emergency and Resuscitation Medicine at Queen Mary University of London. As well as spending his career working in the National Health Service, he also spent 8 years working for Kent Surrey Sussex Air Ambulance. He has authored several peer-reviewed articles and has a special interest in spinal care.

Daniel Cudini is a Clinical Support Officer and Intensive Care Paramedic with Ambulance Victoria (AV), Melbourne, Australia. He is a teaching associate at the department of paramedicine, Monash University and a published author of various research papers in prehospital care. He is an associate investigator of the PASS trial (A phase 2 study of pre hospital blood culture collection and IV ceftriaxone in patients with community acquired sepsis) and other interest areas include management of critical asthma and anaphylaxis.

Luke Dawson is a researcher and cardiologist from Melbourne, Australia previously working at the Alfred and Cabrini hospitals. He is currently undertaking further training in interventional and structural cardiology at Stanford Medicine, California. His main interests are in cardiovascular epidemiology, systems of care, structural and interventional cardiology, and prediction and prognostic modelling. His PhD at the Alfred Hospital and Monash University focusses on improving diagnostic and care pathways in chest pain including for patients with ST elevation myocardial infarction.

Luke De La Rue is an Emergency Physician based in Melbourne, Victoria, with extensive experience in Pre-Hospital and Retrieval medicine. He has worked in Helicopter Emergency Medical Services (HEMS) with LifeFlight in Toowoomba, Queensland, and currently serves as a Retrieval Physician for Adult Retrieval Victoria (ARV). As a Fellow of the Australasian College for Emergency Medicine (FACEM), Luke continues to work as an Emergency Physician at The Royal Melbourne Hospital (RMH), one of Australia's largest major trauma services. He holds postgraduate qualifications in Aeromedical Retrieval, Disaster Management, and Humanitarian Assistance. Luke's special interests include Clinical Toxicology, Point of Care Ultrasound (PoCUS),and medical education. During his time at Guy's and St Thomas' NHS Foundation Trust in London, he contributed to multiple peer-reviewed publications in Clinical Toxicology. He holds a Certificate of Clinician Performed Ultrasound (CCPU) and is a member of The RMH Ultrasound Steering Group, contributing to clinical governance and training in

About the Editors and Contributors

PoCUS for Emergency Medicine trainees. Luke is actively involved in medical education, having lectured for the Master of Specialist Paramedic Practice program at Monash University. He also teaches on various courses, including Emergency Resuscitation with Ultrasonography (ERUSC), and The Royal Melbourne Hospital's High Acuity Basic Interactive Teaching Sessions (HA-BITS) and Basic Interactive Teaching Sessions (BITS) in Trauma.

Belinda Delardes is an ALS paramedic and clinical instructor with Ambulance Victoria (AV). Following her graduate year with AV, she undertook an Honours degree with Monash University focusing on handovers between paramedics and GPs. After achieving the Monash Department of Paramedicine 2019 Academic Excellence in Research Award for this, Belinda continued on with a PhD to improve the referral process from paramedics to GPs in Victoria, Australia. Belinda has been employed in the position of Resuscitation Officer in the Victorian Ambulance Cardiac Arrest Registry for the past year and is a passionate advocate for improving patient safety.

Mark Durell is a Specialist Paramedic (Critical Care) with South East Coast Ambulance service, Specialist Paramedic Lead at Hampshire and Isle of Wight Air Ambulance, UK, and a Senior Lecturer at The University of Brighton.

Mark Durham qualified with a BSc in Paramedic Science from Hertfordshire in 2005, gaining his MSc in 2013. He has been a Critical Care Paramedic for 13 years and currently specialises in all forms of high acuity care, including obstetric emergencies in Brighton, UK (an area which sees a high number of high-risk community births). He also enjoys teaching and has worked as an instructor on various obstetric/newborn courses.

Tim Edwards BA (Hons), BSc (Hons), PGCert, PGCert HCL, PGCert MSc, MSc, PhD, PGCE, FIMC RCSEd, FHEA, MCPara.

Tim Edwards is a consultant Paramedic. Tim joined the LAS in 1997, qualifying as a paramedic in 2000. He has worked as an operational ambulance and FRU paramedic, HEMS paramedic, paramedic practitioner, clinical team leader and advanced paramedic practitioner (APP) in critical care. He holds a visiting lecturer post at the University of Hertfordshire and is an examiner for the diploma and fellowship examinations in immediate medical care at the Royal College of Surgeons Edinburgh. He holds Masters degrees in cardiology and emergency & resuscitation medicine and a PhD investigating out-of-hospital airway management in cardiac arrest. He continues to undertake regular operational clinical shifts.

Ben Fitzgerald completed medical school at the University of Colorado, emergency medicine residency at the University of Iowa, and EMS fellowship at the University of Washington where he had the opportunity to work with King County EMS and the Seattle Fire Department and flew as a flight physician with Airlift Northwest. He now works as an emergency medicine and emergency medical services physician in Anchorage, Alaska. He is passionate about exceptional care of the critically ill or injured, both in and out of the hospital, particularly with interest in cardiac arrest as well as provider wellness.

Mark Fitzgerald is Director of Trauma Services at The Alfred Hospital; Director of the National Trauma Research Institute; Adjunct Professor, Department of Surgery, School of Translational

About the Editors and Contributors

Medicine, Monash University; and Honorary Professor, School of Information Technology, Faculty of Science, Engineering and Built Environment, Deakin University.

Brad Gander is a Critical Care Paramedic for the South East Coast Ambulance Service. Since starting in patient transport services in 2008 he has worked in a number of emergency operations centre and operational roles. He holds a FdSc in Paramedic Science, BSc in Professional Practice and MSc in Prehospital Critical Care and is currently studying in disaster response. His academic interests include prehospital resuscitation and major incidents.

John Glasheen is a prehospital and retrieval physician at Queensland Ambulance Service and LifeFlight Retrieval Medicine, and an emergency specialist at Logan Hospital in Brisbane. His prehospital career started as a paramedic in Ireland. John has a particular interest in prehospital critical care education, and a research background in emergency airway management.

Eystein Grusd is a Paramedic, Researcher, and Educator from Oslo, Norway. He is an Assistant Professor at Oslo Metropolitan University, Faculty of Health Sciences, Division of Emergency Medical Services. Grusds main interest is emergency medical services provided in austere and remote environments, and he has worked as a paramedic in Oslo, as a mountain guide, in emergency medical teams, and with remote wilderness emergency medicine. Grusd has extensive experience working in austere environments.

Luke Hamilton is a Critical Care Paramedic with South East Coast Ambulance Service delivering enhanced care to the population of Kent, Surrey and Sussex, England. Luke is a member of the Health and Care Professions Council, and also a member of the College of Paramedics. Starting his career in the ambulance service in 2006 as an ambulance technician, progressing to paramedic via St Georges University Foundation degree in Paramedic Sciences in 2012, at the College of Surgeons of Edinburgh a Diploma in Immediate Medical Care was attained in 2017, and then a PGCert in Critical Care at the University of Hertfordshire in 2018. I have a special interest in heart failure and patient experience. I would like to thank everyone involved in this publication for the opportunity to contribute, particularly David Anderson.

Dave Hawkins is a Senior Leader and Critical Care Paramedic for the South East Coast Ambulance Service NHS Foundation Trust. After joining the London Ambulance Service in 2001, he qualified as a Paramedic in 2004 and a Critical Care Paramedic in 2010. Dave has completed a secondment as a HEMS Paramedic on the Kent, Surrey and Sussex Air Ambulance where he continues to practice on an emeritus basis. In 2017 he earned his Masters Degree in Advanced Paramedic Practice and has co-authored a chapter of JRCALC, the UK's national ambulance service clinical guidelines. He has a special interest in resuscitation and pre-hospital critical care.

Justin Hensley is an emergency medicine and retrieval physician in Australia with an interest in remote and austere medicine. He trained in emergency medicine in the US at East Carolina University, and was medical director of multiple EMS agencies in Texas. He moved to Australia to practice prehospital and retrieval medicine, where he worked for CareFlight and New South Wales Ambulance, and he now works for the Royal Flying Doctor Service.

About the Editors and Contributors

Felix Ho is a paramedic and medical practitioner from Darwin, Australia. His main interests are in resource limited health care, major incident health management, road trauma and community volunteerism. He holds undergraduate degrees in health science (paramedic), and training and development; he holds postgraduate degrees in medicine, critical care paramedicine, and public health. Felix is a Lecturer with Flinders University and is an adjunct Associate Professor in Paramedicine at Charles Darwin University

Jack Howard is an Intensive Care Paramedic at Ambulance Victoria in Melbourne, Australia. Jack has been working across Victoria, predominantly in the Northern suburbs of Melbourne, as a front-line Paramedic for the past 13 years. He has special interest on the subjects of education, CPR-Induced Consciousness and addiction. Jack has a BSc in Health Science (Paramedicine) from Victoria University and MSc in Specialist Paramedic Practice from Monash University.

Matthew Humar is an intensive care paramedic with Ambulance Victoria (AV) in Melbourne, Australia where he primarily works as an operational paramedic. In addition to this role, he has held temporary secondments with the Patient Safety and Experience and Education departments within AV. He is also currently a member of faculty in the discipline of paramedicine at Monash University, Australia, and a board member with the interprofessional Safe Airway Society (SAS). His main interests are prehospital airway management (particularly advanced airway management), human factors, patient safety, and the overlay between these three concepts.

Dawn Kerslake is a consultant Midwife and former emergency department nurse within the South East Coast ambulance service. She has an MSc in leadership and service improvement and has recently been part of a small working group which led on the (OOH NLS) out of hospital new-born life support RCUK course. She is also a member of the AACE Maternity Ambulance Leads Group and JRCALC as the pre hospital maternity lead. She continues to practice as a midwife on an honorary contract in the South East.

Tatsu Kuwasaki is a Critical Care Flight Paramedic/Clinical Manager for HEMS New Zealand Ltd, the sole Helicopter Air Ambulance Provider for the South Island of New Zealand. Tatsu holds the paramedic engagement role, which is responsible for ensuring a high-standard credentialing process, designing and delivering clinical education, and overseeing the professional development of all flight paramedics within the organization. Additionally, Tatsu's personal interests have led him to take the lead in implementing a point-of-care ultrasound program for HEMS.

Natalie Lavergne currently works full-time as a critical care paramedic and educator with Ornge in Ontario, Canada. In addition to her clinical role, Natalie is a part-time professor at Algonquin College in the Paramedic Program and the Advanced Care Paramedic Program. Natalie has more than 20 years of experience providing prehospital critical care in both the HEMS and ground critical care environment and has a special interest in the development and delivery of paramedic education.

About the Editors and Contributors

Casey Lewis is a senior critical care paramedic with Queensland Ambulance Service. Over the past 18 years he has worked in various capacities in paramedicine across Australia and the Pacific region including critical care, aeromedical operations, rural and remote care provision as well as aid and development. Casey has also taught into paramedic programs at Queensland University of Technology, Australian Catholic University, and the University of Southern Queensland. Informed by his experience across the sector, Casey is passionate about disaster management, capacity development and systems strengthening and has a particular interest in how these are applied in lower resource settings. He holds a Bachelor of Health Science (Paramedic), a Graduate Diploma of Intensive Care Paramedic Practice and a Master of Health Management (Emergency & Disaster Management).

James Manktelow has always been drawn to the emergency services and qualified as a paramedic in 2023 from Oxford Brookes University. Working for South Central Ambulance Service, he has a particular interest in critical care, a passion he developed working in Addenbrookes Emergency Department prior to studying his degree. James is continuing to develop his skills and interests within Paramedic Sciences and has begun training as a Reserve Paramedic for the Royal Air Force. James wishes to thank Dr Virginia Newcombe for providing him with this opportunity and her ongoing support.

Michael 'Miki' Mann is a firefighter/paramedic in Seattle, Washington USA. He has undergraduate degrees in Economics and Accounting and a Master of Architecture degree. He joined the Seattle Fire Department (SFD) in 1987. In 1989 he began the high-angle rescue team, the Rescue company for the SFD. In 1993 he completed his training at the University of Washington/Harborview Medical Center Paramedic Training (UW/HMC PMT) program to become a certified paramedic. In his 30 years as a firefighter/paramedic, he has trained, mentored, and evaluated hundreds of paramedic students. He also spent 5 years as a CONTOMS- and TCCC-trained SWAT medic and spent several years training fire departments and law enforcement agencies in tactical medicine. He is currently responsible for a multi-year project to restructure the methodology that the SFD uses to respond to large-scale disasters. He is currently the SFD subject matter expert in Active Shooter/Hostile Event Response and Large-scale Disaster Response;. Finally, he developed and currently operates a simulation lab that reinforces Department training objectives and trains fire chiefs and fire officers to manage incidents.

Tegwyn McManamny is an Intensive Care Paramedic and prehospital researcher, and is an Adjunct Senior Lecturer with Monash University's Department of Paramedicine. She holds an Honours Degree in Emergency Health (Paramedicine), a Graduate Diploma in Emergency Health (Intensive Care Paramedicine) and PhD from Monash University, Australia. Her research interests span rural health, patient safety, gerontology and community paramedicine. She is the paramedic representative on Safer Care Victoria's Acute Care Learning Health Network Advisory Group, sits on the Albury Wodonga Health Human Research Ethics Committee and is a passionate advocate for safe and high quality prehospital care.

Michelle Murphy ASM, is an intensive care paramedic with a passion for improving systems of care that lead to improved health outcomes for vulnerable populations. Michelle has undergraduate degrees in Nursing and Paramedicine and a Masters in Emergency Health. Moving from a senior management role in an ambulance service, Michelle currently holds dual appointments. Firstly, as the National Manager for Integrated Care Pathways and Partnerships with ForHealth - the leading Australian provider of Urgent Care Services secondly as the Advocacy & Government Relations lead for the Australasian College of Paramedicine. She has undertaken and published research focusing on Out of Hospital Cardiac arrest and improving health outcomes for vulnerable populations and is passionate about the role paramedics play in the future of health care models in Australia. This passion led to her appointment with the University of Sunshine Coast School of Health and position on the advisory committee into micro-credentialing for Urgent Care and further post graduate studies in public policy.

Ziad Nehme ASM PhD FACPara is the Director of Research and Evaluation at Ambulance Victoria and a practising paramedic with over 16 years clinical experience. Ziad holds appointments as a Heart Foundation Future Leader Fellow at the School of Public Health and Preventive Medicine, Monash University and Adjunct Senior Lecturer at the Department of Paramedicine, Monash University. Ziad is also chair of Ambulance Victoria's Cardiac Arrest and Heart Attack clinical quality registries, Executive Member of the Australasian Resuscitation Outcomes Consortium (Aus-ROC), and Basic Life Support Task Force Member of International Liaison Committee on Resuscitation.

Virginia Newcombe is a Consultant in Neurosciences and Trauma Critical Care and Emergency Medicine based at Addenbrooke's Hospital, Cambridge and University of Cambridge, UK. She is the first female Royal College of Emergency Medicine (RCEM) Professor and holds a National Institute for Health and Care Research (NIHR) Advanced Fellowship. Her research encompasses all severities of TBI from mild to severe and focuses on the integration of neuroimaging, biomarkers and clinical data to understand the pathophysiology of TBI, trajectories of outcome and aid prognostication.

Michael (Mike) Noonan is a consultant in the trauma service at the Alfred Hospital, Melbourne and a PhD candidate with the Department of Surgery at the Monash University Central Clinical School. Mike is a fellow of the Australasian College of Emergency Medicine, holds an Associate Fellowship with the Royal Australasian College of Medical Administrators, has completed a Fellowship in Trauma Surgery and Critical Care at the Alfred Hospital, Melbourne and holds a Masters of Medical Education.

Mike's Ikigai (reasons for being...in his work life at least!) include Trauma Care, Clinical Leadership, Trauma Research and Education. Having worked as both a Physiotherapist and Medical practitioner caring for the injured, Mike understands that Trauma Care is truly a team pursuit. Outside his work pursuits, Mike is a proud father and volunteer surf lifesaver and can be found regularly enjoying activities that have the potential to lead to him becoming a trauma unit inpatient!

Segun Olusanya is an Intensive Care Consultant at St Bartholomew's Hospital, London, with special interests in extracorporeal membrane oxygenation (ECMO), critical care outreach, clinician wellbeing, point of care ultrasound, equality/diversity/inclusion, and online education.

About the Editors and Contributors

Judit Orosz is an Intensive Care Specialist and the Deputy Director (Operations) at The Alfred ICU. She originally trained in Hungary and Ireland in Anaesthesia and Intensive Care Medicine before completing Intensive Care training, ultrasound and echocardiography training in Australia.

Lachlan Parker is a Critical Care Paramedic hailing from Brisbane, Australia. After a short-lived career as a registered nurse in a large metropolitan emergency department, he quickly realised his passion for pre-hospital healthcare and commenced employment with the Queensland Ambulance Service in 1998. Following several years working clinically on-road and as a flight paramedic, he transitioned into an ambulance management position to support frontline clinicians. With over 25 years of pre-hospital experience, Lachlan currently leads the Clinical Policy Unit of the Queensland Ambulance Service, showcasing his commitment to pre-hospital evidence-based guidelines in Australia. His research interests include the pharmacological management of acute behavioural disturbance and the translation of research into clinical practice. He has an undergraduate qualification in nursing and postgraduate qualifications in paramedicine, health science and health services management.

Kieren Pugh works as a Critical Care Paramedic at South East Coast Ambulance Service. He has completed the Diploma in Immediate Medical Care (DIMC) from the Royal College of Surgeons in Edinburgh and has an MSc in Healthcare Practice (Pre-hospital Critical Care) from St George's University of London. Kieren was also involved in publishing a paper in the Journal of Paramedic Practice on proning during the coronavirus pandemic. His professional interests include resuscitation and crew resource management.

Sacha Richardson is an intensive care and prehospital retrieval specialist. His research interests are in the delivery of ECMO-CPR in different hospital and prehospital environments. He has led the CHEER3 pre-hospital ECPR feasibility study for metropolitan Melbourne in conjunction with Ambulance Victoria. He has secured independent research funding and authored several key book chapters on the provision of ECPR. His contributions to the development of ECPR globally have been internationally recognised as the first author of the Extracorporeal Life Support Organisation (ELSO) International Adult ECPR guideline.

Nick Roder is an Intensive Care Flight Paramedic and educator with Ambulance Vicotria. He is also a Teaching Associate with Monash University post graduate studies, specialising in respiratory and retrieval paramedicine. Commencing paramedicine in 1991, he has since gained a Masters in Education, developing curriculum for the vocational and tertiary education domains both nationally and internationally. He still remains operational in the aeromedical field, and continues to develop the next generation of paramedics through mentorship, clinical guideline and educational program development.

Ross Salathiel ASM is the Director of Regional and Clinical Operations (Gippsland Region) for Ambulance Victoria and maintains an operational Critical Care Paramedicine presence. Ross is an Adjunct Senior Lecturer with the Monash University department of Paramedicine and supports the Paramedicine Board as a Clinical Advisor (Paramedicine) to the Australian

About the Editors and Contributors

Health Practitioners Registration Authority (AHPRA). With a master's in specialist Paramedic Practice, Graduate Certificate in Health Service Management and advanced diplomas in business, leadership and management Ross has a keen focus on leading the improvement of access to healthcare in rural and regional communities. Ross was the clinical lead for the design and implementation of 12 lead ECG for Ambulance Paramedics in Victoria and the implementation of Pre Hospital Thrombolysis across Victoria.

Peter Sherren (MBBS, FRCA, FFICM, DRTM RCSed) is a consultant in intensive care medicine and anaesthesia at Guy's and St Thomas' NHS Foundation Trust. He has specialist interest in severe cardiorespiratory failure, extracorporeal membrane oxygenation (ECMO)/mechanical circulatory support (MCS), resuscitation and cardiac anaesthesia. He is also a consultant in pre-hospital care and governance lead Essex and Herts Air Ambulance Trust (EHAAT).'

Toby St Clair is a senior intensive care flight paramedic working for Air Ambulance Victoria. With over a decade working on the ambulance rescue helicopter and 20 years working for Ambulance Victoria, Toby has a strong interest in prehospital trauma care, resuscitation, and advanced airway management. He completed his undergraduate diploma in ambulance paramedic studies in 2007, a graduate diploma in emergency health (MICA paramedic) in 2010, a graduate certificate in emergency health (aeromedical retrieval) in 2014, a Master of Specialist paramedic practice (aeromedical retrieval) in 2020, and advanced diploma in leadership & management in 2023. Toby teaches into the Monash University post graduate program for intensive care paramedics, specialising in aeromedical retrieval and trauma. Toby is the current acting director for Patient Safety at Ambulance Victoria and holds an honorary appointment to the Royal Childrens Hospital Trauma Team as the prehospital trauma affiliate.

Dion Stub is an Interventional Cardiologist at Alfred Hospital, Melbourne Australia and Co-director of Centre Cardiovascular Research and Education in Therapeutics Monash University, with leadership positions on major pre-hospital and hospital cardiac registries in Victoria. Prof Stub is an international leader for his research in cardiac emergencies and structural heart intervention. He currently holds the National Heart Foundation Future Leader and NHMRC Fellowships to support his clinical research, and is cardiology medical advisor to Ambulance Victoria.

Matthew Thornton is an Intensive Care Paramedic with a passion for driving innovation and high-quality education, and an overall focus of delivering exceptional, patient-centred prehospital critical care. He has 15 years' experience as a MICA Paramedic with Ambulance Victoria, and has held sessional lecturer roles in Paramedicine at both Australian Catholic University and Monash University. Most recently, he has devoted his time to the operational setup and provision of both prehospital ECMO and advanced mobile stroke services at Ambulance Victoria. These services are at the cutting edge of prehospital practice; they can only be effectively implemented by working productively with hospital-based expert clinicians, embracing a mindset of quality assurance and continuous improvement, adopting new technologies and incorporating the most up-to-date evidence-based practice. More than this, though, his work is helping to forge a new evidence base which will simultaneously promote better health outcomes and inform future best prehospital practice.

About the Editors and Contributors

Nick Trestrail is a Critical Care Paramedic employed by the South East Coast Ambulance Service. After completing his undergraduate studies at the University of Plymouth, he graduated with a BSc (Hons) Paramedic Practitioner (Community Emergency Health) undergraduate degree. He then joined the South East Coast Ambulance Service in 2015 and worked as a Paramedic, and a Clinical Education Lead looking after the education resuscitation portfolio. Nick subsequently undertook the Royal College of Surgeons Edinburgh Diploma in Immediate Medical Care in 2019, and is currently completing his MSc in Healthcare Practice (Prehospital Critical Care) at St George's University of London.

Scott Wallman is an Advanced Paramedic in Critical Care with East of England Ambulance Service who is currently flying with Essex and Herts Air Ambulance Trust. He joined London Ambulance Service in 2001 which provided exposure to high call volumes and two major incidents. This experience paved the way to a successful secondment as a HEMS Paramedic with London's Air Ambulance, Scott built on this solid foundation to begin his career path in Critical Care. He has recently completed post graduate study at University of Cambridge and has a special interest in Critical Care tasking across the East of England region.

Claire Wilkin is a paediatric emergency physician in Melbourne, Australia. Claire completed medical training in 2002 and has worked extensively in the UK, Uganda and Australia. Claire has a Masters in Aeromedical Retrieval and currently serves as the Paediatric Medical Advisor to Ambulance Victoria. She is also a Field Emergency Medical Officer providing additional medical support to paramedics in the pre-hospital arena.

Todd Wollum is Division Chief of EMS for Shoreline Fire Medic One. After graduating from University of Washington paramedicine program as a Mobile Intensive Care Paramedic in 2007, Todd has served as a line Paramedic, Medical Services Officer, Training MSO, and Division Chief. In addition, he currently serves as a paramedic on the Trauma Critical Care Team of the West Coast. This is one of 3 federal disaster response teams providing ICU and surgical capabilities in the event of a disaster. Todd is actively involved in the Resuscitation Academy (R.A.) and the Global Resuscitation Alliance, serving a Faculty member of the R.A. These efforts focus on bringing awareness to high performance CPR and post resuscitative care, with the goal of improving outcomes of out of hospital cardiac arrest.

James Yates is an advanced paramedic in neonatal retrieval for the South West Neonatal Advice and Retrieval Team and a specialist paramedic in critical care for the Great Western Air Ambulance Charity. He also cohosts the popular emergency medicine podcast, The Resus Room. Holding a BSc in Physiology, an MSc in Prehospital Critical Care and the Diploma in Immediate Medical Care, he has worked internationally as both a clinician and educator. He recently became the first paramedic to instruct on the Resuscitation Council UK, Advanced Resuscitation of the Newborn Infant course and he contributed to the development of their new Out-of-Hospital Newborn Life Support course.

Sarah Yong is an Intensivist at The Alfred Hospital and Adjunct Senior Lecturer for the School of Public Health and Preventative Medicine, Monash University. After graduating from The University of Melbourne, she completed her Fellowship of the Royal Australasian College

About the Editors and Contributors

of Physicians before obtaining her Fellowship of Intensive Care Medicine thereafter. Sarah's areas of interest include education and simulation, having completed a Masters in Clinical Education in non-technical skills in intensive care and she is a reviewer for *Advances in Simulation*. A strong advocate for her peers, Sarah convenes the Victorian Primary Exam Course for CICM, and has held past leadership roles with the CICM Board as the New Fellows' Representative. She is a founding convenor of the ANZICS Women in Intensive Care Medicine Network, with published research on gender balance in critical care. Sarah's clinical interests include cardiothoracic intensive care, resuscitation, and the interplay of human factors and crisis resource management with the critical care environment.

Henry Zhao is a Consultant Neurologist and NHMRC Research Fellow at The Royal Melbourne Hospital, Ambulance Victoria and The University of Melbourne. He graduated MBBS with Honours at The University of Melbourne before returning to complete his PhD in pre-hospital stroke care in conjunction with The Royal Melbourne Hospital Melbourne Brain Centre. He co-founded the Australian-first Melbourne Mobile Stroke Unit ambulance project as medical and clinical lead and created the severity-based stroke triage algorithm used by Ambulance Victoria. He is a board member and chair of the scientific committee of the international Pre-Hospital Treatment Organisation. He is highly active in research having co-authored over 30 papers, reviewed for over 25 international journals and currently supervises PhD and graduate researchers. His specific research interests include acute stroke trials as well as hyperacute and pre-hospital stroke care.

# SECTION 1

Airway

Paramedic-Led Prehospital Rapid Sequence Intubation (RSI)

David Anderson, Ben Meadley and Alexander Olaussen

> **In this chapter you will learn:**
> - The evidence base for paramedic-led RSI
> - Indications and potential complications of RSI
> - Common induction and neuromuscular blocking agents used to facilitate prehospital RSI
> - The benefits of video laryngoscopy in prehospital RSI.

Case Details

Dispatch
47-year-old male, fallen 3 metres, noisy breathing.

History
While cleaning gutters using a ladder, a 47-year-old man fell approximately 3 metres onto concrete. His wife called for an ambulance and advised the call taker that her husband was unconscious with noisy breathing. A double-crewed ambulance, a manager and a critical care paramedic were dispatched.

On Arrival of the First Crew
The scene is safe and the patient is lying in a semi-prone position. His primary survey findings and initial vital signs are:

Airway	Trismus, oral secretions, partially obstructed
Breathing	Laboured, RR 28, SpO_2 82% on room air
Circulation	Peripheral pulses present, HR 110, BP 153/96, warm peripheries
Disability	GCS E2, V2, M4 (8), pupils 4 mm and equally reactive
Environmental	Outdoors, temperate climate, no specific concerns

To assist with airway management, and while instituting spinal precautions, the first paramedic crew on scene have repositioned the patient onto his back. They have also applied high-flow oxygen via a non-rebreather mask. A secondary survey reveals a boggy swelling in the left parietal region and no other obvious injuries.

SECTION 1   Airway

On Your Arrival as the Critical Care Paramedic

The initial paramedic crew are struggling to manage the patient's airway due to the trismus and significant oral secretions. One of the paramedics is applying supplemental oxygen via a bag-valve-mask (BVM) using a two-handed grip, while the other attempts to gain IV access. The patient's SpO_2 has increased slightly to 86%.

AMPLE

The patient has no known allergies and only has a past medical history of hypertension for which he is prescribed candesartan 8 mg daily. He works as a stockbroker and is physically very active.

Allergies	NKDA
Medications	Candesartan 8 mg PO daily
Past history	Hypertension
Last ins and outs	Normal
Events prior	Fall from roof

Decision Point

What are your clinical priorities in this situation?

Due to the patient's decreased GCS, clear evidence of head injury, as well as compromised airway (trismus and secretions) with associated difficulties to correct the oxygen saturations, early consideration for rapid sequence intubation (RSI) is warranted.

Question 1: What is the Evidence Related to Rapid Sequence Intubation (RSI) by Paramedics?

Until the late 1990s, prehospital intubation was largely reserved for patients in cardiac arrest who had no upper airway reflexes and could be intubated without the assistance of medication. Such practice, however, left a large group of patients who paramedics commonly encountered (suffering from, for example, traumatic brain injury (TBI), respiratory failure and altered conscious states) at risk of complications, namely, an inadequately secured airway and/or inadequate ventilation. Furthermore, these patients may require the care of paramedics for some time, yet receive only basic airway management. To mitigate these risks, ambulance services from around the world, particularly those with aeromedical programmes, began to implement rapid sequence induction of anaesthesia into the paramedic skill-set[1] (sometimes referred to as rapid sequence intubation and usually abbreviated as RSI).

    Rapid sequence intubation involves co-administration of an anaesthetic induction agent, followed immediately by a neuromuscular blocking agent (hence the 'rapid sequence' terminology). This aims to not only facilitate optimal intubation conditions in a patient who still has some degree of either consciousness or upper airway reflexes or both, but also to reduce the risk of pulmonary aspiration during airway management. While typically performed by

CHAPTER 1   Paramedic-Led Prehospital Rapid Sequence Intubation (RSI)

anaesthetists in the operating room, RSI is often (and increasingly) performed by emergency doctors in the emergency department (ED) and intensivists in the intensive care unit (ICU) who, like paramedics, may be referred to as 'occasional intubators'.

There is limited published evidence to either support or refute the practice of paramedic-led RSI. For instance, a single-centre study from North America, randomising patients to either RSI or usual care in the setting of TBI, found an increased mortality rate in patients receiving prehospital RSI.[2] Despite these results, the methodology of this trial has been criticised due to potential shortfalls related to RSI training. Additionally, a follow-up study found significant periods of hypoxia and hypotension among the patients who received prehospital RSI.[3] Notwithstanding limitations, this trial has been influential in the prehospital space, and has contributed to the hesitance of many North American ambulance services around introducing paramedic-led RSI.

The regions in which paramedic-led RSI is perhaps most established are Australia and New Zealand. This is best represented by a 2010 prospective randomised controlled trial investigating prehospital RSI of patients with severe traumatic brain injury. In this study, it was not only shown that road-based critical care paramedics (CCPs) can safely and effectively perform RSI (with a 97% success rate), but also that it might improve functional outcomes at six months in this patient group.[4]

In Europe there is more involvement of doctors in prehospital critical care, and while it is normal for paramedics to be performing intubation, it would be more common for a doctor to act as a team leader and take overall responsibility for the care of the patient during RSI. There is some evidence to suggest that doctors have a better first-pass and overall success rate than paramedics; however, this is confounded by the fact that, in European EMS systems, doctors are often experienced specialist anaesthetists, who would logically be expected to be more proficient at intubation than any other craft group. Therefore, it may be simply that the more intubations a clinician has performed, the more proficient they will be – regardless of their professional background.[5]

Question 2: What are the Indications for RSI in the Prehospital Environment?

The indications for prehospital RSI can be broadly divided into four categories:

- Airway protection (typically patients who are unconscious)
- Targeted treatment (for example, CO_2 control in TBI)
- Respiratory failure
- Humanitarian/anticipated clinical course (for example, severe burns or major trauma).

Airway protection is likely the most common indication for prehospital RSI. This indication includes patients presenting unconscious or in an altered conscious state (ACS), who, due to attenuated or lost airway reflexes, are at increased risk of aspiration. An altered conscious state, in and of itself, however, is not always an indication for RSI, as some patients who have an ACS will be able to protect their airway and, thus, may be safely managed with less invasive means.

Targeted treatment refers to optimising ventilation with the goal of preventing secondary brain injury in TBI by maintaining oxygenation and preventing hypercarbia. This is a common

SECTION 1 Airway

indication for prehospital RSI, and applies to patients who have an ACS and are not effectively ventilating, despite the presence of airway reflexes. Careful consideration must be given to whether the time taken to carry out prehospital RSI may increase the time to definitive neurosurgical care.

Respiratory failure is typically managed in a stepwise fashion – starting with high-flow supplemental oxygen, moving on to non-invasive ventilation (NIV), and culminating in intubation and mechanical ventilation. The use of NIV is dramatically increasing in incidence in both the prehospital and in-hospital setting, accelerated a great deal by the COVID-19 pandemic. Many patients, such as those with COPD, asthma and acute pulmonary oedema, will respond well to NIV; however, some will still go on to need intubation. While the availability of modern ventilators has increased the utilisation of NIV in the out-of-hospital environment (especially for in the aeromedical setting), there will still be circumstances where a patient with respiratory failure (or indeed any of the indications for intubation) needs to be intubated simply to facilitate a safe transfer. This could also be considered an indication for intubation.

An important but often understated indication for intubation is the so-called humanitarian or anticipated clinical course indication, which includes patients with severe burns or trauma patients with multiple fractures but without a traumatic brain injury. Along a similar line, humanitarian indications describe a patient presenting with a great deal of pain, who will most likely require a large amount of analgesia, which can lead to ACS, attenuated airway protection and/or respiratory compromise. In these cases, it may be safer to intubate the patient early, not only to facilitate comfort but also to reduce the risk of complications during transport. It is important to note that this will be carried out in the context of a patient who almost certainly is going to be intubated shortly after arrival at hospital, as they are highly likely to require surgical management of their injuries.

Last, it must be mentioned that the patient's pathology, while important, is not the only factor that guides decisions around intubation. The mode of transport (road or air) and distance to hospital is also relevant, and will influence decisions around intubation. In these instances, the benefits of undertaking RSI need to be weighed against the risks of not doing so.

Question 3: What are the Potential Complications of RSI in the Critically Ill Patient?

Prehospital RSI for critically ill patients (that is, those suffering physiological derangement) is a high-risk procedure that is associated with significant complications. These complications, most commonly, include hypoxaemia and hypotension, but also involve unrecognised oesophageal intubation and cardiac arrest.

Hypotension is the commonest complication of RSI in critically ill patients, occurring in 43% of patients who undergo RSI.[6] These data are from a large multicentre observational study conducted in critically ill patients in the intensive care unit (ICU) setting (however, there is no reason to believe that the incidence of hypotension is significantly different in the out-of-hospital setting). Given that hypotension is the commonest complication of RSI, close attention must be paid to perfusion assessment and monitoring, both prior to and throughout the procedure. Regardless of the induction agents used, a push dose vasopressor, such

CHAPTER 1 Paramedic-Led Prehospital Rapid Sequence Intubation (RSI)

as metaraminol, phenylephrine or adrenaline, should be immediately available during prehospital RSI, thereby allowing immediate management of post-intubation hypotension, if encountered. Where required, perfusion management can be further supported by an adrenaline or noradrenaline infusion.

While hypoxaemia and inability to intubate are perhaps the most feared complications of RSI, these are relatively rare. Hypoxaemia occurs in 9% of patients and is usually transient. Loss of airway or inability to manage the airway is extremely rare. Most ambulance services that carry out paramedic-led RSI cite intubation success rates in the high 80–90% range, and almost all cases that cannot be managed with intubation can be rescued with a supraglottic airway or front-of-neck access.

Last, approximately 3% of patients will have cardiac arrest as a result of RSI. Often these will be patients who had unrecognised or recognised but ineffectively managed complications leading up to intubation, commonly severe metabolic acidosis or unrecognised pulmonary hypertension or right heart failure. Hypovolaemic shock can deteriorate into cardiac arrest following induction, as positive intrathoracic pressure limits venous return to the right heart. It is also important to be mindful of the possibility of tension pneumothorax as a cause of cardiac arrest after RSI, although this is quite uncommon.

Question 4: What Drugs Should be Used to Induce Anaesthesia in the Prehospital Environment?

While there is no perfect medication regimen for prehospital RSI, many ambulance services are standardising their induction regimens to facilitate patient and procedural safety. The following information will primarily focus on the most commonly used induction regimen for prehospital RSI: ketamine, rocuronium and fentanyl.

- **Ketamine** is an anaesthetic induction agent that acts as an NMDA receptor antagonist. Unlike other induction agents, such as propofol or thiopentone, ketamine has a lower incidence of hypotension and, in fact, may have a slight sympathomimetic effect. This potentially makes it the ideal induction agent for patients presenting with shock or patient cohorts where hypotension may worsen outcomes, such as TBI. The standard dose is 1–2 mg/kg, with a lower dose being appropriate in a hypertensive patient and a higher dose indicated in the setting of normotension or for a patient with a high GCS.
- **Fentanyl** is a potent short-acting opioid that is often added to an induction regimen at a dose of 1–3 mcg/kg to blunt the sympathetic response to laryngoscopy and intubation. Adding fentanyl to RSI may be particularly beneficial in the patient with impaired cerebral autoregulation, where further increases in blood pressure may be deleterious to intracranial pressure. However, as previously mentioned, the addition of fentanyl has been shown to increase the incidence of significant hypotension in patients with low or borderline blood pressure. In these instances, it should be omitted.[12]
- **Rocuronium** is a non-depolarising muscle relaxant which, at large doses (1.2–1.5 mg/kg), can provide an onset of favourable intubating conditions within 45–60 seconds.

Based on emerging evidence, many ambulance jurisdictions have adopted a three-tiered induction regimen wherein:

SECTION 1 Airway

- A patient who has a higher GCS and higher blood pressure will receive a combination of fentanyl, ketamine and rocuronium
- A patient who has borderline blood pressure or is mildly hypotensive will receive a standard dose of ketamine and rocuronium alone
- A patient who is profoundly shocked will receive a lower dose of ketamine and a higher dose of rocuronium.

With regard to shock state, a reduced dose of ketamine and higher dose of rocuronium is rationalised by the varying pharmacokinetics of each medication. For instance, as the effective circulating blood volume decreases, and with that the transit time of drugs from the injection point to the site of action is decreased, a lower dose of an anaesthetic agent will have a more profound effect, but a higher dose of muscle relaxant is required to allow the same onset of action. Given that there is little risk in administering a higher dose of muscle relaxant, it is becoming increasingly standard to administer 1.5–2.0 mg/kg (or simply 150–200 mg) of rocuronium to all patients undergoing prehospital RSI.

Push dose vasopressors must be immediately available when inducing anaesthesia. Metaraminol is an indirect pure alpha-1 agonist that is commonly used in the UK, Australia and New Zealand. A dose of 0.5–1.0 mg is usually sufficient to reverse moderate hypotension. Because it has no beta effects, metaraminol may be associated with a reflex bradycardia. Phenylephrine is more commonly used in North America. It is a direct acting alpha-1 agonist that also may be associated with bradycardia as it has no beta effects. A dose of 50–200 mcg is standard, repeated every three to five minutes.

If neither of these agents is available, then adrenaline is appropriate; however, in a patient who is not profoundly hypotensive, small boluses should be used (for example, 10–20 mcg). In a very shocked or peri-arrest patient, higher doses of 100–200 mcg are appropriate.

Table 1.1 Summary of commonly used prehospital RSI drugs

Medication	Pros	Cons	Notes
Ketamine	Rapid loss of consciousness, haemodynamically stable Cardiovascular stability Familiarity Multiple indications Can be used for DSI	Transient hypertension and tachycardia Slower onset of action than other commonly used induction agents	Although ketamine is associated with emergence phenomena, this is not relevant when long-term anaesthesia is planned. Although historically contraindicated in head injury, ketamine is now considered ideal for TBI patients.

CHAPTER 1   Paramedic-Led Prehospital Rapid Sequence Intubation (RSI)

Medication	Pros	Cons	Notes
Fentanyl	Potent analgesia More haemodynamically stable than other opioids	May cause hypotension	Fentanyl may offset some of the sympathomimetic effects of ketamine. In severely shocked patients relying on sympathetic drive, even a small dose may cause sympatholysis and haemodynamic collapse.
Rocuronium	Long duration of action, excellent intubating conditions	Slower onset than suxamethonium (45 versus 30 sec) Anaphylaxis Needs to be refrigerated	Rocuronium is considered the 'gold standard' paralytic for induction and post-intubation paralysis in prehospital TBI RSI.

Source: Based on Kellyn Engstrom, Caitlin S. Brown, Alicia E. Mattson, Neal Lyons, Megan A. Rech, Pharmacotherapy optimization for rapid sequence intubation in the emergency department, *The American Journal of Emergency Medicine*, 2023;70:19-29.

Question 5: Does Video-Laryngoscopy Improve Intubation Success and Outcomes during Prehospital RSI?

Since its introduction, laryngoscopy in adults has been predominantly performed with a Macintosh curved blade. Commonly referred to as 'direct laryngoscopy', laryngoscopy with a Macintosh blade aims to create a *direct* line of sight to the vocal cords through manipulation of the tongue and placement of the tip of the blade in the vallecula. Over the past two decades, however, video laryngoscopes with a small camera placed at the tip of the laryngoscope blade and a screen have increased in popularity, negating the need to create a direct line of sight to view airway structures. In general, there are three main types of video laryngoscopes (VL):

1. Macintosh-style (with a similar shape to the traditional laryngoscope)
2. Hyperangulated (more curved than other laryngoscopes, generally between 60 and 90 degrees)
3. Channelled (with a groove to guide the breathing tube).

SECTION 1 Airway

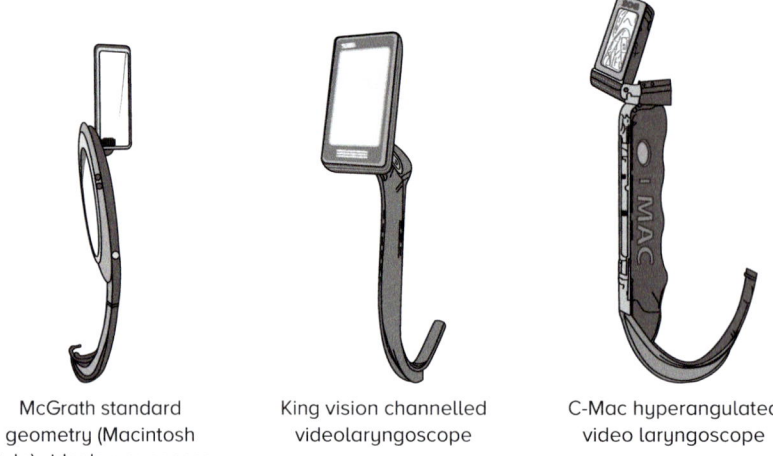

McGrath standard geometry (Macintosh style) videolaryngoscope

King vision channelled videolaryngoscope

C-Mac hyperangulated video laryngoscope

Figure 1.1 Video laryngoscopes.

PRACTICE TIP

 For critically unwell patients who are haemodynamically unstable, an important philosophy when undertaking RSI is:

RESUSCITATE, THEN INTUBATE

Recently evidence has emerged that leaves little doubt about the superiority of VL in critically ill patients. Such evidence includes observational studies, multicentre RCTs, meta-analyses and a Cochrane review, all concluding that VL is consistently associated with increased first-pass success and improved glottic visualisation.[7–10] These findings have led to a view among experts that 'there is no longer a rational debate about whether VL has greater efficacy than DL',[11] and that Macintosh VL should be the default intubation technique for all airway operators, including occasional intubators, such as CCPs. Furthermore, the benefits of VL are not limited to patient care, and extend to education – where the ability of more than one person to see what the intubator is seeing affords better teaching opportunities – and human factors – through fostering teamwork and communication.

PRACTICE TIP

 For the occasional intubator, the evidence suggests to:

GO WITH THE VIDEO

Intubating conditions encountered in the prehospital environment are different from those in the ED, ICU or operating room. Bright sunlight, limited ability to position the patient and commonly intubating patients in cardiac arrest (with CPR in progress) or multi-trauma patients (requiring manual inline stabilisation) mean that evidence from in-hospital studies may not be generalisable to the prehospital setting. Despite these challenges, the evidence that has thus far been collected in the prehospital setting also suggests that critical care paramedics have higher first-pass success with VL, especially when combined with a endotracheal tube introducer (bougie).

CHAPTER 1   Paramedic-Led Prehospital Rapid Sequence Intubation (RSI)

Key Evidence

Systematic Review/Meta-Analyses

von Elm E, Schoettker P, Henzi I et al. Pre-hospital tracheal intubation in patients with traumatic brain injury: systematic review of current evidence. *British Journal of Anaesthesia*. 2009 Sep;103(3):371–386.

von Vopelius-Feldt J, Wood J, Benger J. Critical care paramedics: where is the evidence? A systematic review. *Emergency Medicine Journal*. 2014 Dec;31(12):1016–1024.

Bossers SM, Schwarte LA, Loer SA et al. Experience in prehospital endotracheal intubation significantly influences mortality of patients with severe traumatic brain injury: a systematic review and meta-analysis. *PloS One*. 2015;10(10):e0141034.

Savino PB, Reichelderfer S, Mercer MP et al. Direct versus video laryngoscopy for prehospital intubation: a systematic review and meta-analysis. *Academic Emergency Medicine*. 2017 Aug;24(8):1018–1026.

Randomised Controlled Trials

Denninghoff KR, Nuño T, Pauls Q et al. Prehospital intubation is associated with favorable outcomes and lower mortality in ProTECT III. *Prehospital Emergency Care*. 2017 Oct;21(5):539–544.

Garner AA, Fearnside M, Gebski V. The study protocol for the Head Injury Retrieval Trial (HIRT): a single centre randomised controlled trial of physician prehospital management of severe blunt head injury compared with management by paramedics. *Scandinavian Journal of Trauma, Resuscitation and Emergency Medicine*. 2013 Sep 14;21:69.

Bernard SA, Nguyen V, Cameron P et al. Prehospital rapid sequence intubation improves functional outcome for patients with severe traumatic brain injury: a randomized controlled trial. *Annals of Surgery*. 2010 Dec;252(6):959–965.

Self-Reflection Questions

1. Consider the pros and cons of paramedic-led RSI. Do you think the evidence supports its use?
2. What are five strategies you can use to maximise operator success and patient safety during prehospital RSI?
3. Patients who have undergone RSI are complex and require a detailed handover when you arrive at hospital. Using the table below, prepare a handover of the patient described in the scenario at the start of this chapter using the IMIST AMBO format.

Introduction	
Mechanism	
Injuries	
Symptoms	
Treatment	
Allergies	
Medications	
Background history	
Other information	

SECTION 1 Airway

References

1. Murphy-Macabobby M, Marshall WJ, Schneider C et al. Neuromuscular blockade in aeromedical airway management. *Annals of Emergency Medicine*. 1992 Jun; 21(6):664–668.
2. Davis DP, Hoyt DB, Ochs M et al. The effect of paramedic rapid sequence intubation on outcome in patients with severe traumatic brain injury. *Journal of Trauma*. 2003 Mar;54(3):444–453. Available at: https://pubmed.ncbi.nlm.nih.gov/12634522/
3. Dunford JV, Davis DP, Ochs M et al. Incidence of transient hypoxia and pulse rate reactivity during paramedic rapid sequence intubation. *Annals of Emergency Medicine*. 2003 Dec;42(6):721728. Available at: https://pubmed.ncbi.nlm.nih.gov/14634593/
4. Bernard SA, Nguyen V, Cameron P et al. Prehospital rapid sequence intubation improves functional outcome for patients with severe traumatic brain injury: a randomized controlled trial. *Annals of Surgery*. 2010 Dec;252(6):959–965. Available at: https://pubmed.ncbi.nlm.nih.gov/21107105/
5. Crewdson K, Lockey DJ, Røislien J et al. The success of pre-hospital tracheal intubation by different pre-hospital providers: a systematic literature review and meta-analysis. *Critical Care*. 2017;21:31. Available at: https://ccforum.biomedcentral.com/articles/10.1186/s13054-017-1603-7
6. Russotto V, Myatra SN, Laffey JG et al. Intubation practices and adverse peri-intubation events in critically ill patients from 29 countries. *JAMA*. 2021 Mar 23;325(12):1164–1172. Available at: https://pubmed.ncbi.nlm.nih.gov/33755076/
7. Trent SA, Kaji AH, Carlson JN et al. Video laryngoscopy is associated with first-pass success in emergency department intubations for trauma patients: a propensity score matched analysis of the National Emergency Airway Registry. *Annals of Emergency Medicine*. 2021 Dec;78(6):708–719. Available at: https://pubmed.ncbi.nlm.nih.gov/34417072/
8. Prekker ME, Driver BE, Trent SA et al. Video versus direct laryngoscopy for tracheal intubation of critically ill adults. *New England Journal of Medicine*. 2023;389:418–429. Available at: https://www.nejm.org/doi/full/10.1056/NEJMoa2301601
9. Jiang J, Kang N, Li B et al. Comparison of adverse events between video and direct laryngoscopes for tracheal intubations in emergency department and ICU patients – a systematic review and meta-analysis. *Scandinavian Journal of Trauma, Resuscitation and Emergency Medicine*. 2020;28:10. Available at: https://sjtrem.biomedcentral.com/articles/10.1186/s13049-020-0702-7
10. Hansel J, Rogers AM, Lewis SR et al. Videolaryngoscopy versus direct laryngoscopy for adults undergoing tracheal intubation. *Cochrane Database of Systematic Reviews*. 2022 Apr 4;4(4):CD011136. Available at: https://pubmed.ncbi.nlm.nih.gov/35373840/
11. Cook TM. Evidence, default video laryngoscopy and which mode of laryngoscopy would your patient choose? *Anaesthesia*, 2023;78: 791–792. Available at: https://doi.org/10.1111/anae.16004
12. Ferguson I, Buttfield A, Burns B et al. Fentanyl versus placebo with ketamine and rocuronium for patients undergoing rapid sequence intubation in the emergency department: The FAKT study – a randomized clinical trial. *Academic Emergency Medicine*. 2022 Jan 22. Available at: https://pubmed.ncbi.nlm.nih.gov/35064992/

The Physiologically Difficult Airway

2

Jonathan Begley and Ben Meadley

In this chapter you will learn:
- The definition of a physiologically difficult airway
- How you can predict a physiologically difficult airway
- What strategies can be used to minimise patient risk
- Best practice when performing medication-facilitated endotracheal intubation in a patient with a physiological instability
- What strategies should be employed in the post-intubation phase of care.

Case Details

Dispatch
56-year-old female, chest pain, shortness of breath.

History
A 56-year-old female was discharged home from hospital yesterday after a 10-day admission for pneumonia. This morning she had complained of chest pain and ongoing shortness of breath. Although she insisted on an ambulance not being called, she has since become drowsy and sweaty, and her husband had difficulty rousing her. He has called an ambulance after speaking with the medical team at the hospital from which she was just discharged.

On Arrival of the First Crew
The scene is safe, and the patient is sitting semi-recumbent in a recliner chair. Her primary survey findings and initial vital signs are:

Airway	Patent
Breathing	RR 32, SpO_2 79% on room air, laboured, bilateral coarse crackles
Circulation	Peripheral pulses weak, HR 125, irregular, BP 85/45, cool, clammy peripheries
Disability	GCS E1, V2, M5 (8), pupils midpoint and reactive, BGL 6.3 mmol/L
Environmental	Temp 38.8 °C, indoors, no other environmental concerns

SECTION 1 Airway

The first paramedic crew to arrive position the patient upright and apply high-flow oxygen via a non-rebreather mask. They attempt to rouse her further, but her conscious state does not change. The crew set up for IV access and obtain a 12-lead ECG.

On Your Arrival as the Critical Care Paramedic

The initial paramedic crew are managing the patient well and have gained IV access. One of the paramedics is applying the 12-lead ECG electrodes, but they keep sliding off the patient's skin due to excessive diaphoresis. You assist with acquisition of the 12-lead ECG (**Figure 2.1**). The patient's SpO_2 has increased slightly to 85%. The crew remind you that the nearest hospital is 50 minutes away.

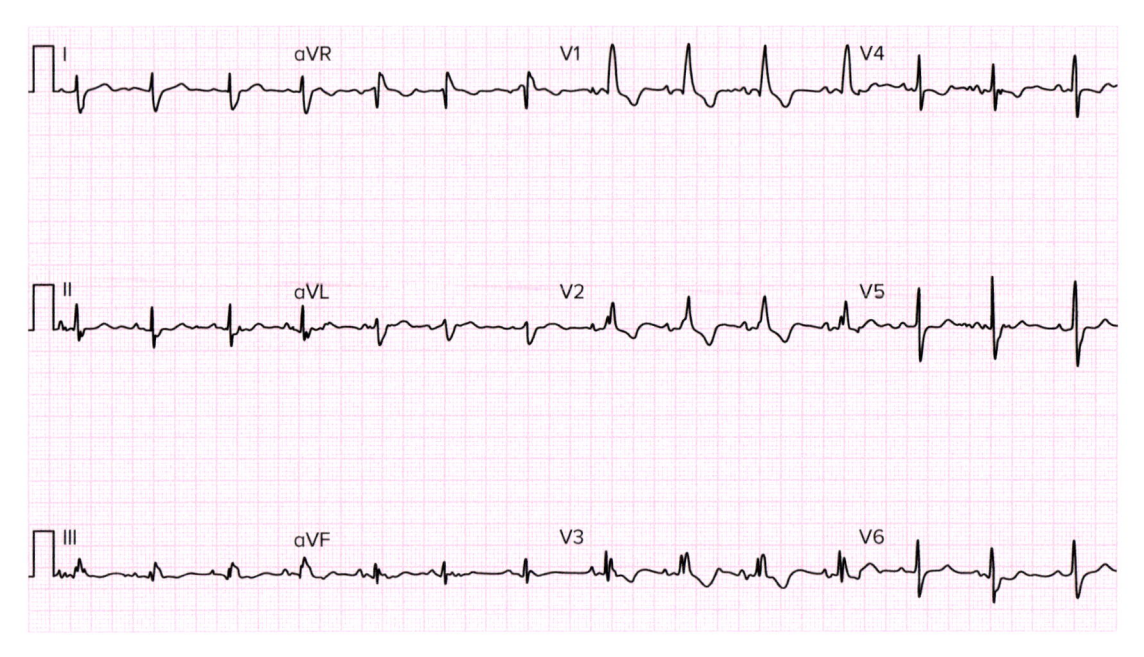

Figure 2.1 A 12-lead ECG for a 56-year-old female with chest pain and shortness of breath.

AMPLE

The patient has a past medical history of hypertension, type 2 diabetes, hyperlipidaemia, cigarette smoking (15 per day) and recent COVID-19 infections (the most recent was the third infection in three years, and she has had three vaccinations). She is morbidly obese, with an estimated body mass index of 40 kg/m².[1] Her medication list is extensive (listed below), and she has no known allergies. She is unemployed and lives a sedentary lifestyle.

CHAPTER 2 The Physiologically Difficult Airway

Allergies	NKDA
Medications	Irbesartan 150 mg PO daily
	Gliclazide 320 mg PO daily
	Aspirin 100 mg PO daily
	Insulin glargine 10 units once daily
	Metformin 500 mg PO daily
	Rosuvastatin 20 mg PO daily
	Metoprolol 50 mg PO twice daily
Past history	Hypertension, T2DM, COVID-19 x 3, hypertension, hyperlipidaemia
Last ins and outs	Has not eaten since discharge from hospital 24 hours ago
Events prior	Chest pain and shortness of breath this morning

Decision Point
What are your clinical priorities in this situation?

With significant myocardial injury, cardiogenic shock, decreased conscious state, clear evidence of refractory hypoxia and respiratory failure, urgent cardiovascular and respiratory support is critical. CPAP and BiPAP are contraindicated due to the patient's low conscious state, therefore medication-facilitated intubation will be required.

Question 1: What is the Physiologically Difficult Airway?

As mentioned in Chapter 1: Paramedic-led prehospital rapid sequence intubation (RSI), peri-intubation cardiac arrest is concerningly common; some patients are at particular risk of collapse post intubation. Whereas a 'difficult airway' has traditionally described an anatomical or physical characteristic that makes airway management difficult, the physiologically difficult airway 'is one in which physiologic derangements place the patient at higher risk of cardiovascular collapse with intubation and conversion to positive pressure ventilation'.[2]

At least five types of physiologically difficult airway have been defined (**Figure 2.2**), which are:

1. Hypoxia
2. Hypotension
3. Severe metabolic acidosis
4. Right heart failure
5. Head or neurological injury.

It is worth noting that the combination of a physiologically and anatomically difficult airway places the patient at particularly high risk of complications, as difficulty with the physical procedures of airway management may prolong or exacerbate the physiological derangements. Even if the anatomy and procedures are easy and quick, the physiologically difficult airway still poses a serious risk and challenge in its own right.

SECTION 1 Airway

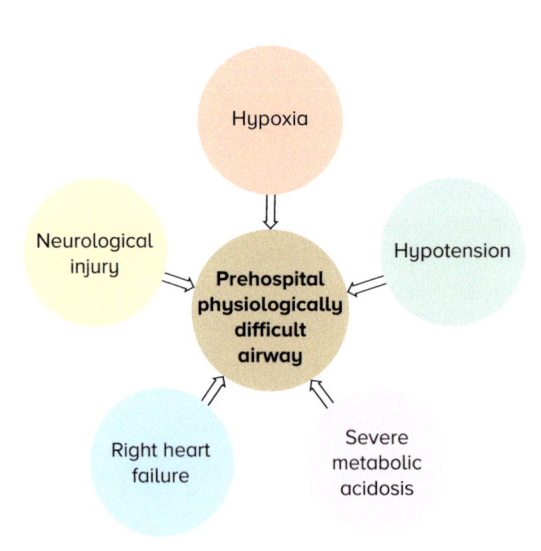

Figure 2.2 Conceptual diagram identifying different types of physiologically difficult airway.

Why is Intubation Physiologically Challenging for the Patient?

Although the concept of the physiologically difficult airway may apply to all elements of airway management, it is usually discussed around the process of intubation because this typically causes several rapid and complex changes to the patient's physiology, which may precipitate cardiovascular collapse. These changes include the following.

- Induction agents commonly cause vasodilation, myocardial depression and hypotension; ketamine can cause tachycardia (increasing myocardial work) and hyper- or hypotension.
- Laryngoscopy, cricoid pressure and passage of the tube are very stimulating and can cause tachycardia, hypertension, raised ICP and increased myocardial work. In infants and small children, however, this reflex can cause bradycardia.
- The patient's own sympathetic response (which may have been keeping their heart rate and blood pressure up) is often reduced.
- The change from normal negative pressure breathing to positive pressure ventilation transmits pressure to the pulmonary capillaries, great vessels and heart. This has complex effects, reducing venous return, increasing resistance to blood flow through the lungs and increasing work and strain on the right ventricle, but it often helps a failing left ventricle.
- Any apnoea or reduction in minute ventilation will increase the CO_2, potentially causing acidosis and pulmonary vascular constriction, increasing further resistance to blood flow through the pulmonary circulation. Any hypoxia may also increase pulmonary vascular constriction. Both can also cause a reflex sympathetic response.
- Suxamethonium has complex effects and can cause bradycardia, especially in children.
- In addition, any complication such as bronchospasm or allergic reaction will challenge the patient's physiology in its own way.

CHAPTER 2 The Physiologically Difficult Airway

Question 2: How can You Predict the Physiologically Difficult Airway?

In general, a potentially physiologically difficult airway should be assumed in all patients who are intubated outside the elective surgery setting. In the majority of cases, the underlying reason for intubation is some sort of physiological compromise. As highlighted in Chapter 1: Paramedic-led prehospital rapid sequence intubation (RSI), up to 40% of intubations in critically ill patients are complicated by some form of physiological compromise, typically hypotension, but also hypoxia and potentially cardiac arrest.

The VAPOUR mnemonic (originally described by Levitan[3] and modified by Nickson[4]) can be used to assess the patient for factors that may increase the risk of physiologically difficult intubation.

Ventilation	Hyperventilation suggests metabolic acidosis with the risk of cardiovascular collapse; hypoventilation suggests potential respiratory acidosis that should be corrected before RSI if possible.
Acidaemia	Extreme care should be taken, and potentially RSI avoided altogether, in the patient with known or strongly suspected severe metabolic acidosis (for example, DKA). Respiratory acidosis should be corrected prior to RSI if possible.
Pressure	There are many pressures to consider: blood pressure (systemic hypotension or pulmonary hypertension); airway pressures (for example, asthmatics who may need very high airway pressures and also have the risk of hypotension); gastric pressures from over-vigorous BVM or ventilation via SGA, increasing the risk of aspiration.
Oxygenation	Any patient with hypoxaemia preceding RSI is at high risk of hypoxaemia during and post RSI.
Underlying disease	Some conditions in particular may significantly increase the risk of physiological compromise with RSI (for example, ischaemic heart disease, heart failure, interstitial lung disease).
Regurgitation	The risk of aspiration is always greater in a critically ill patient compared with a fasted patient undergoing elective surgery.

Question 3: What Strategies can be Used to Minimise Patient Risk?

While they share many of the same principles, management depends on the type of physiologically difficult airway present. Guidelines have been recently published on this topic.[5] As discussed in Chapter 1: Paramedic-led prehospital rapid sequence intubation (RSI), the decision of whether to intubate on scene or transfer is a complex judgement call taking into account several factors; however, the presence of a physiologically difficult airway may push the decision towards transporting unintubated if other factors (such as distance to destination) also make transporting unintubated a reasonable decision.

SECTION 1 Airway

Hypoxia

Head-up positioning

Head-up positioning usually improves FRC and oxygenation. When not contraindicated (for example, a patient in full spinal precautions), pre-oxygenation should be performed head-up (30–45 degrees); it may be necessary to reduce the head-up position somewhat immediately prior to intubation to successfully perform the procedure (for example, to 20 degrees).

Pre-oxygenation

Careful pre-oxygenation lengthens the time until desaturation. There are many valid techniques for pre-oxygenation, but it is important to pay attention to details in this technique. If using a bag-valve-mask (BVM), it is important that a tight seal is maintained for a full 3–5 minutes to prevent any indrawing of nitrogen-rich air. Applying nasal prongs under the mask may improve pre-oxygenation and is useful for apnoeic oxygenation also.

Apnoeic oxygenation

Providing oxygen to the airway during periods of apnoea also reduces desaturation. Practically, this can be delivered with standard oxygen nasal prongs at 10–15 LPM. Pre-oxygenation facilitates apnoeic oxygenation; if the lungs are filled with oxygen prior to the apnoeic period, more oxygen will be drawn in from the upper airway during this period.

PEEP or NIV

The above techniques cannot directly address collapsed alveoli and shunt; however, positive end-expiratory pressure (PEEP) or non-invasive ventilation (NIV) can. If hypoxia is caused by shunt, it may be possible to partly reverse the process prior to intubation using a PEEP valve or NIV, if available. Even in a case such as the one presented, where NIV is classically contraindicated, it may be reasonable to use NIV for a short time (under close supervision) for the purpose of optimising pre-oxygenation. If the conscious state allows, pre-oxygenation via a laryngeal mask airway (LMA) may provide excellent PEEP prior to intubation. These techniques should be considered especially if the patient remains hypoxic (SpO$_2$ <94%) despite pre-oxygenation with other techniques.

Delayed-sequence intubation (DSI)/sedation-facilitated pre-oxygenation

DSI describes using procedural sedation to perform pre-oxygenation in a patient who cannot be pre-oxygenated due to agitation or delirium.[6,8] Doses of 10–20 mg of ketamine at a time are recommended. While ketamine has a favourable safety profile, it can cause complications including apnoea and airway obstruction; the clinician must be immediately ready to proceed to intubation if this occurs.

Hypotension

IV access and fluid resuscitation

Wide-bore IV or IO access must be established. The patient should be assessed for fluid-responsiveness and, if fluid-responsive, should receive fluid resuscitation prior to and during

CHAPTER 2 The Physiologically Difficult Airway

intubation; hypovolaemic patients are at particular risk of peri-intubation hypotension. The mantra 'resuscitate, then intubate' reminds clinicians of the importance of investing time in resuscitation, even though intubation may be delayed. A useful manoeuvre is to have someone raise the patient's legs, especially if unexpected hypotension follows intubation; doing so quickly increases the blood volume of the great vessels (more rapidly than a fluid bolus can be administered). The legs can be held in that position while a fluid bolus or vasopressors are administered and, unlike a fluid bolus, the manoeuvre is reversible (by lowering the legs again).

Vasopressors

Vasopressors may be indicated in patients who are at risk of peri-intubation hypotension and are not fluid responsive. Starting an infusion pre-intubation is often ideal and allows rapid titration as required. Alternatively, bolus dose vasopressors can be very useful. Metaraminol, phenylephrine, noradrenaline and adrenaline may all be appropriate, each with its own relative advantages and disadvantages. Vasopressors can also provide time for fluid to be administered, as they are typically much faster in onset than the time taken to administer a fluid bolus.

Choice and dosing of induction agent

All induction agents have the potential to cause determinantal haemodynamic changes, although several are more prone to this. Benzodiazepines and opioids can cause vasodilation and myocardial depression to some extent. Ketamine is commonly used for prehospital intubation as it is relatively haemodynamically stable, but its effects are still somewhat unpredictable: its sympathomimetic effects cause tachycardia, increased cardiac output and increased blood pressure; however, it also has a myocardial depression effect and can cause hypotension. Etomidate is used in some regions but is not available in Australia. Propofol, used extensively for anaesthesia, is a particularly vasodilating drug and is rarely used prehospital. Regardless of the agent chosen, in general, the dose should be reduced somewhat in haemodynamically at-risk patients.

Right Heart Failure

Identification and assessment

Diagnosis and assessment of right heart failure is particularly challenging prehospital. Acute right ventricular infarction and pulmonary emboli are the classic prehospital presentations, but patients with chronic pulmonary hypertension will often present with acute deteriorations also. Assessing fluid responsiveness is also challenging, and fluid boluses may worsen the situation. Again, raising the patient's legs is a reasonable way of testing fluid responsiveness, and can be reversed if required.

Fluid and vasopressor resuscitation

These should be conducted carefully; 250 mL fluid boluses with reassessment are likely to be safer than larger boluses. Some patients will benefit from diuresis, but this will be difficult to assess prehospital. Vasopressors may improve the situation but can also raise pulmonary arterial pressure, potentially reducing cardiac output.

SECTION 1 Airway

Principles of intubation

It is important that the systemic blood pressure be maintained (to continue right ventricular perfusion). Hypercapnia and hypoxia will cause pulmonary vasoconstriction, worsening strain on the right ventricle, and must be avoided. Positive airway pressure also increases pulmonary arterial pressure; as much as possible, high airway pressures should be avoided. The result of all this is a complex and precariously balanced induction and intubation; the merits and risks of deferring intubation until arrival in hospital (where echocardiography and pulmonary vasodilators may be available) should be considered. Avoiding intubation is often the best approach; NIV also has the problems associated with positive pressure, but is reversible.

Severe Metabolic Acidosis
Identification and assessment

The classic cause of severe metabolic acidosis presenting in the prehospital setting is diabetic ketoacidosis. The patient is breathing hard and fast, but they have normal lung function; the respiratory effort is the patient's attempt to lower their CO_2 to compensate for their metabolic acidosis. Conceptually, it helps to think of CO_2 as being an acid: if the minute ventilation is reduced, the patient will become more acidotic. Acidosis, among other things, causes myocardial depression, which can then worsen the acidosis, causing a spiral towards cardiac arrest. Other causes include salicylate (aspirin) or metformin overdose, or ischaemic bowel, for example. Metabolic acidosis also commonly occurs with trauma, sepsis or any other severe illness, but this can be harder to identify without blood gas testing equipment.

Non-invasive ventilation

NIV supports respiration and reduces the patient's work of breathing, while still allowing them to maintain their own minute ventilation. Note the minute ventilation (if the device displays this) in case intubation is required.

Principles of intubation

The greatest risks with intubation are the apnoeic period, and the possibility that a bag-valve-mask or mechanical ventilator will not be able to maintain the same minute ventilation that the patient was generating (for example, 40 L per minute). Any rise in CO_2 will worsen the acidosis and potentially cause cardiac arrest. Therefore, all efforts should be made to avoid intubation in patients with very high ventilatory requirements. If intubation is necessary, the apnoeic period must be as short as possible (for example, by maintaining positive pressure ventilation after induction), and the high minute ventilation must be maintained (note the respiratory rate prior to intubation). A higher minute ventilation may be achieved with the patient spontaneously breathing, for example using pressure support mode (so a short-acting NMBD such as suxamethonium may be ideal). Awake intubation could be considered but is presently only available on doctor-led services.

Head or Neurological Injury

This is a slightly different physiologically difficult airway to those discussed above. Here, we are less concerned about cardiorespiratory deterioration, but the physiological challenge is

CHAPTER 2 The Physiologically Difficult Airway

to preserve cerebral perfusion pressure and prevent increases in intracranial pressure (see also Chapter 16: Severe traumatic brain injury).

> **PRACTICE TIP**
>
> The physiologically difficult airway presents a high degree of patient safety risk. Remember to:
>
> RESUSCITATE, THEN INTUBATE

Question 4: What is Best Practice when Performing Medication-Facilitated Endotracheal Intubation in a Patient with Physiological Instability?

Physiological Goals of Intubation

Hypotension and hypoxia seem to be particularly harmful in these patients; many of the same elements of the 'hypoxia' and 'hypotension' physiologically difficult airways can be applied here to avoid this. CO_2 should be maintained in the normal range (or low–normal range, for example, $EtCO_2$ 35–40 mmHg) by maintaining minute ventilation. PEEP increases intracranial pressure, so minimal PEEP should be used. Laryngoscopy and intubation cause a sympathetic response and can increase ICP. Fentanyl or lignocaine have been used to ablate this but risk hypotension (which is a greater concern) and should only be utilised if the clinician is confident in their use. Ketamine may cause hypertension and it is reasonable to use alternate agent(s) if the patient is severely hypertensive (for example, >180 mmHg systolic). Checklists that include prompts on physiological optimisation may improve outcomes, as seen in some hospital-based studies.[7]

Human Factors

Wherever possible, the most experienced intubator should perform laryngoscopy if there is a high risk of physiological decompensation. However, it must be emphasised that teamwork is a key element of prehospital RSI, and critical care paramedics (CCPs) must be comfortable acting as the intubator or team leader and also acting as a solo senior clinician or as part of team including doctors or other CCPs. Use of a checklist is key to ensuring that RSI is a standardised procedure regardless of the makeup of the team and, as above, checklists should ideally include some prompts on physiological derangement.

> **PRACTICE TIP**
>
> A team approach is essential for treating these critically unwell patients. Ensure all clinicians have a:
>
> SHARED MENTAL MODEL

SECTION 1 Airway

Question 5: What Strategies Should be Employed in the Post-Intubation Phase of Care?

In the immediate post-intubation period, particular vigilance must be paid to any physiological deterioration. Adequate analgesia and sedation are necessary, while ensuring hypotension is avoided (vasopressors must be immediately available). A post-intubation checklist may be a useful tool to ensure that all required actions are carried out, while avoiding cognitive overload. Hypotension may be due to the direct effects of induction agents, the transition from negative to positive pressure ventilation (particularly in a shocked patient) or directly related to underlying pathology, such as pulmonary hypertension, asthma or tension pneumothorax. While not directly related to airway management, this is a good time to check that venous outflow is not impaired, by ensuring the jugular areas are free of pressure and sitting the patient 30-degrees head-up if possible.

Key Evidence

Jabaley, C.S., 2023. Managing the physiologically difficult airway in critically ill adults. *Critical Care*, *27*(1), pp. 1–7.
Mosier, J.M., Joshi, R., Hypes, C. et al., 2015. The physiologically difficult airway. *Western Journal of Emergency Medicine*, *16*(7), p. 1109.
Kornas, R.L., Owyang, C.G., Sakles, J.C. et al., 2021. Evaluation and management of the physiologically difficult airway: consensus recommendations from Society for Airway Management. *Anesthesia & Analgesia*, *132*(2), pp. 395–405.
Mosier, J.M., 2020. Physiologically difficult airway in critically ill patients: winning the race between haemoglobin desaturation and tracheal intubation. *British Journal of Anaesthesia*, *125*(1), pp. e1–e4.
Myatra, S.N., Divatia, J.V., Brewster, D.J., 2022. The physiologically difficult airway: an emerging concept. *Current Opinion in Anaesthesiology*, *35*(2), pp. 115–121.
Dean, P.N., Hoehn, E.F., Geis, G.L. et al., 2020. Identification of the physiologically difficult airway in the pediatric emergency department. *Academic Emergency Medicine*, *27*(12), pp. 1241–1248.
Fonseca, D., Graça, M.I., Salgueirinho, C. et al., 2023. Physiologically difficult airway: How to approach the difficulty beyond anatomy. *Trends in Anaesthesia and Critical Care*, p. 101212.

Self-Reflection Questions

1. How many people do you think you would need at the scene to safely care for the patient described in this chapter? What roles would you allocate to each of them?
2. Thinking of the service or organisation you work in, develop a list of the essential items you would prepare to care for this patient (for example, the type of laryngoscope, the medications you would use, and other technical and clinical equipment).
3. Assuming you have 360-degree access to this patient, draw a layout of where you would position the patient, personnel, medications and equipment to ensure rapid and safe execution of critical procedures.
4. Write down an example of the 'briefing' that you would give to other staff at the scene to ensure all roles are allocated and the team has a shared mental model of what is about to happen. Read it out to a colleague and seek their feedback.
5. Create a simple flowchart or a concept map showing how you would want this case to run. Consider that many parts of the patient care will be concurrent rather than consecutive.

CHAPTER 2 The Physiologically Difficult Airway

References

1. Wellens, R.I., Roche, A.F., Khamis, H.J. et al., 1996. Relationships between the body mass index and body composition. *Obesity Research, 4*, pp. 35–44.
2. Mosier, J.M., Joshi, R., Hypes, C. et al., 2015. The physiologically difficult airway. *Western Journal of Emergency Medicine, 16*, pp. 1109–1117.
3. Levitan, R.M., 2015. Timing resuscitation sequence intubation for critically ill patients. *ACEPNow*. Available at: https://www.acepnow.com/article/timing-resuscitation-sequence-intubation-for-critically-ill-patients/
4. Nickson, C., 2020. Peri-intubation life threats, *Life in the Fast Lane*. Available at: https://litfl.com/peri-intubation-life-threats/
5. Kornas, R.L., Owyang, C.G., Sakles, J.C. et al., 2021. Evaluation and management of the physiologically difficult airway: consensus recommendations from Society for Airway Management. *Anesthesia & Analgesia, 132*, pp. 395–405.
6. Weingart, S.D., 2011. Preoxygenation, reoxygenation, and delayed sequence intubation in the emergency department. *Journal of Emergency Medicine, 40*, pp. 661–667.
7. Jabaley, C.S., 2023. Managing the physiologically difficult airway in critically ill adults. *Critical Care, 27*(1), pp. 1–7.
8. Weingart, S.D., Trueger, N.S., Wong, N. et al., 2015. Delayed sequence intubation: a prospective observational study. *Annals of Emergency Medicine, 65*, pp. 349–355.

3

The Anatomically Difficult Airway

Jason Bendall and Matt Humar

In this chapter you will learn:
- The definitions of a 'difficult airway' and 'anatomical difficult airway'
- Anatomical features that can increase the difficulty of airway management with face-mask ventilation, supraglottic devices, tracheal intubation and cricothyroidotomy
- How an airway assessment can inform decisions about a safe and appropriate prehospital airway strategy.

Case Details

Dispatch
57-year-old male, collapsed, vomiting with agonal breathing.

History
While at home, a 57-year-old man had a witnessed collapse to the floor. Family members immediately rendered assistance and called for an ambulance. During the phone call, the patient suffered a brief, self-resolving seizure and started vomiting. The patient is now suspected to be in cardiac arrest. An emergency medical response is activated, and an advanced life support paramedic team as well as a dual critical care paramedic team are dispatched.

On Arrival of the First Crew
The scene is safe and the patient is found lying in a supine position with firefighters performing effective CPR. A primary survey confirms the patient is unconscious, apnoeic and pulseless. He also has a large amount of vomit in and around his airway. Monitoring through defibrillation pads shows a coarse VF, and the patient is defibrillated. The crew then move to decontaminate the airway and insert a supraglottic airway device (SAD). Following the fourth defibrillation, the patient has a ROSC.

On Your Arrival as the Critical Care Paramedic
The first crew have successfully decontaminated the airway and are now providing adequate ventilation and oxygenation through the SAD. Despite this, you decide RSI is indicated as it will secure the patient's airway, provide controlled ventilation, and facilitate safe transport.

CHAPTER 3 The Anatomically Difficult Airway

Based on several anatomical features, however, you predict that tracheal intubation, and other rescue airway techniques, may be difficult.

Airway	Maintained with SGA
Breathing	RR 12 (manual ventilations), SpO$_2$ 95% on FiO$_2$ 1.0
Circulation	Peripheral pulses weak, HR 110, regular, BP 136/82, cool peripheries
Disability	GCS E1, VT, M1 (3), pupils midpoint and reactive, BGL 8.3 mmol/L
Environmental	Temp 35.6 °C, indoors, no other environmental concerns

AMPLE

The patient has an extensive past medical history. He is also a heavy smoker, requires a CPAP device overnight and has a large beard. You estimate he weighs between 130 and 140 kg.

Allergies	NKDA
Medications	Symbicort, irbesartan, methotrexate, aspirin, salbutamol
Past history	Hypertension, rheumatoid arthritis, obstructive sleep apnoea (OSA), alcohol use disorder, COPD, neck surgery (cancer)
Last ins and outs	Unknown
Events prior	Complaining of intermittent chest pain and sweating prior to collapse today

Decision Point 1
What aspects of the patient's history and assessment increase the risk of difficult airway management?

The patient has several known risk factors of difficult airway management. Although at times unreliable, anatomical features that are associated with difficult, or impossible, airway management must be assessed.

Decision Point 2
How does an airway assessment inform safe and appropriate airway management?

In conjunction with patient history, an airway assessment will evaluate the potential risks associated with airway management. This information will then guide decisions on performing or withholding prehospital advanced airway management and will aid development of a safe and appropriate airway strategy.

SECTION 1 Airway

Question 1: What is a Difficult and Anatomically Difficult Airway?

The difficult airway is an intuitive concept to understand but not an easy one to define. A definition needs to incorporate several variables, such as airway operator experience and skill, while also specifically describing what qualifies or quantifies difficulty, or failure, with each individual airway technique. A definition also needs to include both anticipated ('I believe this patient's airway *will be* difficult to manage for these reasons') and encountered difficulty ('The patient's airway *was* difficult for these reasons'). To further confound this matter, it has been suggested that 'the difficult airway does not exist ... (but rather) it is a complex situational interplay of patient, practitioner, equipment, expertise and circumstances'.[1] It is perhaps not surprising then that a universal definition of a difficult airway is wanting.

An example of a contemporary definition of the difficult airway can be found in the 2021 Canadian Airway Focus Group (CAFG) airway management guidelines, which state:

> A difficult airway exists when an experienced airway manager anticipates or encounters difficulty with any or all of laryngoscopy or tracheal intubation, face-mask ventilation, supraglottic airway use, or emergency front of neck access.[2]

With consideration of what defines a difficult airway, an anatomically difficult airway is simply one where anatomical or physical features either cause, or are likely to cause, challenges to the success of airway management. Put another way, and as defined by Brown and Walls,[3] an anatomically difficult airway can be defined as:

> Physical attributes that are likely to make airway management more difficult than would be the case in an ordinary patient without those attributes.

This definition will form the basis for the information discussed in this chapter.

PRACTICE TIP
All tracheal intubations performed in the prehospital environment are high risk and should be approached as being potentially difficult.

Question 2: What Clinical History and Anatomical Features Increase the Risk of Difficult Tracheal Intubation?

Before performing tracheal intubation, it is prudent for prehospital clinicians to appreciate the clinical history and anatomical features that *may* increase difficulty. This is especially important when undertaking rapid sequence intubation (RSI), where airway reflexes, airway patency and spontaneous respiratory effort are abolished. Analogous to anaesthetic practice, a prehospital airway assessment aims to prospectively identify the *risk* of difficulty with tracheal intubation, and in conjunction with physiological and contextual factors, guide the optimal approach to successful and safe airway management.

CHAPTER 3 The Anatomically Difficult Airway

> **PRACTICE TIP**
>
> An airway assessment involves evaluating risk for not only tracheal intubation, but all airway techniques.

There is an array of anatomical features associated with difficult tracheal intubation, including dentition, facial, mouth and neck structures. Assessment of many of these features can be challenging for prehospital clinicians, mainly due to unconscious and uncooperative patients. To assist with overcoming some of these challenges, several bespoke airway assessment tools have been developed. A well-known example of these is the LEMON mnemonic (see **Table 3.1**). Although limited in some aspects, this mnemonic nonetheless provides a structured, rapid and easy to remember approach to assessing and predicting difficulty with tracheal intubation.

Table 3.1 LEMON mnemonic for predicting difficult tracheal intubation

Criteria	Explanation
Look externally	Based on an external look, do you 'feel' the patient's airway will be difficult to manage?
Evaluate 3-3-2	Evaluates ability to create a direct line of sight from outside the mouth to the glottis (see **Figure 3.1**): • **3:** Assesses interincisor distance and mouth opening: a normal patient can accommodate three (of their own) fingers between the upper and lower incisors. • **3:** Assesses hyoid–mentum distance and length of the mandibular space: a normal patient can accommodate three (of their own) fingers between the tip of the mentum and hyoid bone. • **2:** Assesses hyoid–thyroid distance and the position of the glottis in relation to the base of the tongue: a normal patient can accommodate two (of their own) fingers between the hyoid bone and the thyroid notch
Mallampati score*	Assess mouth opening and relative size of the tongue and oropharynx, which defines access through the oral cavity.
Obstruction/**O**besity	Upper airway obstruction and obesity can increase the difficulty with laryngoscopy, glottic visualisation and tube delivery.
Neck mobility	Pathology or management (for example, manual in-line stabilisation) that interferes with optimal patient positioning impedes laryngoscopy and tracheal intubation.

* Mallampati score can be excluded where impractical.
Source: Based on Brown III, C.A. and Walls, R.M. 2018. The emergency airway algorithms. In: Brown III, C.A., Sakles, J.C. and Mick, N.W. (eds) *The Walls Manual of Emergency Airway Management*, 5th edn. Philadelphia: Wolters Kluwer.

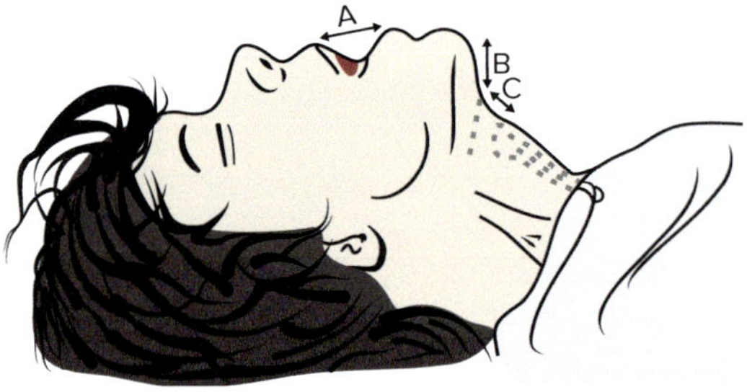

Figure 3.1 The LEMON score: Evaluate 3-3-2: (A) interincisor distance, (B) hyoid–mentum distance, (C) hyoid–thyroid distance.

The HEAVEN criteria (see **Table 3.2**)[27] provide another tool for predicting difficulty with prehospital tracheal intubation or RSI. Although less prescriptive than the LEMON mnemonic in terms of anatomical data, the HEAVEN criteria look beyond anatomical features and integrate physiological considerations that may contribute to difficulty. They have also been validated for both direct and video laryngoscopy.[4] With either of these tools, the presence of more criteria is associated with increased difficulty.

Table 3.2 HEAVEN criteria for predicting difficult tracheal intubation

Criteria	Explanation
Hypoxaemia	Oxygen saturation value ≤93% at the time of initial laryngoscopy
Extremes of size	Paediatric patient (≤8 years of age) or clinical obesity
Anatomic challenge	Includes trauma, mass, swelling, foreign body or other structural abnormality limiting laryngoscopic view
Vomit/blood/fluid	Clinically significant fluid noted in the pharynx/hypopharynx prior to/at the time of laryngoscopy
Exsanguination	Suspected anaemia that could potentially accelerate desaturation during RSI-associated apnoea
Neck mobility issues	Limited cervical range of motion

Source: Davis, D.P. and Olvera, D.J. 2017. HEAVEN criteria: derivation of a new difficult airway prediction tool. *Air Medical Journal*, 36, 195–197.

In addition to the patient's anatomical features, a clinical history can also reveal essential information with regard to airway difficulty. For example, a history of previous difficulty with intubation, if available, is a strong predictor for subsequent difficulty.[5] Medical conditions that alter the airway and/or neck anatomy, such as airway pathologies or previous therapy/surgery, inflammatory arthritis and obstructive sleep apnoea, can also cause or compound difficulty with airway management.[6]

CHAPTER 3   The Anatomically Difficult Airway

Question 3: What Anatomical Features Increase the Risk of Difficulty with Face-Mask Ventilation and Supraglottic Airway Devices?

Both face-mask ventilation (FMV) and supraglottic airway devices (SADs) are primary airway techniques of oxygenation within prehospital care. They are also embedded in difficult airway guidelines, and as such are essential for the provision and maintenance of oxygenation in cases of difficult tracheal intubation. Akin to tracheal intubation, there are several anatomical features that increase the risk of difficulty with FMV and SADs.

Difficult Face-Mask Ventilation

Landmark studies in anaesthesia have identified several anatomical features that are risk factors for difficult or impossible FMV (**Table 3.3**).[7,8,26] More recent studies confirm these earlier results and have also identified that neck changes associated with radiation therapy can be associated with difficult FMV.[9] Broadly speaking, these risk factors – which can be recalled using the mnemonic OBESE (obese, bearded, elderly, snorer and edentulous)[10] – contribute to difficult FMV by either disrupting the face-mask seal and/or increasing upper airway obstruction. Factors that decrease respiratory compliance and/or increase resistance to ventilation can also contribute to difficulty.[11]

Table 3.3   Risk factors for difficult or impossible face-mask ventilation

Difficult	Impossible
Obesity (body mass index >30 kg/m^2)	History of snoring
Presence of a beard	Short thyromental distance (<6 cm)
Mallampati score III or IV	
Age >57 years	
Limited jaw protrusion	
History of snoring	

Source: Kheterpal, S., Han, R., Tremper, K.K. et al. 2006. Incidence and predictors of difficult and impossible mask ventilation. *Anesthesiology*, 105, 885–891.

It is important to highlight here that, although infrequently encountered, difficult FMV has been associated with an increased risk of difficulty with tracheal intubation, which probably represents an overlap between risk factors of these two airway techniques.[11]

Difficulty with Supraglottic Airway Devices

Currently, there is no research specific to prehospital or emergency medicine that has evaluated anatomical predictors of difficulty with SADs. In anaesthesia, however, risk factors that are associated with difficult ventilation via a SAD, as well as the efficacy and safety of

SECTION 1 Airway

these devices, is well defined. Largely derived from South-East Asian patients, four factors for difficult insertion or ventilation through SADs have been identified.[12]

- Male sex
- Age greater than 45 years
- A short thyromental distance
- Limited neck movement

To rationalise these risk factors, Saito et al. suggest that males have a higher incidence of upper airway resistance due to airway narrowing and OSA, as well as less favourable airway mechanics during sleep (or when unconscious).[12] Similarly, age-related changes to airway dimensions may explain why increased difficulty is seen in patients aged over 45 years. Last, a short thyromental distance and limited neck movement, and associated changes to the oral cavity configuration, have been found to interfere with insertion and positioning of SADs.

Question 4: What Anatomical Features Increase the Risk of Difficult Cricothyroidotomy?

Oxygen delivery by means of tracheal intubation, FMV or a SAD will be effective in most episodes of airway management. There will be situations, however, where these airway techniques are unsuccessful or perhaps unfeasible. This is commonly referred to as a 'can't intubate, can't oxygenate' or CICO (pronounced ky-kho) situation.[13] In a CICO situation, cricothyroidotomy is the last resort to re-establish oxygenation and, in turn, avoid hypoxic brain damage and death. On account of this, anatomical features that could make cricothyroidotomy difficult or impossible should be identified and factored into decisions prior to airway management.

Whether using a needle (narrow or wide bore) or surgical technique, accurate location of the cricothyroid membrane (CTM) is fundamental to the success of cricothyroidotomy. It is also vital in avoiding iatrogenic injury to surrounding neck structures. This, however, is often a task easier said than done, as even practising anaesthetists in controlled hospital settings frequently misidentify the CTM while using palpation techniques.[14]

As might be expected, patient factors that affect the depth, location, prominence or access to the CTM are associated with misidentification. These broadly include:

- **Smaller or less prominent laryngeal structures**, such as those seen in females[15] and infants/paediatrics
- **A high BMI or large neck circumference**, which, due to fat accumulation in the neck, increases the CTM depth and impacts tactile sense of cartilaginous landmarks[16]
- **Neck pathologies or trauma,** where airway anatomy is either fixed, disrupted or deviated, or indistinguishable.[17]

Furthermore, non-patient factors can also impact the success of CTM identification. These won't be covered in detail here, but include landmarking the CTM before induction of anaesthesia (opposed to during an airway crisis), marking the CTM while the patient is in an extended-neck position (not the sniffing position)[18] and use of the laryngeal handshake method for CTM identification (**Figure 3.2**).[19,28]

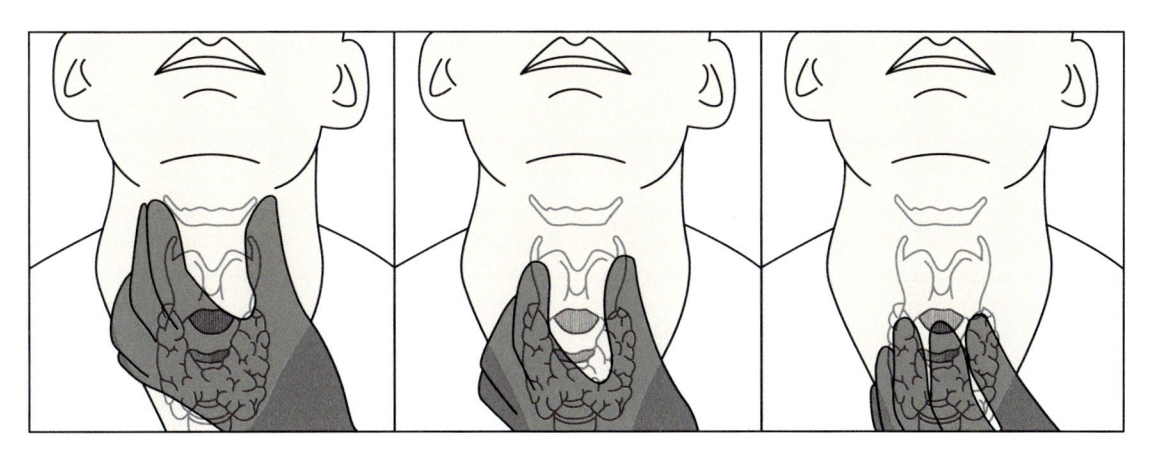

Figure 3.2 The laryngeal handshake method for identification of the cricothyroid membrane.

Point-of-care ultrasound (POCUS) is increasingly available to prehospital clinicians. Research within anaesthesia and emergency medicine has shown ultrasound use for CTM identification to be reliable and accurate, particularly when airway anatomy is impalpable.[20] Use of POCUS would be more appropriate before a predicted difficult intubation, to pre-identify landmarks, rather than as part of a failed airway drill, where time is of the essence.

Question 5: How Does an Airway Assessment Assist Decisions About Prehospital Airway Management?

The goal of an airway assessment is to identify, as effectively as possible, anatomical feature(s) that may hinder or preclude maintenance of oxygenation during airway management. As outlined, this involves an evaluation of the risk of encountering difficulty for each individual airway technique. It is important to highlight that an airway assessment cannot predict difficulty with absolute certainty,[21] which supports the argument that all prehospital airways should be considered potentially difficult. Definitive prediction of difficulty is not, however, the purpose of an airway assessment.[22] Rather, the purpose is to inform a risk–benefit analysis on prehospital advanced airway management and to aid the development of a safe and appropriate airway strategy.

> **PRACTICE TIP**
>
> An airway strategy is required for all prehospital RSIs:
>
> FAILING TO PLAN, IS PLANNING TO FAIL

Risk–Benefit Analysis

A risk–benefit analysis essentially aims to answer the question: Is prehospital advanced airway management necessary, safe and likely to be successful? This analysis is particularly important when undertaking high-risk procedures such as RSI, where airway reflexes, airway patency and spontaneous respiratory effort are abolished. On account of this, prehospital clinicians must not only assess difficulty and the likelihood of success with tracheal intubation, but also with other airway techniques.

Based on patient anatomy alone, the decision to perform RSI is relatively straightforward when an airway assessment reveals no apparent difficulty. The opposite is also true when extreme difficulty is predicted, or when success with intended and other airway techniques is deemed impossible. The challenge, therefore, arises in patients that sit in the middle of these two extremes. As described by Brown and Walls, the decision to perform RSI on a patient with a potentially difficult airway largely hinges on two factors:[23]

1. The confidence that gas exchange can be maintained by FMV or a SAD if tracheal intubation is unsuccessful
2. Whether intubation is likely to be successful, despite the difficult airway attributes.

Although not an absolute contraindication to RSI, the ability to perform a cricothyroidotomy should also be factored into this decision. Naturally, factors such as procedural urgency, patient frailty, underlying clinical conditions and distance to hospital, among others, must also be considered when formulating a risk–benefit analysis.

Development of an Airway Strategy

In addition to informing a risk–benefit analysis, an airway assessment will help develop a safe and appropriate airway strategy. The term 'airway strategy', as opposed to 'airway plan', is preferred here, as it implies a 'series of coordinated plans'[24] beyond the intended airway technique. Therefore, an airway strategy not only outlines the intended plan for airway management, but also answers the question: 'What is the plan if that plan fails?'[22] Represented by a difficult airway algorithm (**Figure 3.3**), and commonly applying a four-step A-B-C-D approach, an airway strategy aims to both optimise success with airway management and minimise complications associated with perseverance, poor communication and loss of situational awareness.[29]

Plan A – tracheal intubation

Within most difficult airway algorithms, tracheal intubation is the intended airway technique; for the most part, this is also true in the prehospital environment, although exceptions do exist.[25] In terms of developing an airway strategy, patient factors, such as anatomy, as well as non-patient factors, such as equipment availability, operating procedures and clinician skill set, will all guide decisions around a best effort at tracheal intubation.

Plan B/C – rescue techniques

Face-mask ventilation and supraglottic airway devices are commonly referred to as 'rescue techniques' – rescuing oxygenation and 'buying time' if attempts at tracheal intubation are unsuccessful. Within an airway strategy, the ordering of rescue techniques is generally guided by standard operating procedures. However, ordering can also be influenced by an airway assessment and predicted difficulty, and in some instances – such as the case

CHAPTER 3 The Anatomically Difficult Airway

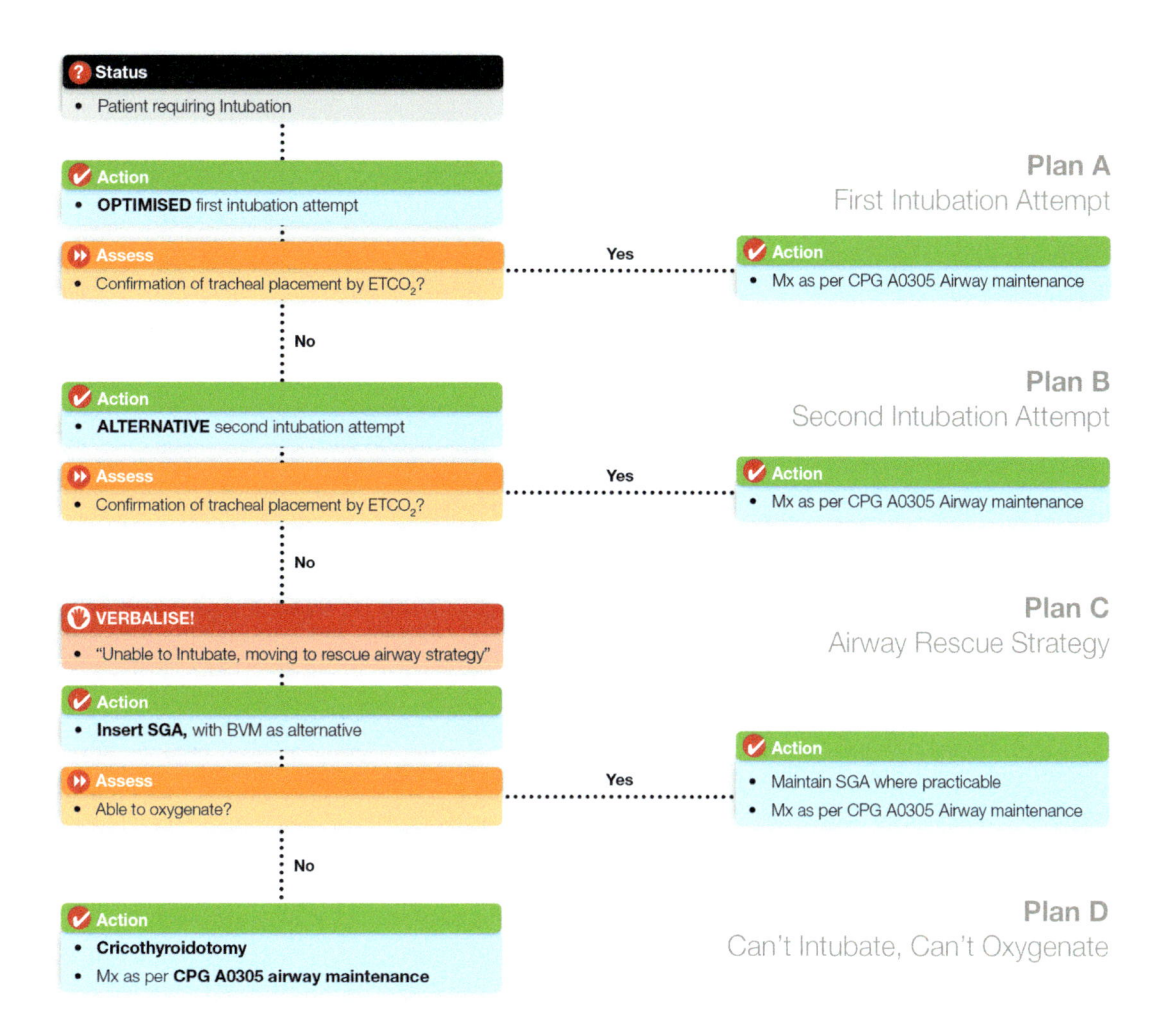

Figure 3.3 Difficult airway guideline from Ambulance Victoria ambulance service.
Source: Ambulance Victoria Clinical Practice Guidelines. Reproduced with permission.

study at the start of this chapter – the success of these techniques prior to induction of anaesthesia.

Plan D – cricothyroidotomy

Whether an anatomically difficult airway is predicted or not, an airway strategy must include a plan for a CICO situation. In the prehospital environment this plan – the last resort to rescue oxygenation – almost exclusively involves cricothyroidotomy. Cricothyroidotomy may also be used as the primary, and perhaps only, feasible airway technique, where tracheal intubation, FMV and SAD have a high likelihood of failure (for example, massive facial trauma).

SECTION 1 Airway

Key Evidence

Bradley, W.P.L. and Lyons, C. 2022. Facemask ventilation. *BJA Education,* 22, 5–11.

Brown III, C.A. and Walls, R.M. 2018. Identification of the difficult and failed airway. In: Brown III, C.A., Sakles, J.C. and Mick, N.W. (eds). *The Walls Manual of Emergency Airway Management, 5th edn.* Philadelphia: Wolters Kluwer.

Chrimes, N. and Fritz, P. 2016. The vortex approach to airway management [Online]. Melbourne, Australia. Available at: http://vortexapproach.org/planning

Price, T.M. and McCoy, E.P. 2019. Emergency front of neck access in airway management. *BJA Education,* 19, 246–253.

Nausheen, F., Niknafs, N.P., Maclean, D.J. et al. 2019. The HEAVEN criteria predict laryngoscopic view and intubation success for both direct and video laryngoscopy: a cohort analysis. *Scandinavian Journal of Trauma, Resuscitation and Emergency Medicine,* 27.

Reardon, R.F., Robinson, A.E., Kornas, R. et al. 2022. Prehospital surgical airway management: an NAEMSP position statement and resource document. *Prehospital Emergency Care,* 26, 96–101.

Self-Reflection Questions

1. Why is it difficult to universally define the term 'difficult airway'?
2. What prehospital-specific factors (not related to patient anatomy) can increase the incidence of difficult airway management?
3. List five anatomical features that may increase the risk of difficult airway management for FMV, SAD *and* tracheal intubation.
4. From a human-factors perspective, why is it important to clearly articulate an airway strategy prior to tracheal intubation? How does this aid teamwork and support decision-making when difficulty is encountered during airway management?
5. How does marking the CTM prior to RSI potentially improve the technical and non-technical performance of cricothyroidotomy?

References

1. Huitink, J.M. and Bouwman, R.A. 2015. The myth of the difficult airway: airway management revisited. *Anaesthesia,* 70, 244–249.
2. Law J.A., et al. Canadian Airway Focus Group. 2021. Canadian Airway Focus Group updated consensus-based recommendations for management of the difficult airway. *Canadian Journal of Anaesthesia,* 68(9), 1373–1404.
3. Brown III, C.A. and Walls, R.M. 2018. The emergency airway algorithms. In: Brown III, C.A., Sakles, J.C. and Mick, N.W. (eds), *The Walls Manual of Emergency Airway Management,* 5th edn. Philadelphia: Wolters Kluwer.
4. Nausheen, F., Niknafs, N.P., Maclean, D.J. et al. 2019. The HEAVEN criteria predict laryngoscopic view and intubation success for both direct and video laryngoscopy: a cohort analysis. *Scandinavian Journal of Trauma, Resuscitation and Emergency Medicine,* 27.
5. Detsky, M.E., Jivraj, N., Adhikari, N.K. et al. 2019. Will this patient be difficult to intubate? The Rational Clinical Examination Systematic Review. *JAMA,* 321, 493–503.
6. Hagberg, C.A., Zheng, G. and Diemunsch, P. 2021. Pre-anaesthetic airway assessment. In: Cook, T. and Kristensen, M. (eds), *Core Topics in Airway Management,* 3rd edn. Cambridge: Cambridge University Press.
7. Langeron, O., Masso, E., Huraux, C. et al. 2000. Prediction of difficult mask ventilation. *Anesthesiology,* 92, 1229–1236.
8. Kheterpal, S., Han, R., Tremper, K.K. et al. 2006. Incidence and predictors of difficult and impossible mask ventilation. *Anesthesiology,* 105, 885–891.

9. Lundstrøm, L.H., Rosenstock, C.V., Wetterslev, J. et al. 2019. The DIFFMASK score for predicting difficult facemask ventilation: a cohort study of 46,804 patients. *Anaesthesia*, 74, 1267–1276.
10. Crawley, S. and Dalton, A. 2015. Predicting the difficult airway. *BJA Education*, 15, 253–258.
11. Bradley, W.P.L. and Lyons, C. 2022. Facemask ventilation. *BJA Education*, 22, 5–11.
12. Saito, T., Liu, W., Chew, S.T.H. et al. 2015. Incidence of and risk factors for difficult ventilation via a supraglottic airway device in a population of 14,480 patients from South-East Asia. *Anaesthesia*, 70, 1079–1083.
13. Chrimes, N. and Cook, T.M. 2017. Critical airways, critical language. *British Journal of Anaesthesia*, 118, 649–654.
14. Siddiqui, N., Yu, E., Boulis, S. et al. 2018. Ultrasound is superior to palpation in identifying the cricothyroid membrane in subjects with poorly defined neck landmarks: a randomized clinical trial. *Anesthesiology*, 129, 1132–1139.
15. Campbell, M., Shanahan, H., Ash, S. et al. 2014. The accuracy of locating the cricothyroid membrane by palpation – an intergender study. *BMC Anesthesiology*, 14, 108.
16. Gadd, K., Wills, K., Harle, R. et al. 2018. Relationship between severe obesity and depth to the cricothyroid membrane in third-trimester non-labouring parturients: a prospective observational study. *British Journal of Anaesthesia*, 120, 1033–1039.
17. Baker, P.A., Duggan, L.V. and Enk, D. 2021. Front of neck airway (FONA). In: Cook, T. and Kristensen, M.S. (eds), *Core Topics in Airway Management*, 3rd edn. Cambridge: Cambridge University Press.
18. Dixit, A., Ramaswamy, K.K., Perera, S. et al. 2019. Impact of change in head and neck position on ultrasound localisation of the cricothyroid membrane: an observational study. *Anaesthesia*, 74, 29–32.
19. Drew, T. and McCaul, C.L. 2018. Laryngeal handshake technique in locating the cricothyroid membrane: a non-randomised comparative study. *British Journal of Anaesthesia*, 121, 1173–1178.
20. Rai, Y., You-Ten, E., Zasso, F. et al. 2020. The role of ultrasound in front-of-neck access for cricothyroid membrane identification: a systematic review. *Journal of Critical Care*, 60, 161–168.
21. Nørskov, A.K., Rosenstock, C.V., Wetterslev, J. et al. 2015. Diagnostic accuracy of anaesthesiologists' prediction of difficult airway management in daily clinical practice: a cohort study of 188 064 patients registered in the Danish Anaesthesia Database. *Anaesthesia*, 70, 272–281.
22. Chrimes, N. and Fritz, P. 2016. *The vortex approach to airway management* [Online]. Melbourne, Australia. Available at: http://vortexapproach.org/planning
23. Brown III, C.A. and Walls, R.M. 2018. Identification of the difficult and failed airway. In: Brown III, C.A., Sakles, J.C. and Mick, N.W. (eds), *The Walls Manual of Emergency Airway Management*, 5th edn. Philadelphia: Wolters Kluwer.
24. Cook, T.M., Woodall, N. and Frerk, C. 2011. Major complications of airway management in the UK: results of the Fourth National Audit Project of the Royal College of Anaesthetists and the Difficult Airway Society. Part 1: anaesthesia. *British Journal of Anaesthesia*, 106(5), 617–631.
25. Braude, D., Dixon, D., Torres, M. et al. 2020. Brief research report: prehospital rapid sequence airway. *Prehospital Emergency Care*, 25, 1–5.
26. Bradley, P., Chapman, G., Crooke, B. et al. 2016. Airway assessment [Online]. Australian and New Zealand College of Anaesthetists (ANZCA). Available at: https://www.anzca.edu.au/resources/incident-reporting-docs/airway-docs/pu-airway-assessment-20160916v1
27. Davis, D.P. and Olvera, D.J. 2017. HEAVEN criteria: derivation of a new difficult airway prediction tool. *Air Medical Journal*, 36, 195–197.
28. Oh, H., Yoon, S., Seo, M. et al. 2018. Utility of the laryngeal handshake method for identifying the cricothyroid membrane. *Acta Anaesthesiologica Scandinavica*, 62, 1223–1228.
29. Whitten, C. 2018. 10 rules for approaching difficult intubation [Online]. Anesthesiology News. Available at: https://www.anesthesiologynews.com/Review-Articles/Article/08-18/10-Rules-for-Approaching-Difficult-Intubation/52456?sub=F97448B936B214B941CA9DB6B95A2523FA8DBAD93E5BB177C7934CC7A&enl=true#:~:text=10%20Rules%20for%20Approaching%20Difficult%20Intubation%201%201.,3%203.%20Teamwork%20and%20Communication%20Are%20Essential%20

SECTION 2

Breathing

Mechanical Ventilation

4

Tim Byrne and Nick Roder

In this chapter you will learn:

- How to describe the benefits of prehospital mechanical ventilator application
- How to detail the basic settings of a mechanical ventilator within the principles of lung protection strategies
- How to discuss the management of common problems associated with mechanical ventilation
- How to differentiate between restrictive and obstructive lung pathology and to detail how the mechanical ventilator would be set up.

Case Details

Dispatch
60-year-old male, cardiac arrest.

History
A 60-year-old man collapsed unconscious in front of his wife this afternoon after complaining of feeling 'unwell' for the past 24 hours. A neighbour commenced CPR while waiting for the ambulance.

On Arrival of the First Crew
The patient is found in cardiac arrest, CPR is continued, ventricular fibrillation (VF) identified, and two DC countershocks performed prior to the critical care paramedic's arrival.

On Your Arrival as the Critical Care Paramedic
The patient has now been in cardiac arrest for 20 minutes. High-quality CPR is being performed; however, the airway is heavily soiled with vomitus. A third defibrillation for VF is initiated at the two-minute pause. Without interrupting external compressions, the patient is intubated to obtain a more reliable airway, with concurrent suctioning of both the endotracheal tube (ETT) and oropharynx. A pulse is identified at the subsequent two-minute check. External compressions are ceased, a complete reassessment is initiated and manual ventilation is continued in the apnoeic patient.

After establishing post return of spontaneous circulation (ROSC) management, the team elect to commence mechanical ventilation prior to extricating the patient. Upon connection to the patient, the ventilator immediately alarms 'High Peak Inspiratory Pressure',

SECTION 2 Breathing

and the patient rapidly desaturates. The primary survey findings and vital signs post ROSC are:

Airway	Intubated
Breathing	RR 10, SpO$_2$ 92% on FiO$_2$ 1.0, no spontaneous effort
Circulation	Peripheral pulses strong, HR 53, BP 110/60, cool peripheries
Disability	GCS E1, Vt, M1 (3), pupils 4 mm and reactive, BGL 8.0
Environmental	Temp 36.3 °C. Other comments: nil relevant

AMPLE

The patient has a past medical history of mild COPD, having ceased smoking around four years ago. He is able to undertake the activities of daily living, requiring occasional use of his inhaled respiratory medications. His hypertension is managed with diet and medication.

Allergies	NKDA
Medications	Salbutamol inhaler Atrovent inhaler Irbesartan/hydrochlorothiazide tablet
Past history	Mild COPD Hypertension
Last ins and outs	Normal
Events prior	Unremarkable. At home, feeling generally unwell.

Decision Point 1
What is the paramedic response to the immediate alarming of the mechanical ventilator?

Decision Point 2
What does the early application of a mechanical ventilator offer this patient in the context of this setting?

Decision Point 3
What is the likely cause of the high pressures in a patient with this presentation, and how can this be effectively managed?

CHAPTER 4   Mechanical Ventilation

Question 1: What does Mechanical Ventilation Offer in this Case Context?

Early initiation of mechanical ventilation offers several benefits to the patient in a prehospital setting:

- Ventilation tailored to the patient's respiratory physiology
- Alarms to provide warnings of patient deterioration or circuit disconnection
- Establishment of therapeutic momentum in the out-of-hospital phase
- Accurate monitoring of respiratory parameters
- Logistical and ergonomic assistance to facilitate safe, rapid transfer to hospital, particularly when extricating from awkward environments.

Respiratory Parameters and Targets

Moving to mechanical ventilation in the out-of-hospital environment provides valuable insight into the patient's clinical presentation, in addition to the accurate titration of ventilation volumes, pressures and gas targets such as PO_2 and PCO_2 normalisation in the post-arrest patient. All ventilators report pressures of ventilation, while many also include assessment of intrinsic PEEP and plateau pressure. In addition, perfusion management is critical in the post-arrest patient, and the presence of accurate respiratory values may provide the clinician with an understanding of how ventilation affects perfusion.[1]

Alarms

Alarms associated with patient monitoring, such as ECG or oxygen saturation, are frequent, often erroneous or the result of artefact, and can bring about clinician 'alarm fatigue'.[2] While not all alarms generated by a mechanical ventilator require immediate attention, they provide a valuable insight into the effectiveness of breathing, evolving problems or, in this case, a concerning elevation of the pressures of inspiration.[3]

Therapeutic Momentum

Prehospital management is part of a continuum of care that often establishes the precedent for in-hospital management. The effective and patient-centred initiation of prehospital mechanical ventilation can positively influence the continued in-hospital care of the patient and is becoming the recommended standard for ventilation once a prehospital advanced airway has been established.[4,5]

Lung Protective Ventilation Strategy

Prolonged exposure to inappropriate ventilation pressures or volumes can result in acute lung injury (ALI), with lung injury from large tidal volumes occurring within 20 minutes.[6,7] While safe ventilation can be attempted with gentle manual-bag ventilation, the lack of objective values often results in high pressures, higher respiratory rates and varying tidal volumes. Conversely, the early establishment of accurate ventilation parameters has been shown to reduce the likelihood of ALI.[8–11]

SECTION 2 Breathing

Logistical and Ergonomic Assistance

Early application of the mechanical ventilator offers the team a substantial advantage when extricating a patient in a logistically complex situation. Safely securing the ventilator within the patient extrication packaging removes the need for a paramedic to awkwardly attend to manual ventilation, while also providing best-care ventilation strategy without interruption.[12]

Once in transit, the application of mechanical ventilation effectively creates another critical care team member, dedicated to delivering precise breathing, alerting the team to changes while providing continuous monitoring of respiratory values. This reduces cognitive workload, enables attention to other critical tasks and reduces the likelihood of missed adverse events due to distraction.

Question 2: How Would You Choose Initial Ventilator Settings?

The pathway to initiating patient-relevant mechanical ventilation settings benefits from two fundamental insights.

1. **The 'tactility' of the BVM** experienced prior to the transition to mechanical ventilation.

   The 'feel' of the BVM provides the clinician with tactile insights into the pressures and clinical response to ventilation that can inform both the subsequent mechanical ventilation settings and the likely challenges once commenced.

> **PRACTICE TIP**
>
> Once a patient is on the mechanical ventilator, make sure that a bag-valve-mask is within arm's reach at all times.

2. **Categorising the patient's lung pathology** as either *normal* (or absence of lung pathology), *obstructive* or *restrictive* disease pattern within the context of their clinical condition.

   A compact algorithm that neatly limits the settings into three categories simplifies the commencement of mechanical ventilation by grouping settings according to clinical condition. **Figure 4.1** illustrates this principle. Once a category is selected, a range of setting parameters is offered, providing the clinician with some flexibility in tailoring the initial settings to the patient's clinical condition, severity and prehospital context.

   It should be noted that these represent commencement settings, with subsequent 'tweaking' by the clinician in response to the patient's evolving clinical trajectory and/or ventilator feedback.

> **PRACTICE TIP**
>
> Follow a systematic approach to ventilator setup, using the logical sequence of your particular device.

CHAPTER 4 Mechanical Ventilation

	Obstructive lung	Normal lung	Restrictive lung
	Acute bronchospasm, COPD, asthma		Pneumonia, aspiration, ARDS, bariatric, COVID
Mode	SIMV, volume-control			
FiO$_2$	1.0 — Titrate to SPO$_2$ >94% (minimum FiO$_2$ 0.4) once *clinically stable, stationary and the ventilator/ETT is secure.*		
Tidal volume	6–8 mL/kg	6–8 mL/kg	6 mL/kg
Rate	6–8/min — Titrate to blood pressure, AutoPEEP, EtCO$_2$ and PIPs	12–15/min — Titrate rate first, then V$_T$ to target EtCO$_2$ 30–35 mmHg	>18/min — Titrate rate first, then V$_T$ to target EtCO$_2$ 30–35 mmHg
	**Rate** is usually the primary method for adjusting minute volume. **Blood gas analysis** should be used to guide ventilation settings where possible.		
PEEP	<5 cm H$_2$O	5 cm H$_2$O	5–15 cm H$_2$O
	Titrate to SpO$_2$ >94%		
I : E	1 : 6–8	1 : 2–3	1 : 1–1.5
Inspiratory time	1–1.5 seconds		Titrate to above I : E
Considerations	**PIPs** may exceed 40–60 cm H$_2$O, particularly in acute asthma. **Accept hypercapnia.** Aim for a slow reduction in EtCO$_2$. **Monitor TPT** in the setting of persistent poor perfusion.	**Many critical patients are acidotic.** Does the patient require respiratory compensation and higher MVs? **EtCO$_2$ target** may change for specific conditions, such as TCA overdose.	**Avoid unnecessary disconnection/suctioning** Optimal lung recruitment depends on continuous airway pressure. **Mild hypercapnia** is acceptable in restrictive lung patients without brain injury. **Severe multi-trauma:** With combined TBI and chest injury, blood pressure preservation outweighs normalisation of EtCO$_2$ or blood gases.
Spontaneously ventilating	**Ensure** triggering and sensitivity accurately captures breaths. **Sedation must be adequate to avoid asynchrony.** **Pressure support (5–10 cm H$_2$O)** titrated to expected V$_T$ and compliance. **Monitor** for ventilator synchrony and MV.		

Figure 4.1 Prehospital mechanical ventilation settings guide.
Source: Ambulance Victoria Clinical Practice Guidelines. Reproduced with permission.

SECTION 2 Breathing

Question 3: What is the Paramedic Response to High Pressure Alarms Upon Connection?

In general, when high pressure alarms are triggered early in the application of mechanical ventilation, it is reasonable for the team to reflect on the ventilator's settings, relative to the patient's lung condition. Having a low threshold for immediately moving back to manual ventilation while the team deliberates on the cause provides time for consideration while attending to settings adjustment, and is a safe redundancy strategy associated with ventilator application. This is particularly relevant where rapid desaturation occurs.

In contrast, high pressure alarms that arise after prolonged, uncomplicated mechanical ventilation are often associated with a change to the patient's clinical status, including analgesia or sedation wearing off post intubation (ventilator asynchrony), airway secretions or an evolving lung pathology.

> **PRACTICE TIP**
>
> Never ignore alarms!
>
> ACKNOWLEDGE – CONFIRM – RESOLVE

Question 4: What are Common Sources of High Ventilation Pressures and How can they be Managed?

Obstructive Lung Pathology

Obstructive lung pathology occurs when there is high resistance to airflow in either the patient's airways or the circuit. Common patient clinical problems that can cause this are listed in **Table 4.1**.

Restrictive Lung Pathology

Restrictive lung pathology occurs due to increased elastance (stiffness) of the lungs or problems relating to chest wall/diaphragmatic expansion. It can also occur due to extrinsic compression on the lung, such as pneumothorax or haemothorax.

Table 4.1 Causes of restrictive and obstructive defects

Obstructive pathologies	Restrictive pathologies
Asthma	Acute respiratory lung disease
COPD	Pneumonia
Anaphylaxis (bronchospasm)	COVID-19
ETT or large airway obstruction (such as sputum plugging)	Pneumo/haemothorax
	Lung tissue injury
	Obesity

CHAPTER 4 Mechanical Ventilation

Airway Secretions

A common cause of elevated pressures of ventilation is the accumulation of secretions in the large airways, particularly the ETT. Targeted suctioning will assist in excluding this as a source; however, prolonged suctioning can quickly induce hypoxia, particularly where alveolar recruitment has been challenging.

Ventilator–Patient Asynchrony

The ventilator 'mode' establishes the ventilator's relationship with the patient to ensure a co-operative delivery of breaths, while accommodating spontaneous respiration. Synchronised intermittent mandatory ventilation (SIMV) aims to ensure a targeted minute volume, while accommodating the patient's desire to breathe spontaneously. When a mechanical ventilator and the patient's spontaneous respiration 'clash', high ventilation pressures (possibly progressing to failed ventilation) often result. This is known as ventilator–patient asynchrony. Ensuring spontaneous breaths are identified by the ventilator and captured (triggering) and are adequately supported (pressure support) will aid ventilator–patient synchrony.

Ventilator settings are clinician set, but patient evaluated. Therefore ventilator–patient asynchrony management should begin with the ventilator settings. Ensure triggering is effective and sufficient flow during spontaneous ventilation is provided. However, if ventilator–patient asynchrony persists, ensure patient comfort by increasing sedation, progressing to the administration of paralysis if sedation alone proves inadequate.

Question 5: What Ventilator Manoeuvres can be Used to Help Diagnose the Cause of High Airway Pressures?

Lung protective strategies are a collection of ventilation parameters that reduce the pro-inflammatory effects of positive pressure ventilation.[3,13] They typically involve:

- Limiting the tidal volume to 6–8 mL/kg
- Maintenance of alveolar inflation by the provision of a minimum PEEP 5 cm H_2O
- Limiting the pressures of ventilation to below plateau 30 cm H_2O
- Reducing the exposure to high-concentration oxygen.

In addition to auscultation of the chest, inspiratory and expiratory hold manoeuvres (when available on the ventilator being used) can assist in diagnosing the pathology causing high airway pressures.

An inspiratory hold manoeuvre is performed by closing the expiratory valve on the ventilator at the end of the inspiratory phase of the respiratory cycle and 'holding' the breath in the patient/circuit. This is usually performed using a dedicated button or menu item on the ventilator. A brief period of observation with the valve closed is required as pressures equilibrate through the circuit and patient's respiratory system. Once a steady state of pressure is reached, airflow has stopped. The observed pressure in the circuit at this point is known as the plateau pressure. This pressure is generally equivalent to the pressure in the patient's alveoli.

SECTION 2 Breathing

If the plateau pressure is high, this indicates that the patient's respiratory system has a restrictive pattern. In this case the plateau pressure is generally only slightly lower than the peak pressure.

If the plateau pressure is normal in the setting of a high peak pressure, this suggests an obstructive pathology leading to high resistance in the airways. In this setting a high airway pressure is required to drive gas through narrow, resistant airways, but once airflow stops, the lungs do not require a high pressure to remain expanded. This also implies that alveoli are not being exposed to dangerously high pressures despite a high PIP.

In the context of this post-arrest patient, the high pressures of ventilation may have two possible causes. The history of COPD implies the potential for bronchospasm, creating restrictive airflow. Alternatively, the presence of possible aspiration and prolonged CPR may suggest an evolving restrictive lung pattern. Understanding the plateau pressure may assist in differentiating the cause and providing an appropriate treatment pathway.

Question 6: What are the Steps to Manage High Airway Pressures due to Obstruction?

1. Attempt to diagnose and treat underlying causes (for example, suctioning or bronchodilators).
2. Accept high peak pressures (up to 60 cm H_2O or higher) if plateau pressures are 'safe' (<30 cm H_2O).
3. Increase expiratory time by setting:
    a. A slow respiratory rate (6 breaths/min)
    b. A long I:E ratio (between 1:3 and 1:6).
4. Accept a high $EtCO_2$ if oxygenation is adequate.
5. Consider PEEP <5 cm H_2O (avoid intrinsic or 'AutoPEEP').

When combined, the settings detailed above will often result in a low minute ventilation and high peak airway pressures. This is an acceptable trade-off, as the aim of this ventilation strategy is to allow adequate time in expiration to prevent gas trapping (AutoPEEP) and dynamic hyperinflation of the thoracic cavity.

Question 7: What are the Steps to Manage High Airway Pressures Due to Restriction?

1. Attempt to diagnose and treat underlying causes (for example, deepening sedation/paralysis; exclude pneumothorax).
2. Aim to keep plateau pressures <30 cm H_2O.
3. Low tidal volumes (5–6 mL/kg) with a high respiratory rate may be required to achieve adequate minute volume while ensuring a plateau pressure <30 cm H_2O.
4. Prolonged inspiration, I:E ratio (1:1.0–1.5).
5. Higher PEEP (10–15 cm H_2O) may improve oxygenation.

CHAPTER 4 Mechanical Ventilation

Smaller tidal volumes exert less lung stretch, reducing the driving pressure of ventilation in the restrictive pathology. However, this compromise may result in a low minute ventilation, elevating PCO_2. In the setting of anoxic head injury post arrest, this strategy should be used cautiously. An acceptable trade-off is the aim to minimise further lung injury by avoiding excessive inspiratory pressure.[1]

Key Evidence

Brower RG, Matthay MA, Morris A et al. Ventilation with lower tidal volumes as compared with traditional tidal volumes for acute lung injury and the acute respiratory distress syndrome. *New England Journal of Medicine*. 2000 May 4;342(18):1301–1308. Available at: https://pubmed.ncbi.nlm.nih.gov/10793162/

Stephens RJ, Siegler JE, Fuller BM. Mechanical ventilation in the prehospital and emergency department environment. *Respiratory Care*. 2019 May 1;64(5):595–603.

Wilcox S, Richards J, Fisher D et al. Initial mechanical ventilator settings and lung protective ventilation in the ED. *American Journal of Emergency Medicine*. 2016;34(8):1446–1451.

Self-Reflection Questions

1. What are the benefits of applying mechanical ventilation in the prehospital setting?
2. What are the principles of lung protective strategy and how can these be applied when establishing mechanical ventilation?
3. What are the two general types of lung pathology that complicate mechanical ventilation and what are the appropriate settings for each?
4. How can the clinician identify and differentiate between these two lung pathologies?
5. What are some of the considerations when mechanically ventilating the post-arrest patient?

References

1. Battaglini D, Pelosi P, Robba C. Ten rules for optimizing ventilatory settings and targets in post-cardiac arrest patients. *Critical Care*. 2022 Dec 17;26(1):390. Available at: https://pubmed.ncbi.nlm.nih.gov/36527126/
2. Scott J, De Vaux L, Dills C et al. Mechanical ventilation alarms and alarm fatigue. *Respiratory Care*. 2019 Oct;64(10):1308–1313. Available at: https://pubmed.ncbi.nlm.nih.gov/31213570
3. Brower RG, Matthay MA, Morris A et al. Ventilation with lower tidal volumes as compared with traditional tidal volumes for acute lung injury and the acute respiratory distress syndrome. *New England Journal of Medicine*. 2000 May 4;342(18):1301–1308. Available at: https://pubmed.ncbi.nlm.nih.gov/10793162/
4. Stephens RJ, Siegler JE, Fuller BM. Mechanical ventilation in the prehospital and emergency department environment. *Respiratory Care*. 2019 May 1;64(5):595–603.
5. Davis D, Bosson N, Guyette F et al. Optimizing physiology during prehospital airway management: a NAEMSP position statement and resource document. *Prehospital Emergency Care*. 2022;26(1):72–79.
6. Fuller BM, Ferguson IT, Mohr NM et al. lung-protective ventilation initiated in the emergency department (LOV-ED): a quasi-experimental, before-after trial. *Annals of Emergency Medicine*. 2017 Sep;70(3):406–418.e4. Available at: https://pubmed.ncbi.nlm.nih.gov/28259481/
7. Fuller BM, Page D, Stephens RJ et al. Pulmonary mechanics and mortality in mechanically ventilated patients without acute respiratory distress syndrome: a cohort study. *Shock*. 2018 Mar;49(3):311–316. Available at: https://pubmed.ncbi.nlm.nih.gov/28846571/
8. Dumont TM, Visioni AJ, Rughani AI et al. Prehospital ventilation in severe traumatic brain injury increases in-hospital mortality. *Journal of Neurotrauma*. 2010;27(7):1233–1241.
9. Elling R, Politis J. An evaluation of emergency medical technicians' ability to use manual ventilation devices. *Annals of Emergency Medicine*. 1983 Dec;12(12):765–768.

SECTION 2 Breathing

10. Siegler J, Kroll M, Wojcik M et al. Can EMS providers provide appropriate tidal volumes in a simulated adult-sized patient with a pediatric-sized bag-valve-mask? *Prehospital Emergency Care*. 2017;21(1): 74–78. Available at: https://pubmed.ncbi.nlm.nih.gov/27690714/
11. Turki T, Young M, Wagers S et al. Peak pressures during manual ventilation. *Respiratory Care*. Mar 2005;50(3):340–344.
12. Weiss SJ, Ernst AA, Jones R et al. Automatic transport ventilator versus bag valve in the EMS setting: a prospective, randomized trial. *Southern Medical Journal*. 2005 Oct;98(10):970–976. Available at: https://pubmed.ncbi.nlm.nih.gov/16295811/
13. Moloney E, Griffiths J. Protective ventilation of patients with acute respiratory distress syndrome. *British Journal of Anaesthesia*. 2004; 92(2):261–270.

Respiratory Failure

5

Daniel Cudini and Segun Olusanya

In this chapter you will learn:
- Contemporary respiratory failure assessment and management in accordance with current guidelines, recommendations, and evidence
- Common aetiologies and the prevalence of prehospital respiratory failure presentations
- Challenges relating to paramedic respiratory failure care and recognition.

Case Details

Dispatch
72-year-old female, severe respiratory distress, drowsy.

History
A 72-year-old female has been experiencing lethargy, myalgia, productive cough and hot/cold episodes over the past 48 hours. Today she has experienced worsening shortness of breath, which has been unresponsive to her own Ventolin administration. Her husband called, as she is now becoming drowsy. A double-crewed ambulance and a critical care paramedic are dispatched.

On Arrival of the First Crew
The scene is safe, and the patient is sitting upright in a lounge chair. Her vital signs are:

Airway	Patent
Breathing	RR 36, SpO_2 82% on room air, laboured, bilateral coarse crackles
Circulation	Peripheral pulses weak, HR 122, irregular, BP 145/90, cool, clammy peripheries
Disability	GCS E3, V4, M5 (12), BGL 6.3 mmol/L
Environmental	Temp 38.3 °C, indoors, no other environmental concerns

SECTION 2   Breathing

The first paramedic crew arrive, leave the patient in the upright position, and apply high-flow oxygen via a non-rebreather mask. Their secondary survey reveals clubbing of the fingers and pursed-lipped breathing. The patient is pale, diaphoretic and leaning forward in a tripod position.

On Your Arrival as the Critical Care Paramedic

One of the paramedics is inserting an 18g IV in the right forearm, and upon observing the patient, you see she is displaying supraclavicular, suprasternal and intercostal retraction. She is unable to speak any words but appears to obey commands. Further assessment of the patient's cardiovascular state reveals a bulging jugular vein and strong peripheral pulses. The patient's SpO_2 has increased to 91% and nasal $EtCO_2$ is 58 mmHg. No other abnormalities are evident upon performing a 12-lead ECG.

AMPLE

The patient is an ex-smoker, has a past medical history of chronic obstructive airways disease and recurrent respiratory infections. She has type 2 diabetes mellitus and was diagnosed with an NSTEMI twelve months prior. You are only able to locate a handful of medications; Ventolin PMDI, Spiriva and aspirin. The patient has no known allergies and lives with her husband, who assists her by providing care. Her estimated weight is approximately 100 kgs.

Allergies	NKDA
Medications	Salbutamol PMDI PRN Budesonide/formoterol (Symbicort) Aspirin
Past history	COPD, T2DM, NSTEMI, chronic respiratory infections
Last ins and outs	Normal
Events	Worsening shortness of breath precipitated by prodromal infective symptoms

Decision Point
What are your clinical priorities in this situation?

The patient presents with severe respiratory distress due to a likely infective exacerbation of her COPD. Hypercapnic respiratory failure also appears to be present, and commencement of immediate respiratory care is crucial in this setting to prevent further morbidity and patient deterioration. The focus of prehospital care in this patient should be a loading dose of nebulised salbutamol and ipratropium bromide, followed by targeting oxygenation as per defined SpO_2 ranges highlighted in current COPD guidelines (SpO_2 88–92%), administration of IV steroid (e.g. dexamethasone) and, if unresponsive to initial therapy, application of NIV (preferably bi-level).

CHAPTER 5 Respiratory Failure

Question 1: What are the Common Aetiologies and Prevalence of Prehospital Respiratory Failure Presentations?

Acute respiratory failure (ARF) is often encountered by critical care paramedics and develops due to either the inability to maintain normal oxygen delivery to tissues (hypoxia) or the inadequate removal of carbon dioxide from the tissues (hypercarbia).[1] It can be classified as acute or chronic, and can be caused by common cardiac and respiratory conditions, such as myocardial infarction, acute heart failure, pulmonary embolism, asthma, pneumonia, chronic obstructive pulmonary disease (COPD) and sepsis.[1,2] Three main mechanisms occur and when any one of them fails, ARF can ensue:[1]

- Transfer of oxygen across the alveolus
- Transport of oxygen to the tissues by cardiac output
- Removal of carbon dioxide from the blood into the alveolus with subsequent exhalation into room air.

Based on a large American dataset from the mid-1990s, four main aetiologies of prehospital respiratory failure were identified:[1]

1. Cardiogenic pulmonary oedema (16%)
2. Pneumonia (15%)
3. Exacerbations of COPD (13%)
4. 'Other' (including asthma, pulmonary embolism and myocardial infarction) (56%).

This was also highlighted in a UK study by Fuller et al. of 77 patients with ARF, where 32.9% presented with COPD, 32.9% with lower respiratory tract infection, 18.4% with heart failure and 15.7% with other secondary contributory conditions, such as myocardial infarction, sepsis, asthma and pulmonary embolism.[3]

ARF can be diagnosed by significant changes in arterial blood gases or arterial oxygen saturation from normal ranges. This can be challenging as normal levels of PaO_2 and $PaCO_2$ can be affected by factors such as age, environment (living at altitude) and metabolic responses.[1] In addition, patients with chronic respiratory conditions can function with blood gas levels that would be abnormal and dangerous in a physiologically normal person. They develop chronic respiratory failure, which results in the development of physiological mechanisms to compensate for inadequate gas exchange.[4]

An arterial PaO_2 of less than 60 mmHg or an arterial $PaCO_2$ of greater than 45 mmHg generally indicates significant respiratory compromise and likelihood of ARF.[4]

> **PRACTICE TIP**
>
> Any patient who presents with respiratory distress with confirmed aetiology and speaks only in single words, or not at all, is likely to be experiencing respiratory failure. Thorough assessment should support this.

SECTION 2 Breathing

Question 2: What is the Contemporary Approach to Respiratory Failure Assessment and How Could this be Applied to the Prehospital Setting?

This should involve a rapid, concise, focused history, often collateral if the patient is obtunded or short of breath. Nonetheless, this is key and can yield several clues to the aetiology of respiratory failure (and thus guide therapy). Any history of chest pain, syncope, fevers and unwell contacts is crucial as this rapidly allows identification of the top three causes listed above.

A focused examination using an ABCDE approach (airway, breathing, circulation, disability, exposure) should be performed. Specific attention should be paid to the following.

Airway: Any evidence of obstruction, a general assessment for intubation difficulty and facial features affecting adequate mask seal for NIV (for example, beards).
Breathing: Respiratory rate, use of accessory muscles, ability to speak in sentences, cyanosis, wheeze, stridor. Auscultation of the chest may allow the identification of lateralising signs such as bronchial breathing. While appropriately de-emphasised in the diagnosis of tension pneumothorax, in the less time-critical situation, there may still be some value in examining the trachea for potential deviation, as it can be a useful sign of intrathoracic pathology. Pathologies that increase unilateral intrathoracic pressure (like a large pleural effusion) may push the trachea away from the site of embarrassment. Pathologies causing a reduction in unilateral intrathoracic pressure (for example, airway collapse from an obstructing bronchial tumour) may pull the trachea towards the site of embarrassment.
Circulation: Any evidence of shock/hypoperfusion.
Disability: Conscious level, agitation, diaphoresis.
Exposure: Rashes, temperature, any evidence of leg swelling.

Vital signs should be assessed – blood pressure, pulse oximetry and blood glucose. Point-of-care blood gas oximetry can be used if available and can allow the separation of hypoxaemic versus hypercarbic respiratory failure. Capnography can be very helpful here if available.

Point-of-care ultrasound (POCUS) is increasingly being used in the hospital environment. In the emergency department it has demonstrated high sensitivity and specificity for the diagnosis of acute cardiogenic pulmonary oedema and the ability to accurately diagnose different causes of respiratory failure.[5,6] A full assessment involves using the BLUE protocol as developed by Daniel Lichtenstein; this includes assessment of the lungs, focused echocardiography and a brief assessment of the lower limbs for a DVT. Some examples of lung ultrasound images are shown below (**Figures 5.1–5.4**), as well as the BLUE protocol (**Figure 5.5**).

CHAPTER 5 Respiratory Failure

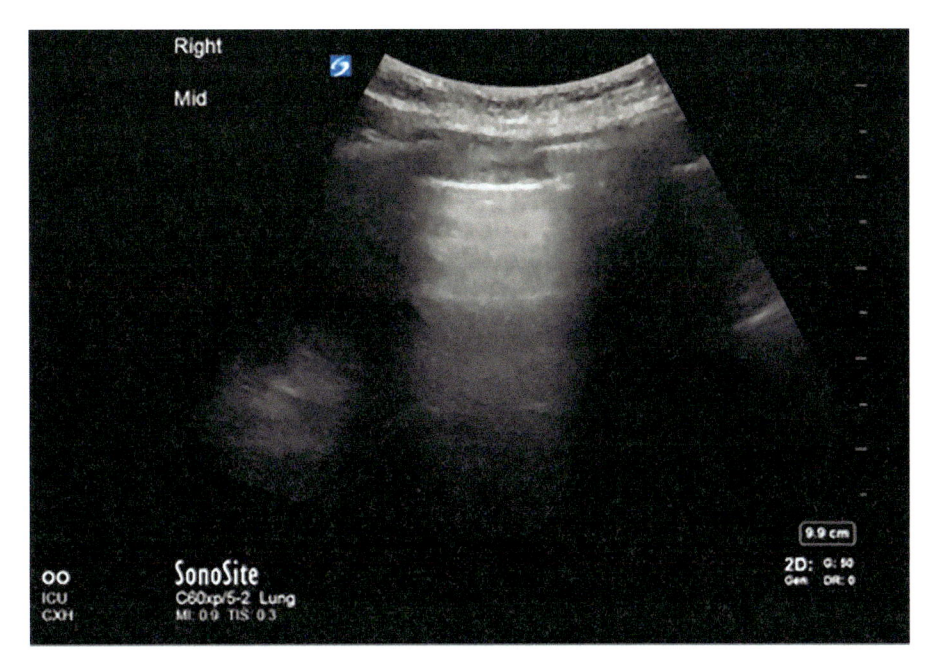

Figure 5.1 An example of normal lung showing multiple A-lines.
Source: Segun Olusanya.

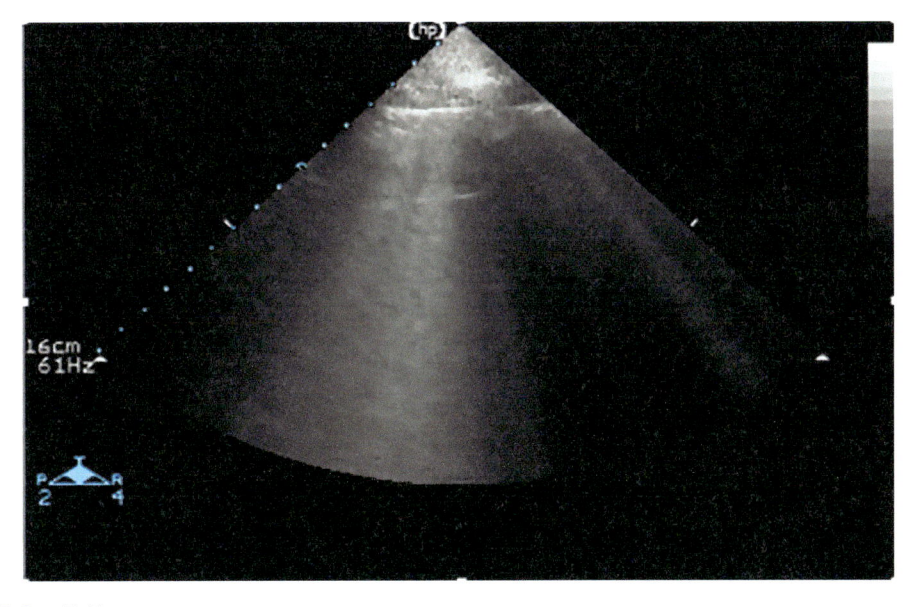

Figure 5.2 B-lines.
Source: Segun Olusanya.

53

SECTION 2 Breathing

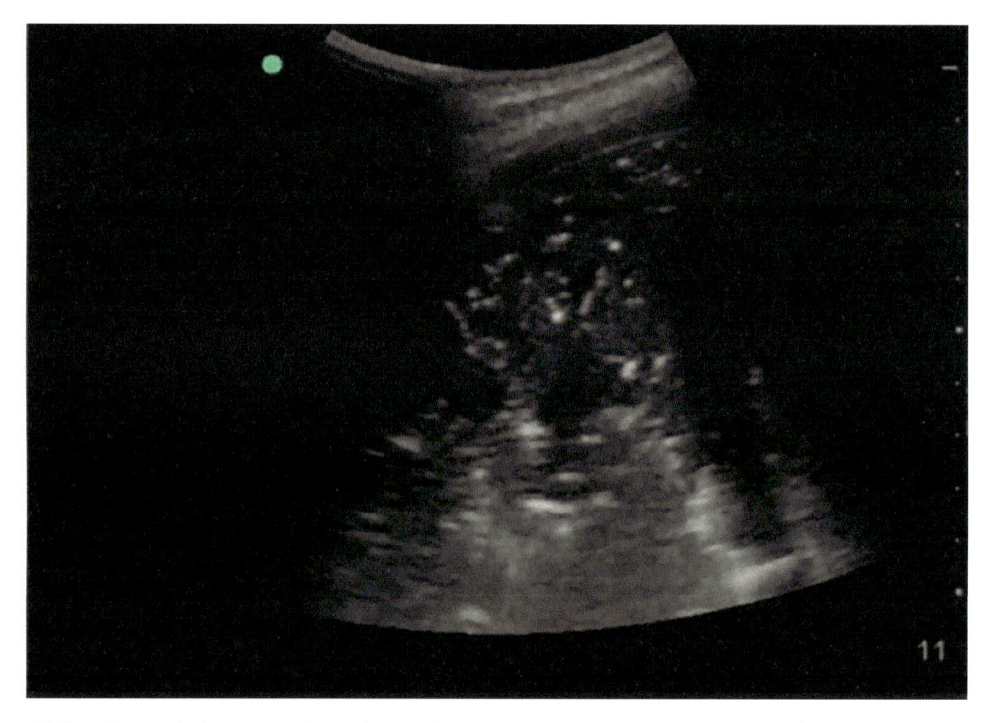

Figure 5.3 Consolidation with air bronchograms.
Source: Segun Olusanya.

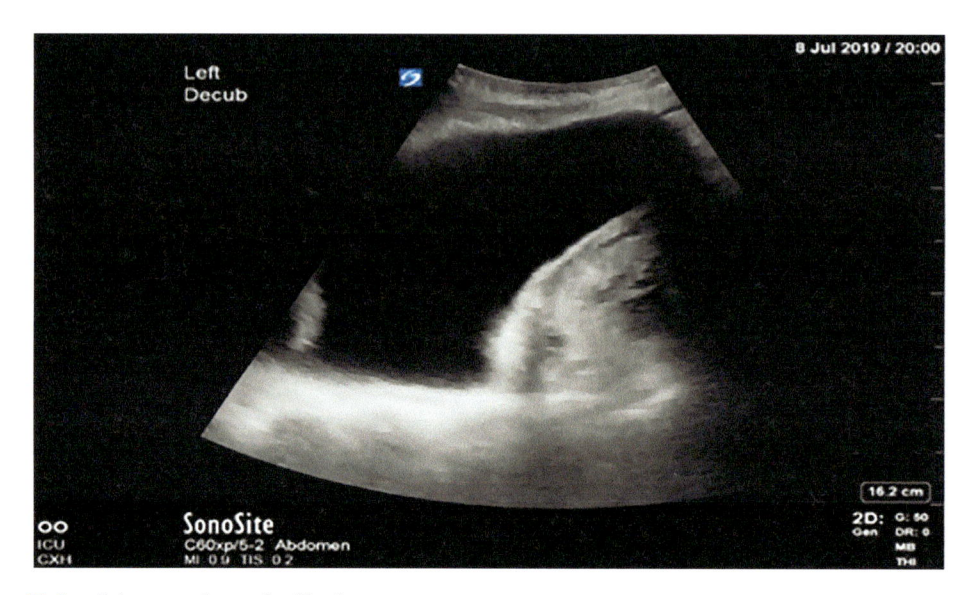

Figure 5.4 A large pleural effusion.
Source: Segun Olusanya.

CHAPTER 5 Respiratory Failure

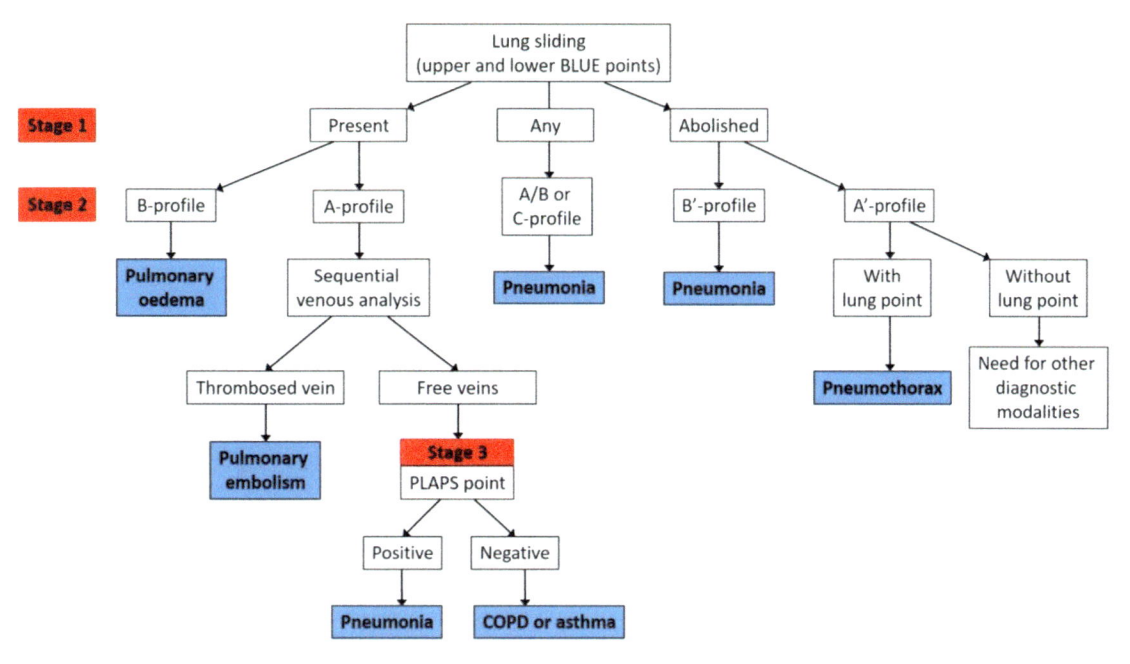

Figure 5.5 The BLUE protocol.
Source: Nick Smallwood; http://famus.org.uk/modules/blue-protocol. Reproduced with permission.
Note: B'-profile is a B-profile without lung sliding. A'-profile is an A-profile without lung sliding.

Studies have demonstrated the feasibility and accuracy of prehospital providers in performing and interpreting POCUS images in the management of respiratory failure; however, a positive impact of POCUS on outcomes has yet to be demonstrated.[7,8]

Question 3: What is the Current Management of Respiratory Failure and How Could this be Applied to the Prehospital Setting?

The mainstay of management involves treating the underlying cause, while providing adequate support (oxygenation and/or ventilatory support) to maintain adequate organ perfusion. This may involve:

- Antibiotics for infection
- Steroids for the management of COPD
- Other therapies, such as adrenaline for anaphylaxis or decompression for pneumothorax.

Hence, timely identification of a cause is imperative. In tandem, supportive therapies, such as oxygen and fluid therapy, should be given. Oxygen should be given in a controlled fashion, titrated to pulse oximetry and to an appropriate target. In the UK, the British Thoracic Society has recommendations for oxygen therapies in different populations.[9] This is in recognition of the fact that oxygen is a drug, with its own risk profile.

55

SECTION 2 Breathing

1. Hyperoxia has been associated with harm in some studies, particularly in individuals with ischaemic heart disease.[10]
2. In some individuals with chronic type 2 (hypercarbic) respiratory failure, aiming for inappropriately high saturations can result in the abolition of a protective lung reflex known as hypoxic pulmonary vasoconstriction; in these people, high-flow oxygen will result in a rise in CO_2 production leading to somnolence, cerebral vasodilation and potential death.

In the prehospital setting, using a saturation probe with a strict oxygen target will improve the safety profile of administering oxygen. Using capnography and point-of-care blood gas assessment can also be helpful, as it may identify individuals with chronic respiratory failure (they will have raised CO_2 and a correspondingly blunted acidosis with a raised bicarbonate).

Oxygen therapy can be delivered via nasal prongs and a non-rebreather mask. Some prehospital teams have the capacity to use high-flow nasal cannulae (HFNC) – specialised humidified circuits that allow the delivery of very high flow rates of oxygen. These have the advantage of increased oxygenation, better patient comfort and humidification, and the delivery of a small amount of positive expiratory pressure.

Other oxygen delivery techniques include the delivery of non-invasive ventilation (NIV) in the form of continuous positive airway pressure (CPAP) or bi-level positive airway pressure (BiPAP). These involve the use of a mechanical ventilator and a specialised mask to deliver extra airway support. CPAP allows the delivery of a continuous external airway pressure; this has multiple advantages of increasing functional residual capacity and is particularly useful in cardiogenic pulmonary oedema. BiPAP involves the delivery of both an inspiratory and expiratory pressure, allowing for both oxygenation and additional ventilation support. BiPAP is particularly effective in hypercarbic respiratory failure, where it allows increased minute ventilation and CO_2 clearance. There is clear evidence showing a mortality benefit from BiPAP in the management of exacerbations of COPD.[11]

COVID-19-induced respiratory failure is an important differential diagnosis. The key initial therapy is targeted oxygen therapy to maintain saturations. Confirming the diagnosis with a lateral flow (rapid antigen) test can be considered, as can lung ultrasound to aid the diagnosis.[12] The mainstay of current therapy in the patient requiring oxygen therapy is corticosteroids; however, it may be prudent to delay giving steroids until a definitive diagnosis can be made and other potential infective causes ruled out.[13]

PRACTICE TIP

If NIV or other high-flow therapies are used, keep a close eye on the patient's minute ventilation. These devices can consume vast amounts of oxygen very quickly, and you need to ensure you have enough supply to transport the patient for further care.

PRACTICE TIP

NIV in a semi-conscious patient is fraught with risk – particularly risk of aspiration. If unsure, consider the pros and cons of intubation straight off.

CHAPTER 5 Respiratory Failure

Question 4: Although not Common, the Prehospital Respiratory Failure Patient with Altered Conscious State Sometimes Requires Intubation. What are the Indications and Considerations for Intubation and Mechanical Ventilation in this Setting?

This is a challenging situation, involving consideration of multiple risks and benefits. As described elsewhere in this text, the indications for prehospital RSI fall generally into four categories:

- Airway protection
- Targeted treatment
- Respiratory failure
- Humanitarian/anticipated clinical course.

Hence, the decision to intubate a patient with respiratory failure will depend on:

- The underlying diagnosis and treatment
- Patient factors (difficult airway, speed of deterioration)
- Operator factors (skill, availability of rescue technologies)
- Means of transport and distance to the receiving facility.

In our patient with an exacerbation of COPD, intubation and mechanical ventilation are rarely required. However, if the patient had septic shock and was peri-arrest, timely controlled intubation with simultaneous resuscitation (either with drugs or fluid) could be lifesaving.

Prehospital application of NIV (CPAP or BiPAP) has been shown to dramatically reduce the need for invasive ventilation (endotracheal intubation and mechanical ventilation) and to provide significant therapeutic benefit.[14,15] Importantly, prehospital NIV has also been associated with a 20% failure in physiological improvement requiring intubation.[14,15] Merlani et al. highlighted predicting factors, such as a GCS <13 (an independent factor) and a pH of <7.35 or respiratory rate >22 after one hour of NIV, which required transition to invasive ventilation.[16]

This is discussed further in Chapter 2: The physiologically difficult airway.

> **PRACTICE TIP**
>
> In order to prevent further patient deterioration or exacerbating respiratory failure, ensure minimal movement and commencement of treatment prior to any extrication and transport. Ideally, NIV should be applied and a period of observation (approximately five minutes) should be allowed to provide respiratory stabilisation prior to any movement, extrication and transport.

Question 5: How do you Differentiate Between Type 1 and Type 2 Respiratory Failure and What Conditions are they Often Associated With?

Type 1 respiratory failure (hypoxic) involves a failure of oxygenation exchange. This is typically seen in conditions such as acute pulmonary oedema, pneumonia and pulmonary embolism and can be characterised clinically by:[17]

- PaO_2 <60 mmHg (profound hypoxia)
- Hypoxaemia refractory to supplemental oxygen (i.e. persistently low O_2 saturations).

SECTION 2 Breathing

Type 2 respiratory failure (hypercarbic) involves failure of oxygenation and ventilation resulting in the inability to remove carbon dioxide. This is typically seen in obstructive conditions such as COPD and asthma. The reduced ability to ventilate the lungs results in build-up of arterial carbon dioxide and can be characterised by:[8]

- $PaCO_2$ >45 mmHg
- Often accompanied by hypoxaemia that corrects with supplemental oxygen.

Type 2 can occur with or without hypoxaemic respiratory failure as many forms of type 1 respiratory failure will progress to type 2. The individual can become exhausted from a continued high work of breathing, such as in a life-threatening asthma attack. However, the most common presentation of type 2 respiratory failure is seen in people with acute-on-chronic respiratory failure, and this is classically seen in patients with exacerbations of chronic lung disease (such as COPD).

Key Evidence

Bakke SA, Botker MT, Riddervold IS et al. Continuous positive airway pressure and noninvasive ventilation in prehospital treatment of patients with acute respiratory failure: a systematic review of controlled studies. *Scandinavian Journal of Trauma, Resuscitation and Emergency Medicine*. 2014;22:69. Available at: https://sjtrem.biomedcentral.com/articles/10.1186/s13049-014-0069-8

Fuller GW, Goodacre S, Keating S et al. The diagnostic accuracy of pre-hospital assessment of acute respiratory failure. *British Paramedic Journal*. 2020 Dec 1;5(3):15–22. Available at: https://pubmed.ncbi.nlm.nih.gov/33456393/

Heidenreich PA, Bozkurt B, Aguilar D et al. 2022 AHA/ACC/HFSA guideline for the management of heart failure: a report of the American College of Cardiology/American Heart Association Joint Committee on Clinical Practice Guidelines. *Journal of the American College of Cardiology*. 2022 May 3;79(17): e263–421. Available at: https://pubmed.ncbi.nlm.nih.gov/35363500/

Lung Foundation Australia. *The COPD-X Plan: Australian and New Zealand Guidelines for the Management of Chronic Obstructive Pulmonary Disease, 2022*. Available at: https://copdx.org.au/wp-content/uploads/2023/07/COPDX-V2-69-DEC-2022_FINAL.pdf

National Asthma Council. Australian asthma handbook: the national guidelines for health professionals [Online] 2022. Available at: https://www.asthmahandbook.org.au/

Prekker ME, Feemster LC, Hough CL et al. The epidemiology and outcome of prehospital respiratory distress. *Academic Emergency Medicine*. 2014 May;21(5):543–550. Available at: https://pubmed.ncbi.nlm.nih.gov/24842506/

Williams TA, Finn J, Perkins GD et al. Prehospital continuous positive airway pressure for acute respiratory failure: a systematic review and meta-analysis. *Prehospital Emergency Care*. 2013;17(2):261–273. Available at: https://pubmed.ncbi.nlm.nih.gov/23373591/

Self-Reflection Questions

1. What are some of the key things to identify when assessing a prehospital respiratory failure?
2. What are the indications and considerations for transitioning from NIV to invasive ventilation (endotracheal intubation and mechanical ventilation) in a prehospital respiratory failure patient?
3. What is the benefit of targeting an SpO_2 range (88–92%) in exacerbations of COPD?
4. What is the benefit of steroid administration (for example, dexamethasone) in exacerbations of COPD?

CHAPTER 5 Respiratory Failure

References

1. Greene KE, Peters JI. Pathophysiology of acute respiratory failure. *Clinics in Chest Medicine*. 1994 Mar;15(1):1–12. Available at: https://pubmed.ncbi.nlm.nih.gov/8200186/
2. Ziliene V, Kondrotas AJ, Kevelaitis E. Uminio kvepavimo nepakankamumo etiologija ir patogeneze [Etiology and pathogenesis of acute respiratory failure]. *Medicina (Kaunas)*. 2004;40(3):286–294. Lithuanian. Available at: https://pubmed.ncbi.nlm.nih.gov/15064552/
3. Fuller GW, Goodacre S, Keating S et al. The diagnostic accuracy of pre-hospital assessment of acute respiratory failure. *British Paramedic Journal*. 2020 Dec 1;5(3):15–22. Available at: https://pubmed.ncbi.nlm.nih.gov/33456393/
4. Matthay MA, Lorraine B. Acute respiratory failure. In: Goldman L, Schafer AI (eds) *Goldman-Cecil Medicine*, Elsevier, 2019.
5. Pivetta E, Goffi A, Lupia E et al. Lung ultrasound-implemented diagnosis of acute decompensated heart failure in the ed: a SIMEU multicenter study. *Chest*. 2015 Jul;148(1):202–210. Available at: https://www.semanticscholar.org/paper/Lung-Ultrasound-Implemented-Diagnosis-of-Acute-in-A-Pivetta-Goffi/2a44d1a3715e5a3b4989dd2077b2219b684a7bb2
6. Lichtenstein DA, Mezière GA. Relevance of lung ultrasound in the diagnosis of acute respiratory failure: the BLUE protocol. *Chest*. 2008 Jul;134(1):117–125. Available at: https://pubmed.ncbi.nlm.nih.gov/18403664/. Erratum in: *Chest*. 2013 Aug;144(2):721.
7. Zanatta M, Benato P, De Battisti S et al. Pre-hospital lung ultrasound for cardiac heart failure and COPD: is it worthwhile? *Critical Ultrasound Journal*. 2018 Sep 10;10(1):22. Available at: https://pubmed.ncbi.nlm.nih.gov/30198053/
8. Becker TK, Martin-Gill C, Callaway CW et al. Feasibility of paramedic performed prehospital lung ultrasound in medical patients with respiratory distress. *Prehospital Emergency Care*. 2018 Mar–Apr; 22(2):175–179. Available at: https://pubmed.ncbi.nlm.nih.gov/28910212/
9. O'Driscoll BR, Howard LS, Earis J et al. British Thoracic Society Guideline for oxygen use in adults in healthcare and emergency settings. *BMJ Open Respiratory Research*. 2017 May 15;4(1):e000170. Available at: https://pubmed.ncbi.nlm.nih.gov/28883921/
10. Cornet AD, Kooter AJ, Peters MJ et al. The potential harm of oxygen therapy in medical emergencies. *Critical Care*. 2013 Apr 18;17(2):313. Available At: https://pubmed.ncbi.nlm.nih.gov/23635028/
11. Osadnik CR, Tee VS, Carson-Chahhoud KV et al. Non-invasive ventilation for the management of acute hypercapnic respiratory failure due to exacerbation of chronic obstructive pulmonary disease. *Cochrane Database of Systematic Reviews*. 2017;7:CD004104. Available at: https://pubmed.ncbi.nlm.nih.gov/28702957/
12. Volpicelli G, Gargani L, Perlini S et al. Lung ultrasound for the early diagnosis of COVID-19 pneumonia: an international multicenter study. *Intensive Care Medicine*. 2021 Apr;47(4):444–454. Available at: https://pubmed.ncbi.nlm.nih.gov/33743018/
13. RECOVERY Collaborative Group, Horby P, Lim WS et al. Dexamethasone in hospitalized patients with Covid-19. *New England Journal of Medicine*. 2021 Feb 25;384(8):693–704. Available at: https://pubmed.ncbi.nlm.nih.gov/32678530/
14. Williams TA, Finn J, Perkins GD et al. Prehospital continuous positive airway pressure for acute respiratory failure: a systematic review and meta-analysis. *Prehospital Emergency Care*. 2013;17(2):261–273. Available at: https://pubmed.ncbi.nlm.nih.gov/23373591/
15. Bakke SA, Botker MT, Riddervold IS et al. Continuous positive airway pressure and noninvasive ventilation in prehospital treatment of patients with acute respiratory failure: a systematic review of controlled studies. *Scandinavian Journal of Trauma, Resuscitation and Emergency Medicine*. 2014;22:69. Available at: https://sjtrem.biomedcentral.com/articles/10.1186/s13049-014-0069-8
16. Merlani PG, Pasquina P, Granier JM et al. Factors associated with failure of noninvasive positive pressure ventilation in the emergency department. *Academic Emergency Medicine*. 2005 Dec;12(12):1206–1215.
17. Gurka DP, Balk RA. Acute respiratory failure. In: Parrillo JE, Dellinger RP (eds). *Critical Care Medicine: Principles of Diagnosis and Management in the Adult*, 3rd edn. Maryland Heights, MO: Mosby, 2008, 773–794.

6

Severe and Life-Threatening Asthma

David Anderson and Tatsu Kuwasaki

> **In this chapter you will learn:**
> - The classification of severe asthma
> - Critical care paramedic drug therapies for severe and life-threatening asthma
> - The role of non-invasive ventilation (NIV) and intubation
> - The principles of mechanical ventilation in a patient with life-threatening asthma.

Case Details

Dispatch
35-year-old male, shortness of breath, history of asthma.

History
A 35-year-old male of Pacific Island descent has chronic asthma and has become severely short of breath. He has used his salbutamol inhaler multiple times with no improvement in symptoms. He calls for an ambulance and advises the call-taker that he has an extensive history of asthma. A double-crewed ambulance and a critical care paramedic are dispatched, due to the known history of brittle asthma. The patient lives in a low socioeconomic part of a small town.

On Arrival of the First Crew
The scene is safe and the patient is found sitting in the tripod position on the stairs leading to the front door of his flat. His primary survey findings and initial vital signs are:

Airway	Patent
Breathing	RR 32, SpO$_2$ 82% on room air, laboured, bilateral expiratory wheeze
Circulation	Peripheral pulses strong, HR 130, regular, BP 165/96, warm peripheries
Disability	GCS E4, V5, M6 (15), BGL 9.3 mmol/L
Environmental	Temp 36.8 °C, outdoors, no specific environmental concerns

The first paramedic crew to arrive finds the patient speaking one word per breath, with bilateral expiratory wheezes on auscultation. They immediately administer salbutamol

CHAPTER 6 Severe and Life-Threatening Asthma

and ipratropium via nebuliser mask and load the patient into the ambulance using a stair chair.

On Your Arrival as the Critical Care Paramedic

The patient is sitting on the ambulance stretcher in the tripod position. He appears distressed and states that he feels fatigued. You have 40 minutes' transport time to a tertiary hospital with ICU facilities.

AMPLE

The patient has a past medical history of brittle asthma with multiple ICU admissions. He is a known IV drug user and is often non-compliant with his medication. He has a food allergy to dairy products, which presents with a facial rash.

Allergies	Dairy food, pollen (hayfever)
Medications	Symbicort (budesonide/formoterol), Ventolin (salbutamol)
Past history	Severe asthma (previously intubated), IVDU
Last ins and outs	Constipated
Events prior	Severe exacerbation of asthma

Decision Point

What are your clinical priorities in this situation?

The patient's previous history, presentation and risk factors all indicate that you need to treat his condition aggressively and do everything to avoid respiratory arrest and/or intubation.

Question 1: How is the Severity of Asthma Classified?

The incidence of life-threatening asthma has decreased over the years, and death from asthma is now relatively rare. A further decline in mortality is expected with increased population access to evidence-based management strategies, therapies and healthcare in general.[1] Paradoxically, though, the overall incidence of asthma in the population is increasing. In Australia, for example, the mortality rate of asthma has had a steady decline over the past decade, with 1.3 deaths per 100,000 population recorded in 2018. There are some exceptions to this trend, though. New Zealand, for example, has seen a gradual increase in asthma mortality since 2010 when the lowest rate was recorded, reaching the highest rate of 2.5 deaths per 100,000 in 2017. Both countries share the same trend of higher mortality rates in people living in rural communities, those in low socio-economic status groups and those from indigenous populations, such as Aboriginal Australians and New Zealand Māori.[2,3]

Preventing death from asthma starts with appropriately identifying the severity of the disease in the individual patient. Many guidelines for both in-hospital and prehospital management of asthma classify asthma exacerbations as mild, moderate, severe and life-threatening. The severity is based on clinical features, and while the details of criteria vary

SECTION 2 Breathing

depending on various local guidelines, they all include key features, such as conscious state, work of breathing, heart rate and ability to speak. Clinically, it may be useful to simplify the classification further into mild to moderate and severe to life-threatening (**Table 6.1**).[4–8]

Table 6.1 Asthma severity summary chart

	Mild to moderate	Severe to life-threatening
Appearance	Calm, mildly anxious, distressed	Distressed, exhausted, anxious, agitated, altered conscious state
Speech	Speaking sentences, clear, steady	Speaking words, unable to speak
Sounds	Quiet, cough, basal crepitations, mild expiratory wheeze	Expiratory/inspiratory wheeze, progressing to silent chest
Respiratory rate	12–25 bpm	<8 or >25 bpm
Rhythm	Normal to slightly prolonged expiratory phase	Marked prolonged expiratory phase
Work of breathing	Normal to moderate increase, accessory muscle use	Marked increase, intercostal retraction, tracheal tugging, poor respiratory effort
Pulse	<120	>120 or <60 (late)
Skin	Pale, sweaty	Sweaty, cyanosis (late)
Conscious state	Alert, altered	Altered, agitated, severely agitated, falling level of consciousness, unconscious
O_2 saturation	90–94%	<88%/rapidly falling

Special notes:
- Despite hypoxaemia being a late sign of deterioration, pulse oximetry should be used. However, this is not a reliable indicator of the severity of asthma and cannot be used to determine improvement in clinical condition.[6,7]
- The patient presenting with acute asthma may improve initially with treatment but can deteriorate rapidly without any warning of sudden clinical decline.[6,7]

To aid risk classification, some guidelines give a summary of risk factors associated with fatal or near-fatal asthma. These risk factors may further guide the critical care paramedic's clinical decision making (**Table 6.2**). (Example shown: *British guideline on the management of asthma: a national clinical guideline* 2019.)

CHAPTER 6   Severe and Life-Threatening Asthma

Table 6.2   Patients at risk of developing near-fatal or fatal asthma

A combination of severe asthma recognised by one or more of:
• previous near-fatal asthma, for example previous ventilation or respiratory acidosis • previous admission for asthma, especially if in the last year • requiring three or more classes of asthma medication • heavy use of β_2 agonist • repeated attendances at ED for asthma care, especially if in the last year.
AND adverse behavioural or psychosocial features recognised by one or more of:
• non-adherence with treatment or monitoring • failure to attend appointments • fewer GP contacts • frequent home visits • self-discharge from hospital • psychosis, depression, other psychiatric illness or deliberate self-harm • current or recent major tranquilliser use • denial • alcohol or drug abuse • obesity • learning difficulties • employment problems • income problems • social isolation • childhood abuse • severe domestic, marital or legal stress.

Question 2: What is the Role for IV Beta Agonists in the Prehospital Environment?

The use of short-acting beta agonists (SABA) as a first-line therapy for asthma exacerbation has strong supportive evidence. Therefore, it makes logical sense to seek an alternative route of beta-2 agonist administration for the silent chest when there may be minimal inhaled SABA reaching beta receptors in the bronchial smooth muscles. The COVID-19 pandemic has also highlighted the potential risk to healthcare workers from aerosolised medication delivery. While IV beta agonists (salbutamol or adrenaline) are commonly recommended for life-threatening asthma that is not responding to inhaled agents, large meta-analyses have failed to show any clear benefit of IV administration over nebulised salbutamol. In addition, IV beta agonists are associated with potentially serious adverse reactions, such as hypo- or hypertension, tachycardia, lactic acidosis and hypokalaemia.[9–11] Due to a lack of strong evidence, there are wide variations of practice, and some hospitals and many emergency medical services (EMS) do not use IV salbutamol at all. The latest National Asthma Council

SECTION 2 Breathing

Australia (NACA) guidelines recommend IV salbutamol as the third-line bronchodilator in life-threatening acute asthma that has not responded to continuous nebulised salbutamol after considering other add-on treatment options, such as magnesium sulphate. NACA also advises that salbutamol's use is limited within the critical care environment, where close monitoring of the patient can be achieved.[12,13] In the United States, where IV salbutamol (albuterol) is not available, terbutaline given via subcutaneous route is common but, along with salbutamol, the literature has not demonstrated an improvement in patient outcomes.[9]

> **PRACTICE TIP**
>
> Early treatment with inhaled beta agonists, and early progression to IV beta agonists in patients with progressive respiratory failure, can be lifesaving.

Instead of IV salbutamol, adrenaline appears to fill the role of the second- or third-line beta-2 agonist in the clinical practice guidelines for most EMS systems in Australasia. Interestingly, IV adrenaline does not feature in many hospital guidelines, and intramuscular (IM) administration may be considered only in the group of patients with anaphylaxis as the cause of asthma. Nevertheless, IV adrenaline is advocated by the Global Initiative on Asthma guidelines for severe exacerbation refractory to the inhaled bronchodilators, and it is the most common beta agonist used where methylxanthines are not recommended, such as in US guidelines.[9,13–15]

While some clinicians may be concerned about adverse cardiovascular or neurological effects of IV adrenaline, the literature has not demonstrated increased incidence of such adverse events, and the benefit of the resulting bronchodilation outweighs the risk.[9]

> **PRACTICE TIP**
>
> Hypotension in a ventilated asthma patient is dynamic hyperinflation or tension pneumothorax until proven otherwise.

Question 3: What is the Evidence for Other Drug Therapies, such as Magnesium and Aminophylline?

Early administration of systemic corticosteroids has been associated with improved patient outcomes. Corticosteroids improve lung function through the upregulation of beta receptors and reduction of airway inflammation. Most guidelines recommend the early administration of corticosteroids for moderate to severe asthma exacerbations, as the clinical effects may take six to twelve hours to take effect. Oral administration is effective, so IV administration can be withheld unless required for another reason. Commonly recommended and used corticosteroids include prednisolone, prednisone, hydrocortisone and dexamethasone.[6–9,13,14,16]

Magnesium and aminophylline (along with IV salbutamol) are commonly recommended second- and third-line bronchodilators.[4,5] Although both drugs have been widely used for many years, their roles remain an active topic of debate.

CHAPTER 6 Severe and Life-Threatening Asthma

Magnesium acts by inhibiting calcium ion transport in the membranes of smooth muscle cells. NACA recommends IV magnesium as a second-line agent. The New Zealand Asthma and Respiratory Foundation guidelines extend the use of intravenous magnesium to prehospital settings. Despite these recommendations, systemic reviews have not shown any benefit of IV magnesium administration for the mild to moderate cohort, but reduction in hospitalisation and improved pulmonary function have been seen in the severe exacerbation subgroup. However, the literature has so far failed to demonstrate any reduction in mortality or need for NIV or intubation with magnesium. Additionally, the latest prospective observational study has found that the administration of IV magnesium in children resulted in a statistically significant worsening of asthma score, greater odds of hospitalisation and no improvements in exacerbation resolution.[9,14,17,18]

Aminophylline, the most widely used methylxanthine in asthma, is a non-selective phosphodiesterase inhibitor, with a narrow therapeutic range requiring close monitoring. The British and NACA guidelines recommend IV aminophylline as the third-line bronchodilator, and it is commonly used in Australian and New Zealand hospitals. However, studies have not shown any further benefit in bronchodilation or the risk of hospital admission, while showing increased incidence of potentially detrimental adverse reactions. Because of the safety profile and superior bronchodilation effects of inhaled beta agonists, the Global Initiative for Asthma (GINA) recommends against the use of IV aminophylline for the treatment of acute asthma exacerbation.[4,5,14,19–21]

In the patient who is already intubated, ketamine may offer multiple beneficial effects, including bronchodilation, anti-inflammation, anti-anxiety, dissociation and anaesthesia. These effects can improve pulmonary functions not only directly, but also indirectly by breaking the cycle of agitation-induced tachypnoea, assisting non-invasive ventilation and facilitating intubation.[14,22]

Question 4: What is the Role of NIV in Asthma?

International guidelines are hesitant in giving a recommendation for the use of NIV in severe asthma due to the lack of evidence.[23–25] Nevertheless, NIV may play an important role in preventing intubation and mechanical ventilation in severe asthma exacerbation. Morbidity and mortality increase dramatically once patients with asthma are intubated; hence preventing intubation is a crucial step in the management of this cohort. While NIV, in combination with drug therapies, may not prevent all patients from being intubated, clinical experience suggests that the number of intubated patients can be reduced. Although the evidence is weak on mortality, a growing body of evidence suggests NIV is safe and effective in patients with severe asthma – including those with altered level of consciousness – improves respiratory physiology and is associated with fewer hospital and ICU admissions and shorter lengths of stay.[9,16,26]

PRACTICE TIP

Careful application of NIV may prevent intubation, but the patient must be continuously and very closely observed for signs of deterioration.

SECTION 2 Breathing

Question 5: What are the Risks of Intubation and Ventilation in a Patient with Life-Threatening Asthma?

Endotracheal intubation is associated with increased morbidity and mortality, with mortality rates as high as 20% among intubated patients admitted to the ICU.[9]

Patients with severe or life-threatening asthma should be considered a physiologically difficult intubation (see Chapter 2: The physiologically difficult airway), due to factors such as poor reserve, respiratory acidosis and haemodynamic instability caused by insensible losses. Post-intubation hypotension is also common and may be due to dynamic hyperinflation, tension pneumothorax hypovolaemia and the effects of sedation. Once intubated and ventilated, a variety of complications, such as tube displacement or obstruction, pneumothorax, barotrauma, equipment failure and breath stacking, may result in rapid decompensation.[9,27,28] Point-of-care ultrasound is a very useful tool to rule out pneumothorax.

Question 6: What are the Principles of Mechanical Ventilation in a Patient with Life-Threatening Asthma?

While the goals for mechanical ventilation in severe asthma patients include oxygenation, supporting work of breathing and improved delivery of inhaled medication, the key strategy is to minimise dynamic hyperinflation to avoid the lethal complications mentioned above. Minimising dynamic hyperinflation is best achieved by reducing minute ventilation and lengthening expiratory time. Applying a low tidal volume of 6–8 mL/kg of ideal body weight, slow respiratory rate of six to ten breaths per minute, high inspiratory airflow rate and increased inspiration to expiration (I:E) ratio of 1:4 or greater is recommended. While still debatable, some authors recommend the use of low-level PEEP (≤5 cm H_2O), which may help reduce the work of breathing by splinting the alveoli, reduce the risk of atelectrauma and reduce the patient's effort required to trigger the ventilator. The degree of hyperinflation needs to be closely monitored using end-inspiratory and end-expiratory holds to limit the plateau pressure (Pplat) and apply the minimum PEEP required. The resulting increase in $PaCO_2$ is inevitable, and reducing the $PaCO_2$ is very much a secondary goal. Instead, allowing high $PaCO_2$ is the important ventilator strategy for the management of severe asthma often described as permissive hypercapnia.[9,16,23]

tV	RR	I:E ratio	PEEP	PPlat	PIP
6–8 mL/kg	6–8/min	>1:4	≤5 cm H_2O	30 cm H_2O	35 cm H_2O

Key Evidence

Demoule, A, Brochard, L, Dres, M et al., 2020, December 1, 'How to ventilate obstructive and asthmatic patients', *Intensive Care Medicine*, 46(12):2436–2449. Available at: https://pubmed.ncbi.nlm.nih.gov/33169215/

Garner, O, Ramey, JS and Hanania, NA, 2022, October 1, 'Management of life-threatening asthma: severe asthma series', *Chest*, 162(4):747–756. Available at: https://pubmed.ncbi.nlm.nih.gov/35218742/

Long, B, Lentz, S, Koyfman, A et al., 2021, 'Evaluation and management of the critically ill adult asthmatic in the emergency department setting', *American Journal of Emergency Medicine*, 44:441–451. Available at: https://pubmed.ncbi.nlm.nih.gov/32222313/

Self-Reflection Questions

1. What clinical features can distinguish moderate asthma from severe asthma?
2. When should IV beta agonists be introduced?
3. What is the role of magnesium sulphate in asthma management?
4. What ventilator settings would you select for a patient with severe asthma?
5. How would you respond to sudden, unexpected hypotension in a ventilated asthma patient?

References

1. Lin MP et al., 2020. Trends and predictors of hospitalization after emergency department asthma visits among US adults, 2006–2014, *Journal of Asthma*, 57(8): 811–819.
2. *Asthma*, 2020, https://www.aihw.gov.au/reports/chronic-respiratory-conditions/chronic-respiratory-conditions/contents/asthma
3. Telfar Barnard, L and Zhang, J, 2021, *The Impact of Respiratory Disease in New Zealand: 2020 Update*, Asthma and Respiratory Foundation NZ, University of Otago. Available at: https://www.asthmafoundation.org.nz/assets/documents/Respiratory-Impact-report-final-2021Aug11.pdf
4. The Royal Children's Hospital Melbourne, 2022, 'Acute asthma', Clinical Practice Guideline. Available at: https://www.rch.org.au/clinicalguide/guideline_index/Asthma_acute/#resources.
5. Starship, 2022, 'Asthma, life threatening', Clinical Guideline. Available at: https://starship.org.nz/guidelines/asthma-life-threatening/.
6. Ambulance Victoria, 2022, Clinical Practice Guidelines. Available at: https://cpg.ambulance.vic.gov.au/#/tabs/tab-0/list.
7. Queensland Ambulance Service, 2020, 'Respiratory/asthma', Clinical Practice Guideline. Available at: https://www.ambulance.qld.gov.au/docs/clinical/cpg/CPG_Asthma.pdf
8. St John New Zealand, 2022, *Clinical Procedures and Guidelines*. Available at: https://www.stjohn.org.nz/globalassets/documents/health-practitioners/clinical-procedures-and-guidelines---comprehensive-edition.pdf
9. Long, B, Lentz, S, Koyfman, A et al., 2021, 'Evaluation and management of the critically ill adult asthmatic in the emergency department setting', *American Journal of Emergency Medicine*, 44: 441–451. Available at: https://pubmed.ncbi.nlm.nih.gov/32222313/
10. Travers, AA, Jones, AP, Kelly, KD et al., 2001, 'Intravenous beta2-agonists for acute asthma in the emergency department', *Cochrane Database of Systematic Reviews*, 2001(2). Available at: https://pubmed.ncbi.nlm.nih.gov/11406055/
11. Travers, AH, Milan, SJ, Jones, AP et al., 2012, 'Addition of intravenous beta(2)-agonists to inhaled beta(2)-agonists for acute asthma', *Cochrane Database of Systematic Reviews*, 12:12. Available at: https://pubmed.ncbi.nlm.nih.gov/23235685/
12. National Asthma Council Australia, 2022, 'Managing acute asthma in clinical settings', *Australian Asthma Handbook*. Available at: https://www.asthmahandbook.org.au/acute-asthma/clinical
13. Powell, CV, 2016, Feb, 'Acute severe asthma', *Journal of Paediatrics and Child Health*, 52(2):187–191. Available at: https://pubmed.ncbi.nlm.nih.gov/27062622/
14. Maselli, DJ and Peters, JI, 2018, 'Medication regimens for managing acute asthma', *Respiratory Care*, 63(6):783–796. Available at: https://pubmed.ncbi.nlm.nih.gov/29794211/
15. Sellers, WFS, 2013, 'Inhaled and intravenous treatment in acute severe and life-threatening asthma', *British Journal of Anaesthesia*, 110(2):183–190. Available at: https://pubmed.ncbi.nlm.nih.gov/23234642/
16. Garner, O, Ramey, JS and Hanania, NA, 2022, 'Management of life-threatening asthma: severe asthma series', *Chest*, 162(4):747–756. Available at: https://pubmed.ncbi.nlm.nih.gov/35218742/
17. Arnold, DH, Gong, W, Antoon, JW et al., 2022, 'Prospective observational study of clinical outcomes after intravenous magnesium for moderate and severe acute asthma exacerbations in children', *Journal of Allergy and Clinical Immunology: In Practice*, 10(5):1238–1246. Available at: https://pubmed.ncbi.nlm.nih.gov/34915226/

18. Erumbala, G, Anzar, S, Tonbari, A et al., 2021, 'Stating the obvious: intravenous magnesium sulphate should be the first parenteral bronchodilator in paediatric asthma exacerbations unresponsive to first-line therapy', *Breathe*, 17(4):210113. Available at: https://pubmed.ncbi.nlm.nih.gov/35035570/
19. Global Initiative for Asthma, 2022, *Global Strategy for Asthma Management and Prevention*. Available at: https://ginasthma.org/wp-content/uploads/2022/07/GINA-Main-Report-2022-FINAL-22-07-01-WMS.pdf
20. Craig, S, Powell, CV, Nixon, GM et al., 2022, 'Treatment patterns and frequency of key outcomes in acute severe asthma in children: a Paediatric Research in Emergency Departments International Collaborative (PREDICT) multicentre cohort study', *BMJ Open Respiratory Research*, 9(1):e001137. Available at: https://pubmed.ncbi.nlm.nih.gov/35301198/
21. Nair, P, Milan, SJ and Rowe, BH, 2012, 'Addition of intravenous aminophylline to inhaled beta(2)-agonists in adults with acute asthma', *Cochrane Database of Systematic Reviews*, 12(12):CD002742. Available at: https://pubmed.ncbi.nlm.nih.gov/23235591/
22. Farkas, J, 2021, 'Asthma', The Internet Book of Critical Care [online]. Available at: https://emcrit.org/ibcc/asthma/
23. Demoule, A, Brochard, L, Dres, M et al., 2020, 'How to ventilate obstructive and asthmatic patients', *Intensive Care Medicine*, 46(12):2436–2449. Available at: https://pubmed.ncbi.nlm.nih.gov/33169215/
24. le Conte, P, Terzi, N, Mortamet, G et al., 2019, 'Management of severe asthma exacerbation: guidelines from the Société Française de Médecine d'Urgence, the Société de Réanimation de Langue Française and the French Group for Pediatric Intensive Care and Emergencies', *Annals of Intensive Care*, 9(1):115. Available at: https://pubmed.ncbi.nlm.nih.gov/31602529/
25. Rochwerg, B, Brochard, L, Elliott, MW et al., 2017, 'Official ERS/ATS clinical practice guidelines: noninvasive ventilation for acute respiratory failure', *European Respiratory Journal*, 50(2):1602426. Available at: https://pubmed.ncbi.nlm.nih.gov/28860265/
26. Guthrie, K, 2019, 'Case of acute severe asthma', Life in the Fast Lane [online]. Available at: https://litfl.com/case-of-acute-severe-asthma/
27. Bond, KRL, Horsley, CAE and Williams, AB, 2018, 'Non-invasive ventilation use in status asthmaticus: 16 years of experience in a tertiary intensive care', *Emergency Medicine Australasia*, 30(2):187–192. Available at: https://pubmed.ncbi.nlm.nih.gov/29131536/
28. Rowell, SE, Barbosa, RR, Holcomb, JB et al., 2019, 'The focused assessment with sonography in trauma (FAST) in hypotensive injured patients frequently fails to identify the need for laparotomy: a multi-institutional pragmatic study', *Trauma Surgery and Acute Care Open*, 4(1):11–16. Available at: https://tsaco.bmj.com/content/tsaco/4/1/e000207.full.pdf

SECTION 3

Circulation

Undifferentiated Shock

7

Andy Celestia and Todd Wollum

> **In this chapter you will learn:**
> - A definition of shock
> - A basic review of physiological terms related to circulatory shock
> - The different categories of shock
> - An out-of-hospital approach to initial stabilisation of a patient with undifferentiated shock
> - An approach to fluid resuscitation
> - The basics of common vasoactive medications used in shock.

Case Details

Dispatch
73-year-old male, difficulty breathing.

History
The patient was diagnosed with COVID-19 two weeks ago and was treated with antiviral medications (nirmatrelvir and ritonavir). He was feeling better until he started developing shortness of breath five days ago. His dyspnoea has been getting progressively worse since then and is now accompanied by chest tightness and a non-productive cough.

On Arrival of the First Crew
The scene is safe. The patient's spouse meets the initial crew (two paramedics) at the door of their home and leads them to the living room.

The primary survey findings and initial vital signs are as follows:

Airway	Patent
Breathing	RR 32, SpO$_2$ 64% on room air, effort: anxious but no increased WOB
Circulation	Peripheral pulses weak, HR 134, BP 84/52, cool peripheries
Disability	GCS E4, V5, M6 (15), BGL 7.2 mmol/L
Environmental	Temp 38.1 °C

The patient is sitting up in an overstuffed chair, gripping the arm rests. He is quite anxious and tachypnoeic.

SECTION 3 Circulation

On Your Arrival as the Critical Care Paramedic

The initial crew has administered supplemental oxygen via a non-rebreather mask at 15 L/min with a minimal improvement in SpO_2 to 72%. The patient still appears to be in distress; he remains tachycardic and tachypnoeic with accessory muscle use, although his lungs are clear to auscultation with good air movement bilaterally.

AMPLE

Allergies	NKDA
Medications	Metformin, empagliflozin, rosuvastatin, lisinopril, metoprolol
Past history	Coronary artery disease, hypertension, T2DM
Last ins and outs	Normal
Events prior	Recent COVID-19 infection treated with antivirals, now with five days of worsening dyspnoea

Decision Point
What are your clinical priorities in this situation?

Given his hypoxia, tachycardia and hypotension, you are concerned about possible imminent cardiovascular collapse. How would you describe his current clinical status? What are some possible aetiologies of his presentation? What can you do to help stabilise him and prevent cardiac arrest?

Question 1: What Is Shock?

Our patient is in shock.

Cells require oxygen to produce energy via aerobic metabolism. In a healthy resting state, the circulatory system is generally able to supply the cells with enough oxygen-rich blood to meet demand. The supply of blood to the tissues is called perfusion.

Shock is a condition in which the circulatory system is unable to maintain adequate perfusion. This deficit results in cellular and tissue hypoxia and can progress quickly to multiorgan system failure and death. Prompt recognition and intervention by healthcare providers is imperative. Clinicians may use the term 'undifferentiated shock' when they recognise that a patient is in shock, but they have not yet determined the aetiology.

> **PRACTICE TIP**
>
> Patients in shock are in a critical condition. Stabilise using the ABC approach and expedite transport to definitive care.

Different types of shock essentially reflect problems with different aspects of the oxygen supply chain and/or changes in oxygen demand. A basic review of some of the relevant physiology is included here to facilitate the discussion of the types of shock and interventions.

CHAPTER 7 Undifferentiated Shock

The rate at which oxygen is delivered from the lungs to the tissues depends primarily on the cardiac output, the haemoglobin concentration and the arterial oxyhaemoglobin saturation.

Cardiac output is a function of the stroke volume and the heart rate. The stroke volume is the amount of blood the heart pumps out of the left ventricle into the systemic circulation with each beat. The stroke volume depends on the contractility of the heart, the preload and the afterload. Contractility refers to the force with which the myocytes (heart muscle cells) contract. This strength of contraction is also known as 'inotropy'.

The term 'preload' refers to the effects of the load applied to the muscle fibres of the left (unless otherwise indicated) ventricle by the blood volume within it just before it contracts (at the end of diastole, just before systole). This loading causes myocytes to stretch as the volume of blood in the left ventricle increases during diastole (the filling period). Technically, preload describes the extent of this stretch. However, as myocyte stretch is not practical to measure in an intact heart, the left ventricular end-diastolic pressure is often used as an indicator of preload instead. The extent to which the muscle fibres stretch depends not only on the load applied to them, but also on the intrinsic properties of the fibres themselves, which differ with disease processes, for example, heart failure.

Among other things, preload is highly dependent on the venous return, that is, the amount of blood delivered back to the right side of the heart from the systemic circulation via the inferior and superior vena cava.

The term 'afterload' refers to the load applied to the muscle fibres of the left ventricle by the blood volume within it while it is contracting (during systole). Afterload is heavily influenced by the systemic vascular resistance. Systemic vascular resistance, in turn, reflects arterial blood pressure, central venous pressure and cardiac output. To simplify, some people think of afterload as the force against which the heart is working to pump blood forwards, and as the blood pressure increases, the heart has to work harder to maintain cardiac output.

If there is not enough oxygen available to support aerobic metabolism, cells are still able to produce a small amount of energy by anaerobic metabolism. Cells produce lactate as a by-product of anaerobic metabolism. Lactate is therefore often measured as an indicator of inadequate perfusion.

Oxygen demand can increase in a variety of conditions, including sepsis.

Question 2: What Are the Different Types of Shock?

There are four types of shock cardiogenic, obstructive, hypovolaemic and distributive (**Figure 7.1**).

Cardiogenic Shock

Cardiogenic shock is the result of the heart not being able to pump enough blood to the peripheral vascular system to maintain adequate oxygen delivery. An acute myocardial infarction is the most common cause of cardiogenic shock but there are many other causes. Cardiomyopathy, impaired preload, valvular disease/disorder or refractory dysrhythmias are other causes.

Obstructive Shock

Obstructive shock results from a mechanical blockage of the forward flow of blood. Tension pneumothorax, cardiac tamponade and pulmonary emboli are examples of obstructive shock.

SECTION 3 Circulation

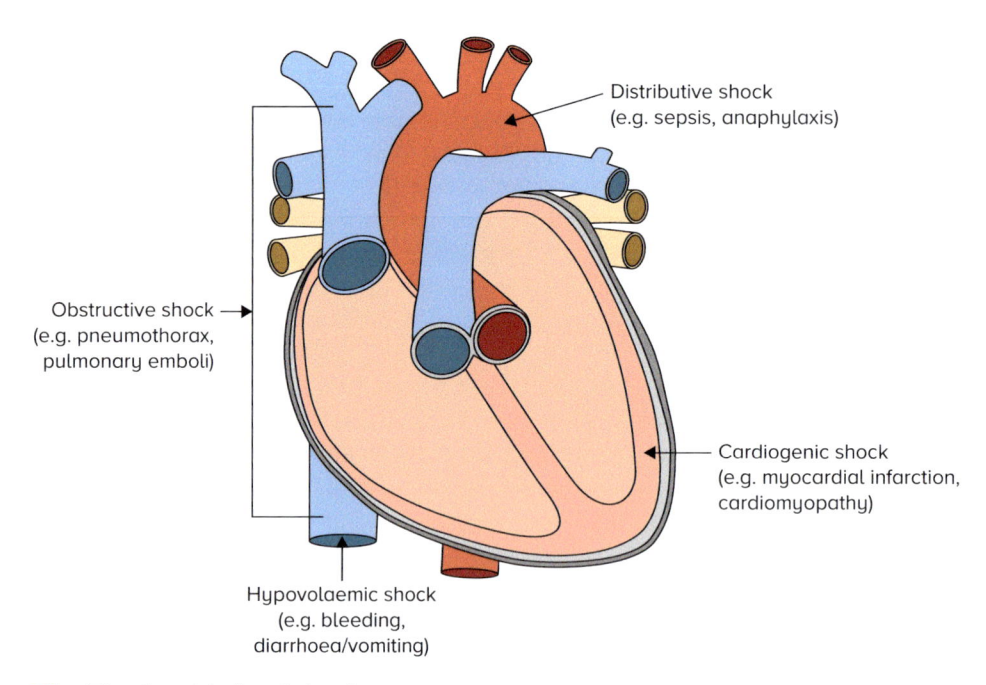

Figure 7.1 The four kinds of shock.

- Distributive shock (e.g. sepsis, anaphylaxis)
- Obstructive shock (e.g. pneumothorax, pulmonary emboli)
- Cardiogenic shock (e.g. myocardial infarction, cardiomyopathy)
- Hypovolaemic shock (e.g. bleeding, diarrhoea/vomiting)

The intrathoracic pressure caused by a tension pneumothorax can compress the heart and collapse the vena cava (in addition to the lung), physically obstructing venous return and thereby decreasing cardiac output.

Note that positive pressure ventilation similarly decreases venous return, thereby decreasing preload. In the setting of shock, this incremental reduction in venous return can be enough to cause cardiovascular collapse and arrest. It may therefore be wise to defer intubation of patients with preload-dependent conditions until they can be stabilised, if possible.

Distributive Shock

Distributive shock occurs when the blood vessels dilate, causing the blood to pool in the vascular beds. This category includes septic, neurogenic and anaphylactic shock. An overwhelming infection causing an activation of the inflammatory response causes sepsis. Neurogenic shock is usually the result of a trauma to the spinal cord resulting in the loss of sympathetic tone. Anaphylaxis causes massive vasodilatation coupled with bronchoconstriction, which results in distributive shock and impaired ventilation.

Hypovolaemic Shock

Hypovolaemic shock results from an inadequate volume of blood in the vascular system and is classified in two ways: haemorrhagic and non-haemorrhagic. The loss of blood, whether internally or externally, is considered haemorrhagic. The loss of intravascular fluid due to perspiration, exhalation, third-spacing (for example, ascites), vomiting or diarrhoea all constitute non-haemorrhagic losses.

CHAPTER 7   Undifferentiated Shock

Question 3: How Does Shock Progress?

Compensated Shock

When the body is still able to maintain an adequate blood pressure by increasing heart rate and increasing respiratory rate and depth, it is considered compensated shock.

Decompensated Shock

As soon as the body is no longer able to maintain the blood pressure, the body is in decompensated shock. Sometimes a decrease in blood pressure is the last indicator that there has been a change.

Irreversible Shock

The body begins to shunt blood away from vital organs and even with aggressive treatment, the damage to organs might be irreversible.

Question 4: What Can I Do in the Out-of-Hospital Setting to Stabilise a Patient in Shock?

A standard EMS primary assessment focuses on quickly finding and treating any immediate life-threatening conditions, prioritising airway, breathing and circulation (ABCs). This approach works well for patients in shock, as they are critically ill and may be altered, hypoxic and hypotensive. If they are unable to protect their own airway due to altered mental status, they may require intubation or a supraglottic airway device. If they are hypoxic or hyperventilating, provide supplemental oxygen or ventilatory assistance with a bag-valve-mask.

Hypotension should be addressed promptly with fluids and vasoactive medications, which are discussed below, in addition to condition-specific interventions (as allowed under local prehospital protocols). For example, a tension pneumothorax is treated with needle, finger or tube thoracostomy. Cardiac tamponade may be treated in hospital with pericardiocentesis. Massive pulmonary emboli may be treated with thrombolysis.

History-taking also starts during the primary assessment. It is important to gather as much information about the patient's illness or injury at the scene, provided this does not interfere with treatment of life threats. EMS clinicians may be the only source of history available to clinicians at the receiving facility.

A secondary assessment is then conducted, which includes a thorough physical examination to ensure that less obvious conditions are not missed, as well as an evaluation of the results of any interventions that have already been performed.

Patients in shock require rapid transport to definitive care.

Question 5: What Is the Role of Fluids in the Management of Shock?

The main goal in the treatment of shock is to restore tissue perfusion as quickly as possible. Fluid administration is critical for many patients in shock. However, fluid overload can also cause serious harm. Ideally, we would like to be able to predict which of our patients will

SECTION 3 Circulation

benefit from fluids before their administration. Expanding intravascular volume should increase venous return and therefore preload (to the right if not the left ventricle, depending on the aetiology of shock). In some cases, but not all, this translates to an increase in cardiac output and improved tissue perfusion.

> **PRACTICE TIP**
>
> Take care with fluid administration. Adequate fluid resuscitation is imperative, but fluid overload can also cause serious harm.

There are a number of strategies used to predict fluid-responsiveness, none of which has yet become a time-tested gold standard. Research on this dilemma is ongoing. Vital signs, history, examination findings and the suspected type of shock should all be considered. Patients with hypovolaemic, septic and anaphylactic shock generally require prompt fluid resuscitation.

If it is not clear that a person will respond well to fluids, you might try a 'fluid challenge', or a small bolus, and then reassess. For an adult, this might be 500 mL, or for a child, 10 mL/kg.

Alternatively, the passive leg raise test is a simple reversible manoeuvre that can be used to determine if cardiac output will improve with fluids without administering a bolus. With this test, the patient begins in a semi-recumbent position and vitals are noted. The provider then changes the angle of the bed so that the patient's torso is horizontal and their feet are at an approximately 30–45 degree incline. Changes in haemodynamic parameters are reassessed. The patient is then returned to the original position and haemodynamics are again noted. The leg raise has been shown to be equivalent to an approximately 300 mL fluid bolus as the blood from the legs flows towards the heart. Unfortunately, one of the best-correlated parameters for predicting fluid responsiveness with this test is cardiac output, which requires specialised monitoring equipment that may not be available in the prehospital environment.[1] An increase in $EtCO_2$ of >2 mmHg can also predict fluid responsiveness in well-controlled ventilated patients.[2]

Reassess the patient carefully after administering a fluid bolus. Findings that suggest that the fluids have been helpful may include improvements in tachycardia, hypotension, mental status and capillary refill. Over longer periods of time, urine output is used as a measure of adequate resuscitation. Additional fluids may then be given if the patient has responded well but there is still room for improvement. Listen to the patient's lungs and monitor their respiratory rate, work of breathing and SpO_2. If they have developed crackles in the lungs, difficulty in breathing or a new or increasing supplemental oxygen requirement, they may have developed pulmonary oedema, and additional fluids may be detrimental. Other signs of fluid overload include pitting oedema in the lower extremities and jugular venous distension. Note that it is easier to give more fluid than it is to remove it from a patient's lungs.

Fluids should be used cautiously in certain patients, especially those with heart failure, cardiogenic shock or end-stage renal disease. If you suspect these patients also have a component of distributive or hypovolaemic shock and you have reason to believe they might benefit from intravascular volume expansion, consider a trial of a small fluid bolus until more information is available.

CHAPTER 7 Undifferentiated Shock

Crystalloids are the most commonly used resuscitation fluids in worldwide. Crystalloid refers to balanced salt solutions such as compound sodium lactate (CSL, also known as lactated Ringer's in North America and Hartmann's solution in the rest of the world) or Plasmalyte-148, or normal saline (NS) A large meta-analysis suggests that resuscitation with CSL may be associated with lower rates of mortality and acute kidney injury than NS in critically ill patients with sepsis.[3] The same study also suggests increased mortality with CSL in patients with traumatic brain injury (TBI). Large quantities of NS can cause hyperchloraemia. Given that sepsis or undifferentiated shock are among the commonest reasons to administer IV fluids, some providers prefer LR to NS, but this preference is not universal and fluid choice in critically ill patients remains an active area of research.

It is important to use isotonic fluids, such as CSL or NS, to expand intravascular volume. Five per cent dextrose or 0.45% normal saline should not be used as boluses for resuscitation. Albumin or other volume expanders are sometimes used for resuscitation but are unlikely to be available in the prehospital setting. Note that CSL, unlike NS, is not compatible with blood products or certain medications; they should not be run through the same IV line simultaneously.

Some prehospital agencies carry blood products – either whole blood or components, such as packed red blood cells and plasma – for the acute treatment of haemorrhagic shock. Resuscitation can be started with crystalloids for volume expansion if blood products are not available, although these patients will likely require replacement of essential elements, such as haemoglobin and clotting factors, as soon as possible as well. The choice of fluids and/or blood products in the prehospital resuscitation of haemorrhagic shock is another area of active research, and several notable studies have been published on this topic with inconsistent results. The PAMPer trial[4] showed a significant reduction in mortality at 30 days when plasma was used in prehospital resuscitation of patients at risk of haemorrhagic shock, whereas the Control of Major Bleeding After Trauma Trial did not show any significant difference.[5] The RePHILL trial did not show any significant difference in 30-day mortality between patients with haemorrhagic shock who received RBCs and plasma versus those who were resuscitated with 0.9% normal saline in the prehospital setting.[6]

The standard fluid bolus for adult patients in septic shock in the hospital setting is 30 mL/kg of crystalloid.[7] Wherever possible and practical, any fluid administered should be warmed (especially blood products which may have been refrigerated before use).

Question 6: How Do I Choose a 'Pressor'?

If a patient continues to have hypotension or inadequate cardiac output despite fluid resuscitation, they may need a vasopressor, inotropic and/or chronotropic medication. Vasopressors (commonly referred to as 'pressors') increase blood pressure via vasoconstriction. Inotropes increase the heart's contractility. Chronotropic drugs increase heart rate. A selection of common vasoactive medications and their effects on the cardiovascular system are shown in **Table 7.1**. Their effects are mediated by the types of receptors to which they bind.

These medications are often titrated to a blood pressure goal, such as a mean arterial pressure (MAP) of 65 mmHg in adults. Remember that normal blood pressure ranges in paediatrics vary by age. More than one vasoactive medication may be needed to achieve perfusion goals.

SECTION 3   Circulation

Table 7.1   Vasoactive medications and their primary effects on the cardiovascular system

Vasoactive agent	Dose	Vasoconstriction	Inotropy	Chronotropy
Noradrenaline	0.05–1 mcg/kg/min	X	X	
Adrenaline	0.05–1 mcg/kg/min	X	X	X
Phenylephrine	0.25–5 mcg/kg/min	X		
Vasopressin	0.01–0.04 units/min	X		
Dopamine	5–10 mcg/kg/min		X	X
Dopamine	10–20 mcg/kg/min	X	X	X
Dobutamine	2.5–20 mcg/kg/min		X	X

Noradrenaline

Noradrenaline increases blood pressure and contractility. Noradrenaline has a strong effect on alpha-1 adrenergic receptors and a moderate effect on beta-1 adrenergic receptors, which mediate contractility and heart rate. Improved contractility generally increases cardiac output. Vasoconstriction, however, though critical in cases of vasodilatory shock, increases afterload, which can decrease cardiac output. When blood pressure drops, the heart attempts to compensate by increasing cardiac output (heart rate x stroke volume) in order to keep the vasculature full and pump enough blood forward to continue to perfuse the tissues. The opposite is also seen. In the case of noradrenaline, the reflexive decrease in heart rate from increased blood pressure is roughly balanced out by chronotropic effects of beta-1 receptor activation. Overall, therefore, noradrenaline does not tend to result in an increased heart rate.

Noradrenaline is recommended as the first-line agent for septic shock in adults by the 2021 Surviving Sepsis Campaign guidelines.[7]

PRACTICE TIP

Noradrenaline is often a good choice in an emergency if you need a vasopressor but you are not sure which to use.

Adrenaline

Adenaline has a strong effect on alpha-1 receptors, a strong effect on beta-1 receptors and a moderate effect on beta-2 receptors. Adrenaline causes vasoconstriction via alpha-1 receptors (increasing blood pressure). Beta-2 effects cause increased contractility and heart rate (increasing cardiac output). Adrenaline also causes bronchodilation. Adrenaline is the first-line treatment for anaphylaxis,[8] and a third-line agent in septic shock in adults.[7] The 2021 Surviving Sepsis Campaign guidelines for paediatrics suggests either adrenaline or noradrenaline as the first-line vasoactive agent in septic shock if the patient is still hypotensive after 40–60 mL/kg of crystalloid. Dopamine is also acceptable if adrenaline and noradrenaline are not available.[9]

CHAPTER 7 Undifferentiated Shock

Phenylephrine

Phenylephrine is an alpha-1 agonist that causes vasoconstriction and is used to increase blood pressure. It does not affect inotropy or chronotropy. Neurogenic shock is an example of excessive vasodilation without cardiac depression, which might respond well to phenylephrine.

Vasopressin

Vasopressin works through a different type of receptor (V1 receptor) and is a potent vasoconstrictor. Vasopressin doses are usually limited to a maximum of 0.04 units/minute, as higher doses may cause adverse ischaemic effects, including ischaemic digits, mesenteric ischaemia or myocardial ischaemia. This vasopressor is currently recommended as the second-line agent for the treatment of septic shock by the 2021 Surviving Sepsis Campaign guidelines.[7]

Dopamine

Dopamine is somewhat unique in that it has different effects at different doses.

At low doses of approximately 0.5–2.0 mcg/kg/min, dopamine has a moderate effect on the dopaminergic receptors and a weak effect on the beta-1 receptors. Low-dose dopamine increases renal blood flow via action on the dopaminergic receptors but is generally not used clinically for this effect or at these doses.

At intermediate doses of approximately 5–10 mcg/kg/min, dopamine has a moderate effect on the dopaminergic receptors, a moderate effect on the beta-1 receptors and a weak effect on the alpha-1 receptors. Intermediate-dose dopamine results in increased contractility and heart rate (and therefore increased cardiac output), as well as a small increase in blood pressure.

At high doses of approximately 10–20 mcg/kg/min, dopamine has a moderate effect on the dopaminergic receptors, a moderate effect on the beta-1 receptors, and a moderate effect on the alpha-1 receptors, resulting in both increased cardiac output and vasoconstriction.

Dopamine is indicated for use primarily in symptomatic bradycardia or AV block. The infusion should be started at 5 mcg/kg/min and titrated to effect to a maximum of 20 mcg/kg/min.

Dopamine should be avoided in patients with cardiogenic shock, post arrest or with heart failure. Dopamine can induce arrhythmias and was associated with higher mortality in patients with cardiogenic shock compared to noradrenaline in the SOAP 2 trial.[10]

Dobutamine

Dobutamine is primarily used in cardiogenic shock in the setting of advanced heart failure. Dobutamine has a strong effect on beta-1 receptors and a moderate effect on beta-2 receptors, and results in increased cardiac output and vasodilation (*decreased* blood pressure).[11] Note that dobutamine can cause tachyarrhythmias.

Key Evidence

Guidelines

Evans L, Rhodes A, Alhazzani W et al. Surviving sepsis campaign: international guidelines for management of sepsis and septic shock 2021. *Intensive Care Medicine*. 2021;47(11):1181–1247. Available at: https://pubmed.ncbi.nlm.nih.gov/34599691/

Muraro A, Worm M, Alviani C et al. EAACI guidelines: anaphylaxis (2021 update). *Allergy*. 2022;77(2):357–377. Available at: https://pubmed.ncbi.nlm.nih.gov/34343358/

SECTION 3 Circulation

Weiss SL, Peters MJ, Alhazzani W et al. Surviving sepsis campaign international guidelines for the management of septic shock and sepsis-associated organ dysfunction in children. *Intensive Care Medicine*. 2020;46(1):10–67. Available at: https://pubmed.ncbi.nlm.nih.gov/32030529/

Trials

Crombie N, Doughty HA, Bishop JRB et al. Resuscitation with blood products in patients with trauma-related haemorrhagic shock receiving prehospital care (RePHILL): a multicentre, open-label, randomised, controlled, phase 3 trial. *Lancet Haematology*. 2022;9(4):e250–e261. Available at: https://pubmed.ncbi.nlm.nih.gov/35271808/

De Backer D, Biston P, Devriendt J et al. Comparison of dopamine and norepinephrine in the treatment of shock. *New England Journal of Medicine*. 2010;362(9):779–789. Available at: https://pubmed.ncbi.nlm.nih.gov/20200382/

Moore HB, Moore EE, Chapman MP et al. Plasma-first resuscitation to treat haemorrhagic shock during emergency ground transportation in an urban area: a randomised trial. *Lancet*. 2018;392(10144):283–291. Available at: https://pubmed.ncbi.nlm.nih.gov/30032977/

Sperry JL, Guyette FX, Brown JB et al. Prehospital plasma during air medical transport in trauma patients at risk for hemorrhagic shock. *New England Journal of Medicine*. 2018;379(4):315–326. Available at: https://pubmed.ncbi.nlm.nih.gov/30044935/

Self-Reflection Questions

1. What signs and symptoms might help you recognise that a patient is in shock?
2. What can you do in the prehospital setting to help prevent circulatory shock from progressing to cardiac arrest?
3. How might you determine if a patient should receive fluids?
4. Which types of fluids and/or blood products are available to you in your agency?
5. Which vasoactive medication(s) might you consider in the following scenarios, and how do they work?
   - Septic shock in an adult
   - Septic shock in a child
   - Cardiogenic shock
   - Neurogenic shock.

References

1. Monnet X, Marik P, Teboul JL. Passive leg raising for predicting fluid responsiveness: a systematic review and meta-analysis. *Intensive Care Medicine*. 2016;42(12):1935–1947. Available at: https://pubmed.ncbi.nlm.nih.gov/26825952/
2. Nassar BS, Schmidt GA. Capnography for monitoring of the critically ill patient. *Clinics in Chest Medicine*. 2022;43(3):393–400. Available at: https://pubmed.ncbi.nlm.nih.gov/36116809/
3. Zampieri FG, et al., Balanced crystalloids versus saline for critically ill patients (BEST-Living): a systematic review and individual patient data meta-analysis. *Lancet Respiratory Medicine*. 2024;12(3): 237–246.
4. Sperry JL, Guyette FX, Brown JB et al. Prehospital plasma during air medical transport in trauma patients at risk for hemorrhagic shock. *New England Journal of Medicine*. 2018;379(4):315–326. Available at: https://pubmed.ncbi.nlm.nih.gov/30044935/
5. Moore HB, Moore EE, Chapman MP et al. Plasma-first resuscitation to treat haemorrhagic shock during emergency ground transportation in an urban area: a randomised trial. *Lancet*. 2018;392(10144):283–291. Available at: https://pubmed.ncbi.nlm.nih.gov/30032977/
6. Crombie N, Doughty HA, Bishop JRB et al. Resuscitation with blood products in patients with trauma-related haemorrhagic shock receiving prehospital care (RePHILL): a multicentre, open-label, randomised,

controlled, phase 3 trial. *Lancet Haematology*. 2022;9(4):e250–e261. Available at: https://pubmed.ncbi.nlm.nih.gov/35271808/
7. Evans L, Rhodes A, Alhazzani W et al. Surviving sepsis campaign: international guidelines for management of sepsis and septic shock 2021. *Intensive Care Medicine*. 2021;47(11):1181–1247. Available at: https://pubmed.ncbi.nlm.nih.gov/34599691/
8. Muraro A, Worm M, Alviani C et al. EAACI guidelines: anaphylaxis (2021 update). *Allergy*. 2022;77(2):357–377. Available at: https://pubmed.ncbi.nlm.nih.gov/34343358/
9. Weiss SL, Peters MJ, Alhazzani W et al. Surviving sepsis campaign international guidelines for the management of septic shock and sepsis-associated organ dysfunction in children. *Intensive Care Medicine*. 2020;46(1):10–67. Available at: https://pubmed.ncbi.nlm.nih.gov/32030529/
10. De Backer D, Biston P, Devriendt J et al. Comparison of dopamine and norepinephrine in the treatment of shock. *New England Journal of Medicine*. 2010;362(9):779–789. Available at: https://pubmed.ncbi.nlm.nih.gov/20200382/
11. Killu K, Sarani B. *Fundamental Critical Care Support*, 6th edn. Mount Prospect, IL: Society of Critical Care Medicine; 2016.

8
Myocardial Infarction (STEMI)

Luke Dawson, Ross Salathiel and Dion Stub

> **In this chapter you will learn:**
> - Potential causes of acute chest pain and diagnosis of myocardial infarction (MI)
> - Potential complications and management of MI
> - The evidence base for paramedic-led prehospital thrombolysis
> - Indications and contraindications for prehospital thrombolysis.

Case Details

Dispatch
55-year-old male, central severe chest pain, diaphoretic.

History
A 55-year-old man developed left arm pain while gardening around 1730 this afternoon. The pain became progressively worse, and the patient developed central chest pain and right arm pain, increasing to 10/10 by 2030, at which time he contacted the ambulance. A double-crewed ambulance and a critical care paramedic are dispatched. The nearest major hospital with 24-hour percutaneous coronary intervention (PCI) cardiac services is more than three hours' drive away.

On Arrival of the First Crew
The scene is safe, and the patient is sitting inside on a chair. He appears diaphoretic. Primary survey findings and initial vital signs are:

Airway	Patent
Breathing	RR 22, SpO$_2$ 95% on room air
Circulation	Peripheral pulses present, HR 108, BP 102/64, cool peripheries
Disability	GCS E4, V5, M6 (15), BGL 8.1 mmol/L
Environmental	Temp 37.1 °C

Six minutes after arriving on scene the first paramedic crew obtains a 12-lead ECG, which indicates inferior ST-segment elevation with reciprocal changes in leads I and aVL (**Figure 8.1**). Their secondary survey reveals that the patient does not have a cardiac murmur on auscultation and that there are normal breath sounds with good air entry bilaterally.

CHAPTER 8   Myocardial Infarction (STEMI)

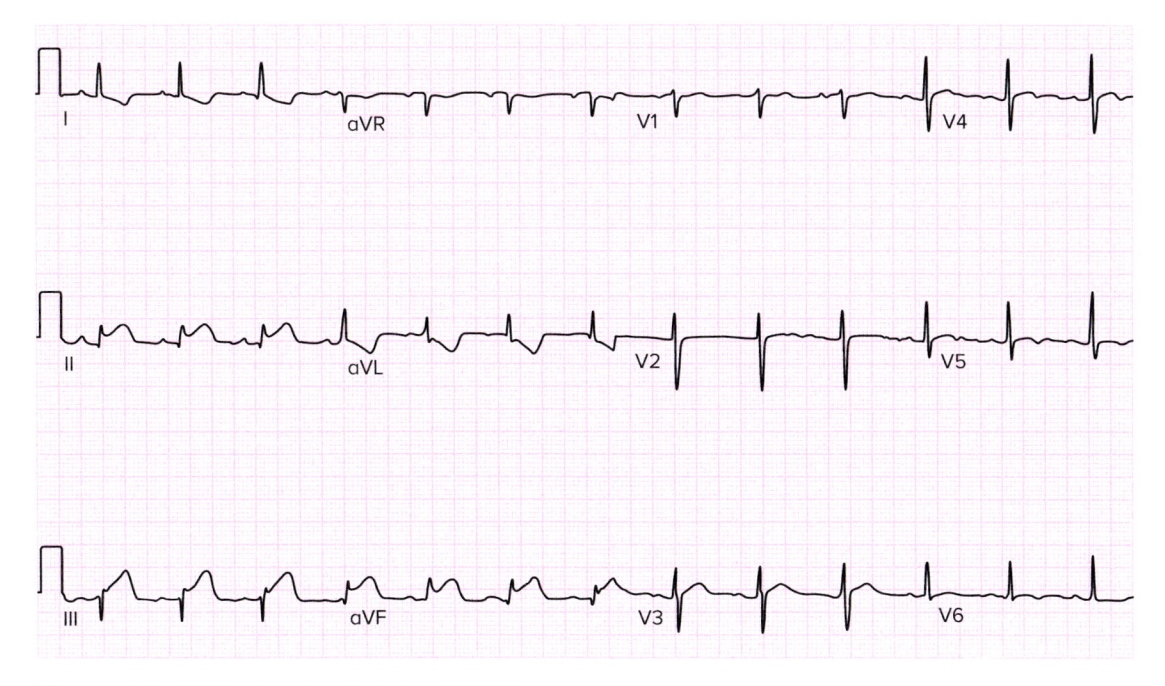

Figure 8.1   ECG showing inferior STEMI.

On Your Arrival as the Critical Care Paramedic

The initial paramedic crew have administered 300 mg aspirin orally and are in the process of placing two large-bore intravenous cannulas into both cubital fossa. During this process the patient develops ventricular fibrillation and loses consciousness. CPR is commenced, and defibrillation pads are placed in the anterior and lateral positions, with a single cardioversion reverting the patient to sinus rhythm. Vital signs following defibrillation are: pulse 102 bpm (regular), blood pressure 108/68 mmHg, RR 24 bpm, SpO_2 94% on room air and GCS 15, with the patient conversing normally but concerned regarding the immediately preceding events.

AMPLE

The patient has a past history of asthma, current smoking and depression. His only medication is sertraline. He has an allergy to shellfish, works as a truck driver and is moderately overweight.

Allergies	Shellfish
Medications	Sertraline 50 mg PO daily
Past history	Asthma, depression, current smoker
Last ins and outs	Dinner three hours prior
Events prior	Onset of ischaemic-sounding chest pain while gardening

SECTION 3   Circulation

Decision Point
What are your clinical priorities in this situation?

With MI and evidence of ongoing ischaemia on the ECG, including complications such as VF, re-establishing coronary perfusion is of the utmost importance. This can be achieved either by primary percutaneous coronary intervention, if this can be achieved in a timely manner (the nearest cardiac centre is more than three hours away in this case), or by intravenous thrombolysis.

Question 1: What are Possible Causes of Acute Chest Pain and the Key Presenting Clinical Features in MI?

Acute chest pain is one of the most common reasons for calling an ambulance, representing approximately one in ten ambulance attendances.[1] The causes of acute chest pain are diverse and while serious and life-threatening conditions underly a proportion of cases, around half of patients presenting with acute chest pain can be discharged safely from hospital after initial investigations with no specific cause identified. The most serious underlying diagnoses can be life-threatening and include MI (~3–4%), pulmonary emboli (~1%) and acute aortic syndromes such as dissection or rupture (<1%), and for this reason, despite the relative low incidence among overall chest pain presentations, urgent care and management is prioritised.

MI most commonly presents with acute chest pain, typically tight, heavy or crushing in nature, sometimes with radiation to either arm or jaw, and frequently associated with other symptoms, such as dyspnoea, diaphoresis, sweating and nausea. It is important to note that the clinical presentation can be diverse and not all patients present with typical symptoms, especially women, who may be less likely to have typical chest pain, and diabetics, who may not have chest pain in the setting of diabetic neuropathy. For this reason, a high index of suspicion is required, and early ECG should be prioritised in suspected MI cases.

Question 2: What are the Priorities of Care and Potential Complications of MI in the Prehospital Setting?

Mortality rates among patients with MI increase progressively with delays to treatment, and therefore rapid diagnosis and transport to definitive management should be the priority. Diagnosis is made through 12-lead ECG, and the use of prehospital 12-lead ECG to guide cardiac catheterisation laboratory activation or thrombolysis has been associated with shorter times to coronary reperfusion. Many regions have systems in place to transmit prehospital ECGs to emergency physicians or on-call cardiologists to confirm the MI diagnosis and guide decisions regarding appropriate reperfusion strategy, that is, either primary PCI or prehospital thrombolysis.

Following diagnosis, current guidelines recommend administration of aspirin (usually 300 mg orally) and a bolus of intravenous heparin or enoxaparin, with pain managed usually using intravenous opioids, such as fentanyl or morphine, and sublingual glyceryl trinitrate. Oxygen therapy is generally reserved for patients that are hypoxic (with oxygen saturations <92%), given that recent randomised studies have demonstrated increased infarct size with oxygen supplementation for patients with MI that are not hypoxic.[2] The conceptual rationale for prehospital thrombolysis is outlined in **Figure 8.2**. Primary PCI (PPCI) is the preferred intervention for STEMI, but in clinical situations where PPCI is unlikely to be feasible within 120 minutes, prehospital thrombolysis is preferred. This would typically be the case in rural or remote areas.

CHAPTER 8 Myocardial Infarction (STEMI)

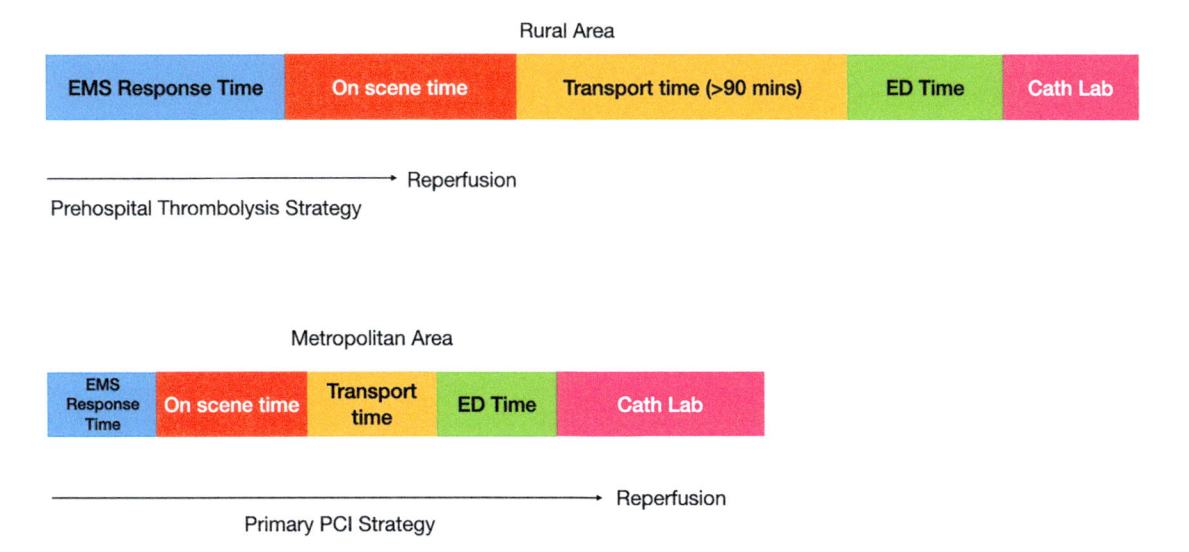

Figure 8.2 Time to reperfusion in prehospital thrombolysis and primary PCI.
Source: Image by David Anderson.

Patients with MI are at high risk for complications during transit to hospital, with the most serious including arrhythmias, such as ventricular tachycardia or ventricular fibrillation and cardiogenic shock. Ventricular arrhythmias (affecting up to 10% of MI patients) should be managed according to standard ALS pathways, with chest compression and cardioversion in the setting of loss of cardiac output or significant hypotension. Ventricular arrhythmias with maintained cardiac output are commonly managed with antiarrhythmic medications, such as an amiodarone or lignocaine bolus. Cardiogenic shock affects approximately 5% of MI patients, more commonly with large anterior infarcts, and is generally managed with inotropes (often adrenaline; however, different EMS providers may have differing preferred inotrope agents, given lack of conclusive evidence). Cardiogenic shock in the setting of an inferior infarct can also be treated with intravenous fluids (500 ml to 1 litre) provided there is no evidence of pulmonary oedema, as the mechanism underlying the hypotension is commonly right ventricular dysfunction, which responds to intravenous filling.

Question 3: What Is the Evidence for Thrombolysis, Including in the Prehospital Setting?

Thrombolysis is well established as a treatment that reduces all-cause mortality for patients with MI both in the prehospital and hospital settings. Prior to PPCI for MI, thrombolysis was the key definitive treatment for MI, improving outcomes if administered within twelve hours of symptom onset. PPCI has since become the preferred treatment, following multiple trials and meta-analyses showing improved outcomes with PPCI compared to thrombolysis, with both improved efficacy and safety of PPCI over thrombolysis. Specifically, reductions in mortality for PPCI compared to intravenous thrombolysis are mainly driven by reduced rates of recurrent MI and intracranial haemorrhage.[3–5] Currently, a large body of evidence supports the use of both PPCI or thrombolysis, with PPCI being the preferred initial management if PCI can be performed within 60–120 minutes from the time of diagnosis.[6] If PCI is unlikely to be performed within 60–120 minutes (for example, due to a rural location of a patient), thrombolysis is the preferred option likely to result in better outcomes.

> **PRACTICE TIP**
>
> Obtaining a prehospital ECG in a timely fashion for patients with suspected acute coronary syndromes is critical to facilitate rapid management of MI. Australian Healthcare Standards recommend a 12-lead ECG should be recorded in patients with acute coronary syndrome symptoms within 10 minutes of first clinical contact.

When thrombolysis is selected as the optimal initial reperfusion strategy, this should be administered as early as feasible. Several studies have demonstrated improved clinical outcomes with early thrombolysis, which extends to using thrombolysis in prehospital settings rather than transporting the patient to a local non-PCI hospital to administer hospital-based thrombolysis. Two meta-analyses have shown shorter time to reperfusion with prehospital thrombolysis compared to hospital thrombolysis,[7,8] and possibly reduced mortality rates.[8] In one study, the relative reduction in mortality was 44% for patients thrombolysed within 0–2 hours, compared to 20% for patients thrombolysed within 2–6 hours after symptom onset.[9] Moreover, rates of left ventricular dysfunction and the size of the myocardial infarct are reduced among survivors if thrombolysis occurs earlier.

Question 4: What Are the Indications and Contraindications for Prehospital Thrombolysis?

While the majority of patients with MI are likely to benefit from early thrombolysis within 12 hours of symptom onset, there are several clinical conditions that could lead to greater net harm rather than benefit, with most of these relating to risk of significant bleeding. To facilitate rapid thrombolysis without the clinician needing to recall a long list of contraindications, most organisations use a checklist, protocol or algorithm to determine each patient's suitability for thrombolysis. **Table 8.1** presents a list of contraindications to the administration of thrombolysis, but each ambulance service generally uses their own specific checklist for contraindications relating to thrombolysis.

Table 8.1 Contraindications to thrombolysis

Contraindications to the administration of thrombolysis (consider expert consultation)
• Blood pressure >180/110 mmHg • Recent trauma/surgery • Gastrointestinal or genitourinary bleeding within previous two to four weeks • Stroke/TIA within twelve months • Prior intracranial haemorrhage at any time • Current anticoagulation or bleeding diathesis (relative contraindication with warfarin).

Source: Adapted from the National Heart Foundation of Australia, *Australian Clinical Guidelines for the Management of Acute Coronary Syndromes*, 2016.

CHAPTER 8   Myocardial Infarction (STEMI)

The indications for thrombolysis are symptoms consistent with MI, ST-elevation on ECG, symptom onset less than 12 hours, and unable to undergo PPCI within 60–120 minutes (with specific timing varying according to jurisdiction). Contraindications include non-modifiable criteria, such as diagnosed allergies to thrombolytic agents, currently taking an anticoagulant (warfarin, dabigatran, apixaban, rivaroxaban), recent bleeding or surgery within four weeks, major stroke within twelve months, pregnancy or delivery within two weeks. Or modifiable criteria such as systolic blood pressure >180 mmHg or diastolic blood pressure >110 mmHg, which could be treated to allow thrombolysis once the patient is less hypertensive.

PRACTICE TIP

Decisions regarding emergency transfers for MI versus prehospital thrombolysis should be made as early as possible. On attending patients with acute chest pain that may be MI, paramedics should be aware of the likely transit times to the nearest 24-hour cardiac catheterisation facility for primary PCI.

Generally, if this transit time is greater than 90 minutes (with a corresponding time to PCI likely to be greater than 120 minutes), then prehospital thrombolysis should be considered.

Question 5: What Are the Potential Complications of Thrombolysis in the Prehospital Setting and What Steps Should be Taken If It is Unsuccessful?

The main potential complications of thrombolysis relate to bleeding or unsuccessful reperfusion. Intracranial bleeding is probably the most devastating complication, with a rate of 0.5–1.0%[10] and up to two-thirds of these patients subsequently dying. Careful screening of contraindication criteria is required to minimise this risk. Non-intracranial bleeding is more common but less likely to lead to death. Allergic reaction is possible but less common with newer non-streptokinase thrombolytic agents (such as tenecteplase and alteplase). Reperfusion arrhythmias (usually accelerated idioventricular rhythms) are common after thrombolysis, occurring in up to 50% of patients and these generally do not require treatment.

Unsuccessful thrombolysis may occur and is more common if there is substantial plaque burden or if there is a delay from symptom onset to thrombolysis. Success rates of thrombolysis are approximately 50–70% in the contemporary literature.[11] Thrombolysis is considered successful if there is resolution of chest pain and a greater than 50% reduction in ST-elevation on ECG at 60–90 minutes after thrombolysis. If there is ongoing chest pain, persistent or worsening ST-elevation or other ongoing evidence of ischaemia, such as haemodynamic instability or worsening heart failure, then thrombolysis is considered to have been unsuccessful and the patient should be urgently transported to a cardiac catheterisation centre for rescue PCI.[12] Rescue PCI is defined as PCI within twelve hours of failed thrombolysis and is associated with improved outcomes compared to conservative management or repeat thrombolysis.[13] Conversely, if thrombolysis is successful, patients should be transported to a cardiac catheterisation centre for PCI within 24 hours (but longer than three hours) after thrombolysis. This is considered the optimal time to reduce bleeding complications related to thrombolysis during the procedure without increasing ischaemic complications by delaying PCI too long (termed a pharmaco-invasive PCI strategy).

SECTION 3 Circulation

Question 6: What Is the In-Hospital Trajectory of Patients with MI?

Patients with MI generally are admitted to hospital for three to five days for uncomplicated presentations, although this period may be substantially longer among patients with complications such as cardiac arrest or cardiogenic shock, or among those that require bypass surgery. The vast majority of patients are managed with immediate reperfusion with either thrombolysis or primary percutaneous coronary intervention. The decision not to reperfuse a patient with MI is relatively rare, but reasons for this include elderly patients with very significant co-morbidities or those presenting very late, where the myocardium is unlikely to be salvageable. In Australia, approximately 90–95% of patients can undergo primary PCI in a timely manner, while the remainder have thrombolysis prior with subsequent angiography and revascularisation ideally 3–24 hours after thrombolysis (or with rescue PCI as soon as possible if thrombolysis fails). Studies have demonstrated that revascularisation for non-culprit vessels improves outcomes in patients with MI,[14] and this is most often done during the same admission, with either PCI or coronary artery bypass surgery. For patients with cardiogenic shock or refractory cardiac arrest, advanced support options include extracorporeal membrane oxygenation (ECMO), or mechanical support devices, such as the Impella axial-flow pump and intra-aortic balloon pumps, which support the patient in the acute setting with the hope that cardiac function improves after revascularisation.

Following revascularisation, patients with MI are commenced on several medications prior to discharge including dual antiplatelet therapy (aspirin and a P2Y12 inhibitor, such as prasugrel, ticagrelor or clopidogrel), high-dose lipid-lowering therapy (statins +/- ezetimibe) and usually a beta-blocker and angiotensin-converting enzyme inhibitor (ACEI) or angiotensin-receptor blocker (ARB). All patients should undergo a transthoracic echocardiogram during admission to assess cardiac function and exclude complications such as ventricular septal defects or left ventricular thrombus. Patients with reduced left ventricular function or heart failure are additionally considered for mineralocorticoid antagonists, either eplerenone or spironolactone, and frusemide to achieve euvolaemia as required. Following discharge, patients should have close cardiology follow-up and risk factor modification, including lifestyle modifications, such as smoking cessation. Most patients are referred for cardiac rehabilitation programmes, which improve survival and reduce recurrent MI through risk factor modification and cardiac-specific exercises.

Question 7: What Are the Contemporary Outcomes for MI and How Does Prehospital Care Contribute to These Outcomes?

Coronary heart disease is the leading single cause of mortality in Australia, accounting for 10% of all deaths, and approximately 40% of cardiovascular deaths in 2020.[15] Rates of death related to coronary disease have fallen by over 80% since 1980, which relates to better risk factor modification and improvements in the management of acute MI.[15] Contemporary MI outcomes have mortality rates of approximately 6% in comparison to untreated mortality rates of approximately 30%.[6] Mortality rates are substantially higher for patients with serious complications of MI, such as out-of-hospital cardiac arrest or cardiogenic shock. Much of the improvement in MI mortality rates over the past three decades relates to rapid coronary reperfusion, which has been achieved by the availability of reperfusion treatments

CHAPTER 8   Myocardial Infarction (STEMI)

(thrombolysis and PCI) and improved systems of care to rapidly facilitate these treatments. These improvements have led to reductions in infarct size and subsequent heart failure complications of MI, and to shortened hospital stays for patients with MI.

Improving prehospital systems of care has played an important part of these improved outcomes. Prehospital ECG and paramedic-activated catheterisation laboratory activation is associated with a reduction in time from symptom onset to coronary reperfusion by approximately 30 minutes and a reduction in mortality rates (adjusted odds ratio 0.94) in one population-based observational study in the UK.[16] Prehospital thrombolysis similarly has been found to improve outcomes, decreasing all-cause hospital mortality compared with in-hospital thrombolysis with an odds ratio of 0.83 (95% confidence ratio 0.70–0.98) in one meta-analysis.[8]

Australian ambulance services vary in their approach to managing transport of post-thrombolysis patients for rescue PCI, with geography being a major factor. Ensuring a system of care that enables unsuccessful thrombolysis patients timely access to PCI (rescue PCI) is an optimal approach; however, in some locations across the vast Australian continent, this is not practicable and relies heavily on aeromedical retrieval. In these instances, a co-ordinated system is needed to ensure time to PCI is minimised as much as possible for best patient outcomes.

Key Evidence

This is the current evidence pool of high-quality studies to guide paramedic/prehospital thrombolysis and prehospital MI management. Search last updated January 2023.

Systematic Review/Meta-Analyses

Huynh T, Perron S, O'Loughlin J et al. Comparison of primary percutaneous coronary intervention and fibrinolytic therapy in ST-segment-elevation myocardial infarction: Bayesian hierarchical meta-analyses of randomized controlled trials and observational studies. *Circulation*. 2009;119(24):3101–3109.

McCaul M, Lourens A, Kredo T. Pre-hospital versus in-hospital thrombolysis for ST-elevation myocardial infarction. *Cochrane Database of Systematic Reviews*. 2014;2014(9):CD010191.

Morrison LJ, Verbeek PR, McDonald AC et al. Mortality and prehospital thrombolysis for acute myocardial infarction: a meta-analysis. *JAMA*. 2000;283(20):2686–2692.

Randomised Controlled Trials

Andersen HR, Nielsen TT, Rasmussen K et al. A comparison of coronary angioplasty with fibrinolytic therapy in acute myocardial infarction. *New England Journal of Medicine*. 2003;349:733–742.

Castaigne AD, Hervé C, Duval-Moulin AM et al. Pre-hospital use of APSAC: results of a placebo-controlled study. *American Journal of Cardiology*. 1989;64(2):30A–33A.

Gershlick AH, Stephens-Lloyd A, Hughes S et al. Rescue angioplasty after failed thrombolytic therapy for acute myocardial infarction. *New England Journal of Medicine*. 2005;353:2758–2768.

Morrow DA, Antman EM, Sayah A et al. Evaluation of the time saved by prehospital initiation of reteplase for ST-elevation myocardial infarction: results of the Early Retavase-Thrombolysis in Myocardial Infarction (ER-TIMI) 19 trial. *Journal of the American College of Cardiology*. 2002;40(1):71.

Schofer J, Büttner J, Geng G et al. Prehospital thrombolysis in acute myocardial infarction. *American Journal of Cardiology*. 1990;66(20):1429–1433.

Wallentin L, Goldstein P, Armstrong PW et al. Efficacy and safety of tenecteplase in combination with the low-molecular-weight heparin enoxaparin or unfractionated heparin in the prehospital setting: the

SECTION 3   Circulation

Assessment of the Safety and Efficacy of a New Thrombolytic Regimen (ASSENT)-3 PLUS randomized trial in acute myocardial infarction. *Circulation*. 2003;108(2):135–142.

Weaver WD, Cerqueira M, Hallstrom AP et al. Prehospital-initiated vs hospital-initiated thrombolytic therapy. The Myocardial Infarction Triage and Intervention Trial. *JAMA*. 1993;270(10):1211–1216.

Self-Reflection Questions

1. What do you think about the evidence base for paramedic-led prehospital thrombolysis?
2. How important do you think prehospital care is in influencing outcomes of emergent clinical conditions such as MI?
3. How critical is getting a prehospital ECG in patients with acute chest pain?
4. When would you make the decision to transfer for primary PCI versus thrombolysis in the acute workup for MI?
5. Using the table below, prepare a handover of the patient described using the IMIST AMBO format.

Introduction	
Mechanism	
Injuries	
Signs and symptoms	
Treatment	
Allergies	
Medications	
Background history	
Other information	

References

1. Dawson LP, Smith K, Cullen L et al. Care models for acute chest pain that improve outcomes and efficiency: JACC state-of-the-art review. *Journal of the American College of Cardiology*. 2022;79:2333–2348.
2. Stub D, Smith K, Bernard S et al. Air versus oxygen in ST-segment-elevation myocardial infarction. *Circulation*. 2015;131:2143–2150.
3. Andersen HR, Nielsen TT, Rasmussen K et al. A comparison of coronary angioplasty with fibrinolytic therapy in acute myocardial infarction. *New England Journal of Medicine*. 2003;349:733–742.
4. Huynh T, Perron S, O'Loughlin J et al. Comparison of primary percutaneous coronary intervention and fibrinolytic therapy in ST-segment-elevation myocardial infarction: Bayesian hierarchical meta-analyses of randomized controlled trials and observational studies. *Circulation*. 2009;119:3101–3109.
5. Keeley EC, Boura JA, Grines CL. Primary angioplasty versus intravenous thrombolytic therapy for acute myocardial infarction: a quantitative review of 23 randomised trials. *Lancet*. 2003;361:13–20.
6. Claeys MJ, de Meester A, Convens C et al. Contemporary mortality differences between primary percutaneous coronary intervention and thrombolysis in ST-segment elevation myocardial infarction. *Archives of Internal Medicine*. 2011;171:544–549.
7. McCaul M, Lourens A, Kredo T. Pre-hospital versus in-hospital thrombolysis for ST-elevation myocardial infarction. *Cochrane Database of Systematic Reviews*. 2014;2014:CD010191.
8. Morrison LJ, Verbeek PR, McDonald AC et al. Mortality and prehospital thrombolysis for acute myocardial infarction: a meta-analysis. *JAMA*. 2000;283:2686–2692.

9. Boersma E, Maas AC, Deckers JW et al. Early thrombolytic treatment in acute myocardial infarction: reappraisal of the golden hour. *Lancet*. 1996;348:771–775.
10. Savonitto S, Armstrong PW, Lincoff AM et al. Risk of intracranial haemorrhage with combined fibrinolytic and glycoprotein IIb/IIIa inhibitor therapy in acute myocardial infarction. Dichotomous response as a function of age in the GUSTO V trial. *European Heart Journal*. 2003;24:1807–1814.
11. Cannon CP, Gibson CM, McCabe CH et al. TNK-tissue plasminogen activator compared with front-loaded alteplase in acute myocardial infarction: results of the TIMI 10B trial. Thrombolysis in Myocardial Infarction (TIMI) 10B Investigators. *Circulation*. 1998;98:2805–2814.
12. Goldman LE, Eisenberg MJ. Identification and management of patients with failed thrombolysis after acute myocardial infarction. *Annals of Internal Medicine*. 2000;132:556–565.
13. Gershlick AH, Stephens-Lloyd A, Hughes S et al. Rescue angioplasty after failed thrombolytic therapy for acute myocardial infarction. *New England Journal of Medicine*. 2005;353:2758–2768.
14. Mehta SR, Wood DA, Storey RF et al. Complete revascularization with multivessel PCI for myocardial infarction. *New England Journal of Medicine*. 2019;381:1411–1421.
15. Australian Institute of Health and Welfare. Heart, stroke and vascular disease: Australian facts. Coronary heart disease [online]. 2022. Available at: https://www.aihw.gov.au/reports/heart-stroke-vascular-diseases/hsvd-facts/contents/all-heart-stroke-and-vascular-disease/coronary-heart-disease
16. Quinn T, Johnsen S, Gale CP et al. Effects of prehospital 12-lead ECG on processes of care and mortality in acute coronary syndrome: a linked cohort study from the Myocardial Ischaemia National Audit Project. *Heart*. 2014;100:944–950.

9 The Management of Unstable Bradycardia

Alan Cowley and Mark Durell

In this chapter you will learn:
- What constitutes an unstable bradycardia
- What causes bradycardia
- What pharmacological options exist in the management of bradycardia
- The methods and challenges of prehospital pacing.

Case Details

Dispatch
72-year-old male, fall at home, unable to get up.

History
A 72-year-old man has fallen in his living room while standing up from his chair. He says he is not injured but feels dizzy and light-headed. He lives in a second-floor apartment in a block without an elevator. A double-crewed ambulance have been dispatched and, on arrival, requested the assistance of a critical care paramedic.

On Arrival of the First Crew
The scene is safe and the patient is lying on the living room floor. His primary survey findings and initial vital signs are:

Airway	Patent
Breathing	RR 18, SpO_2 not recordable due to poor trace
Circulation	Peripheral pulses absent, central pulses present, HR 30, BP 70/40, cool, clammy peripheries
Disability	GCS E4, V5, M6 (15), BGL 6.8 mmol/L
Environmental	Temp 37.1 °C

The first paramedic crew have attempted to assist the patient from the floor to a stair chair so they can move him to the ambulance, but every attempt to move the patient from a supine position causes a syncope. The patient has no obvious injury on primary survey.

CHAPTER 9   The Management of Unstable Bradycardia

On Your Arrival as the Critical Care Paramedic

The crew have applied high-flow oxygen, taken a 12-lead ECG and gained IV access. The 12-lead ECG shows a third-degree heart block (**Figure 9.1**). One of the paramedics has given a single dose of 600 mcg atropine with no change to the patient's heart rate.

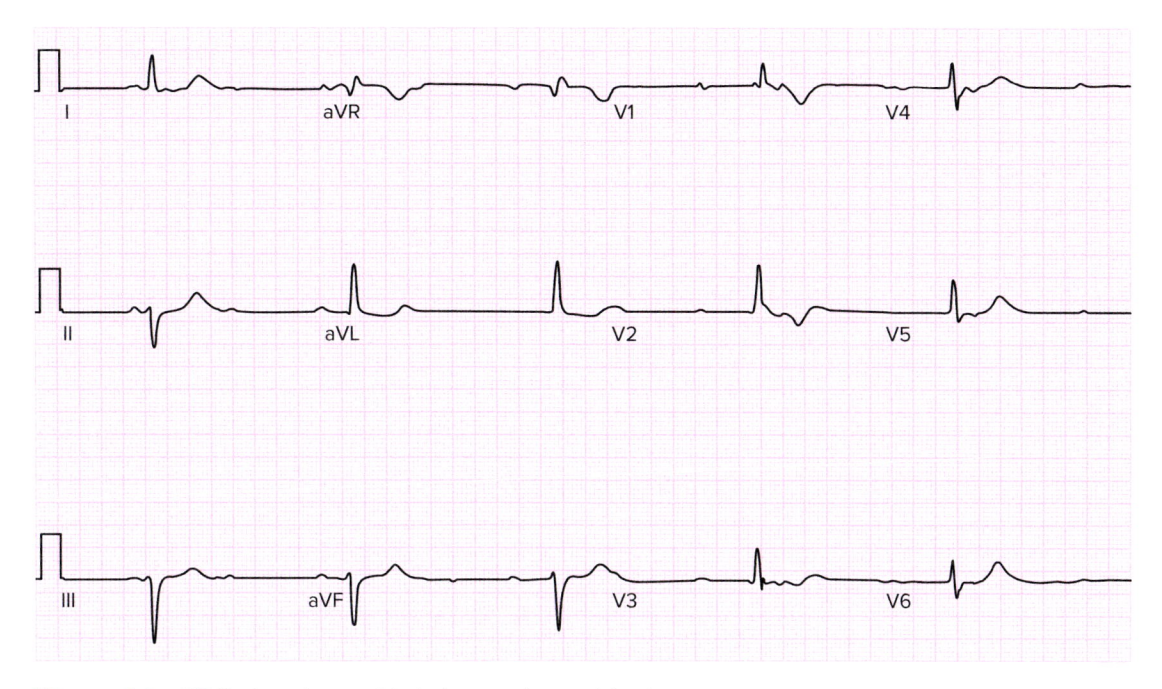

Figure 9.1   ECG showing a third-degree heart block.

AMPLE

Allergies	Penicillin
Medications	Ramipril
Past history	Hypertension
Last ins and outs	Normal
Events prior	Collapse

Decision Point
What are your clinical priorities in this situation?

SECTION 3   Circulation

Question 1: What Constitutes an Unstable Bradycardia?

Bradycardia is defined as a heart rate slower than that which would be considered physiologically normal. In adults this is generally considered to be a rate below 60 beats per minute, although this obviously differs in relation to age and overall physical fitness. A bradycardia is considered unstable or compromised when it has a significant impact on perfusion.[1,2]

Broadly, there are four categories that suggest compromise:

- Syncope
- Heart failure
- Hypotension – generally considered a systolic below 80 mmHg
- Myocardial ischaemia.[3,4]

Syncope is often the primary initial presenting complaint for unstable bradycardias, either in the form of partially resolved collapse or, less commonly, through deep coma. Resolved syncope alone does not indicate the patient has a compromised bradycardia, and transient complaints such as vasovagal syncope should not be immediately disregarded as differentials. Alongside this, coma in the presence of bradycardia doesn't always indicate the patient has a cardiovascular cause for their collapsed state and causes such as raised intracranial pressure should be considered.[5]

Heart failure in this context is not the pre-existing medical history, but the acute clinical findings, such as acute pulmonary oedema and lowered cardiac output, will suggest this. There are occasions, such as a patient with known congestive heart failure or acute conditions such as myocarditis, where the underlying heart failure should be addressed prior to or alongside the treatment of the bradycardia itself.

Hypotension is the most common indicator of compromise in bradycardic patients. Insufficient cardiac rate cannot indefinitely be compensated for with an increase in stroke volume, and so cardiac output decreases. Typically, hypotension is defined as a systolic of 80 mmHg or below, though the individual presentation and history, such as a background of hypertension, may well change the threshold in which intervention is necessary.

Myocardial ischaemia should be considered in acute cardiac chest pain with changes to the ECG indicative of ischaemia. While this subgroup may contain those with existing known stable angina, it is the presence of pain and other features of acute ischaemia that should be used when deciding whether intervention is necessary.

In summary, compromised patients are those in which the bradycardia is affecting their perfusion.

Question 2: What Causes Bradycardia?

The workings of cardiac cells are intricate and interconnected and the heart rate may change if any one of these processes fails. Normal sinus node automaticity, efficient atrioventricular (AV) node and His–Purkinje conduction are necessary for normal cardiac electrical activation. Bradycardia can be brought on by anything that impairs sinus node automaticity, conduction through the AV node and/or His–Purkinje system.[1]

Broadly speaking, the causes of bradycardia can be either intrinsic or extrinsic. Fibrous alterations in the nodal tissue constitute the majority of intrinsic causes. There are a wide

CHAPTER 9 The Management of Unstable Bradycardia

variety, such as natural degenerative processes (for example, ageing), congenital or genetic abnormalities, valvular disease, direct tissue damage (such as hypoxia or surgical trauma), tissue inflammation or infiltration (for example, sarcoidosis, amyloidosis and haemochromatosis), infections and autoimmune disease.[2,3]

Extrinsic causes include exposure to toxins, such as lead or the venom of some spiders, as well as some medications, such as digoxin, beta-blockers, calcium channel blockers, ivabradine or class I or III anti-arrhythmic medications, and abnormal electrolytes, such as hyperkalaemia or acidaemia. Bradycardia can also be brought on by conditions that result in high (intense) vagal tone (activity), which increases the parasympathetic input to the sinus node. These include diarrhoea, micturition, glottis stimulation, vomiting and coughing. Vagal nerve stimulators are among the iatrogenic causes. Bradycardia may also result from neurocardiogenic syncope and hypersensitivity of the carotid sinus. Some causes, including hypothyroidism, electrolyte imbalances and drug-induced conditions, are reversible. Different types of bradycardia, such as the Cushing's reflex, can also be brought on by inferior wall myocardial infarction and raised intracranial pressure.[3,5]

Several bradycardias have been linked to sleep disordered breathing (SDB), which includes obstructive sleep apnoea (OSA), central sleep apnoea and Cheyne–Stokes breathing. Some individuals have only experienced sinus bradycardia, second-degree atrioventricular (AV) block, vagotonic AV block or full heart block while sleeping. The chronic physiological stress brought on by SDB is thought to interact with circadian systems over time to change the way the heart beats and how its electrophysiology works, raising the risk of rhythm problems.[2]

Lev's disease (or Lev–Lenegre syndrome), a generalised conduction system disorder associated with calcification and fibrosis, is the root cause of acquired total heart block. Lev's illness, which most frequently affects older individuals, is often referred to as senile conduction system degeneration.[2]

Bradyarrhythmias are a common symptom of congenital heart disease in adulthood. Arrhythmias are, in fact, the most frequent consequence seen by people with congenital heart disease. This is brought on by irregularities in cardiac conduction or it could also be a result of a surgical procedure.[4]

Rarely, bradycardia may be linked to clinical problems that do not seem to have anything in common. For instance, bradycardia should be taken into consideration in patients with unique syncope presentations or in those who have a history that points to both epilepsy and syncope. Bradycardia is a rare condition that can be linked to epilepsy.[2]

Question 3: What Pharmacological Options Exist in the Management of Bradycardia?

Atropine has long been the starting point for most bradycardia algorithms. Its actions as an anticholinergic oppose the vagal response, making atropine useful in lower-degree heart blocks. There is good evidence to suggest its limited value in the higher-degree blocks, such as third-degree and second-degree type two blocks. Initial doses of 500–600 mcg repeated up to 3 mg total are normally sufficient to see effect. It should be noted that there are cases of profoundly worsening bradycardia on administration of small doses, as this may worsen

SECTION 3 Circulation

infranodal block, and caution should be applied in its use in the presence of ischaemia, as it may worsen myocardial oxygen demand.[6,7]

A further agent of use is adrenaline. With its wide range of alpha and beta effects and its safety when given through peripheral IV, making it a useful chronotrope, 2–10 mcg/min is usually sufficient dosing for increasing heart rate. However, as with atropine, caution should be used in the presence of ischaemia. Isoprenaline or dopamine have similar mechanisms of action, but their longer-term use presents a wider side-effect profile.[8]

Specific reversal agents should be considered in patients with a known or suspected toxic cause of their bradycardia. Consider agents such as calcium for calcium blocker overdose and glucagon for both calcium channel and beta-blocker overdose, though there is only weak evidence to support its widespread use.[8]

Most guidelines advocate for the use of atropine, followed by adrenaline, before moving on to transcutaneous pacing (**Figure 9.2**). Some jurisdictions may also use isoprenaline or dobutamine in addition to or in place of adrenaline.

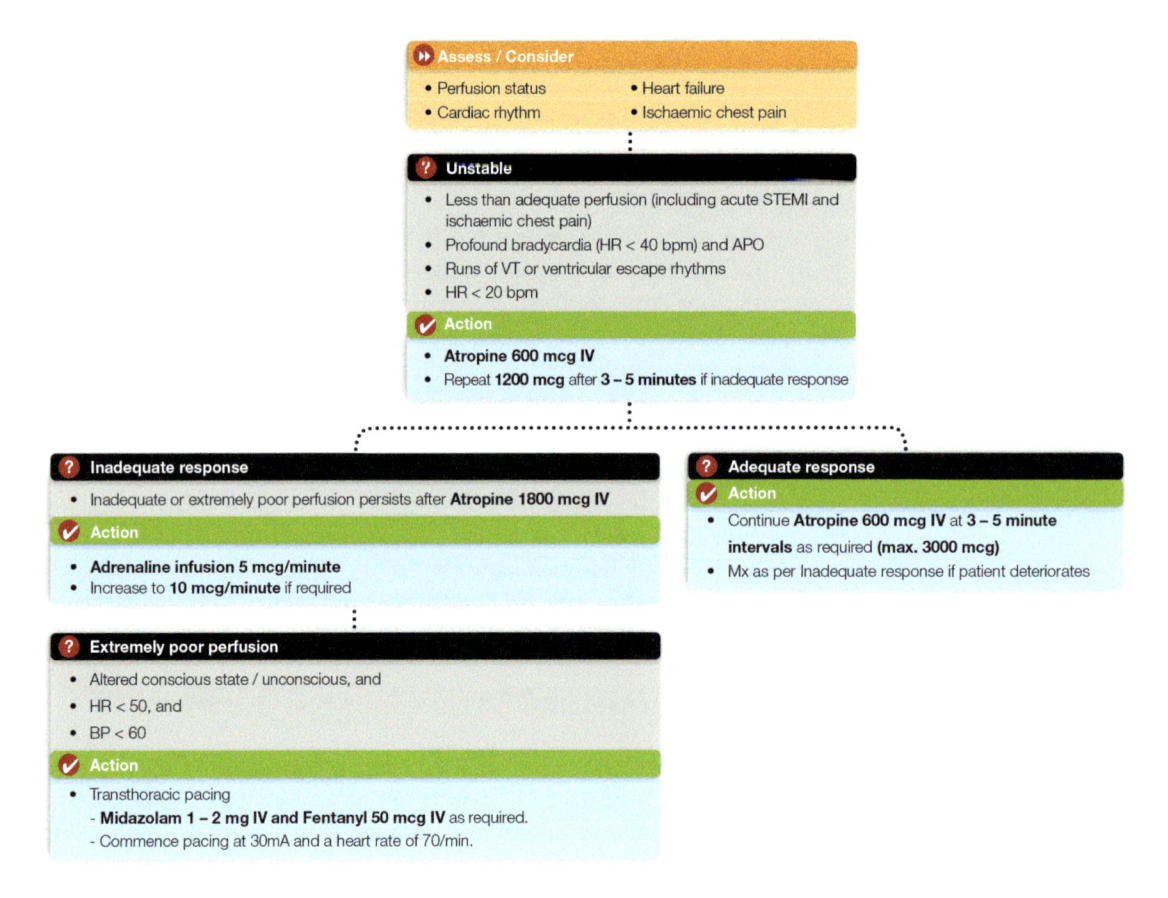

Assess / Consider
- Perfusion status
- Cardiac rhythm
- Heart failure
- Ischaemic chest pain

Unstable
- Less than adequate perfusion (including acute STEMI and ischaemic chest pain)
- Profound bradycardia (HR < 40 bpm) and APO
- Runs of VT or ventricular escape rhythms
- HR < 20 bpm

Action
- Atropine 600 mcg IV
- Repeat **1200 mcg** after **3 – 5 minutes** if inadequate response

Inadequate response
- Inadequate or extremely poor perfusion persists after **Atropine 1800 mcg IV**

Action
- Adrenaline infusion 5 mcg/minute
- Increase to **10 mcg/minute** if required

Adequate response

Action
- Continue **Atropine 600 mcg IV** at **3 – 5 minute intervals** as required **(max. 3000 mcg)**
- Mx as per Inadequate response if patient deteriorates

Extremely poor perfusion
- Altered conscious state / unconscious, and
- HR < 50, and
- BP < 60

Action
- Transthoracic pacing
  - **Midazolam 1 – 2 mg IV and Fentanyl 50 mcg IV** as required.
  - Commence pacing at 30mA and a heart rate of 70/min.

Figure 9.2 Algorithm for managing bradycardia.
Source: Ambulance Victoria. Reproduced with permission.

CHAPTER 9 The Management of Unstable Bradycardia

Question 4: The Methods and Challenges in Prehospital Pacing

Transcutaneous pacing is the primary prehospital therapy for unstable patients who are not responsive to medical therapy.[9] It can be applied rapidly through external electrodes and usually serves as an adjunct to a more permanent solution once at the appropriate facility.[8] In the prehospital environment it should be carried out with a device that is certified for this function. The exact method will depend upon the device itself, and you should always follow local guidance. In almost all devices, you will require the use of the defibrillator pads to deliver the therapy, as well as the monitoring leads to observe the underlying rhythm. Thought should be given to the pad placement and you should have a low threshold for adopting an 'anterior–posterior' configuration, since air ('the lungs') is a poor conductor of electricity (**Figure 9.3**). An appropriate starting heart rate is 80 beats per minute, but the required energy levels will vary widely.[8]

Anterior **Posterior**

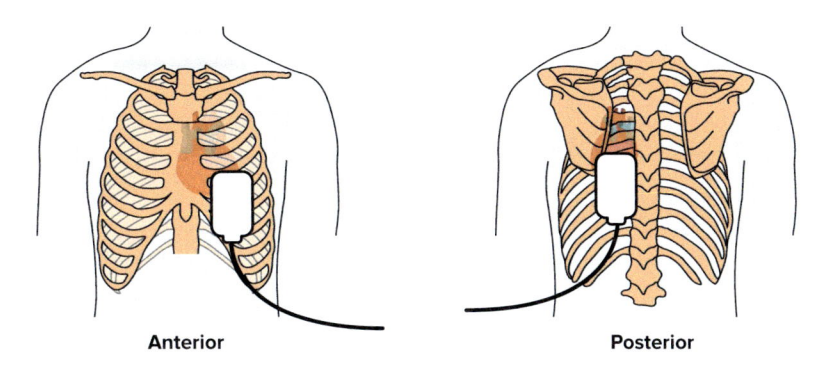

Figure 9.3 Anterior–posterior pad position for transcutaneous pacing.

There is no consensus on a starting energy level and, indeed, whether the current should be dialled up or down in order to obtain mechanical capture. Anecdotally, it may be wise in the peri-arrest patient to start with a high current in order to guarantee early capture (and then dial down), as opposed to the more stable patient, where a low current and dialling up may be more appropriate.[10]

> **PRACTICE TIP**
>
> When sedating patients for transcutaneous pacing, remember that all agents will have a much slower onset time; don't rush and inadvertently compromise the patient.

Both mechanical and electrical capture should be obtained to benefit the patient, and while the presence of pulses is often used to measure mechanical capture, the clinician should be aware that the muscle contractions generated by the therapy can make assessment of pulses unreliable. Improved blood pressure, level of consciousness and skin colour should be considered alongside pulses to confirm mechanical capture. Pulse oximetry waveform showing a pulse that *matches* that of the pacemaker can also be effective. Once both forms

SECTION 3 Circulation

of capture are achieved, the 'ideal' current is generally considered to be 1.25 times that required for capture, but 10–20 mA above is also acceptable.[10]

In all but the most obtunded patients, adequate analgesia and/or sedation must be considered. Few patients can tolerate currents of more than 50 mA without this. Even in patients where sedation is initially deemed unnecessary, a plan should be in place, as levels of consciousness may rise rapidly once mechanical capture is obtained. The exact agents and levels of analgosedation may be limited by the patient's instability. Though deep sedation (even with intubation) may be appealing, the instability caused by this procedure may outweigh the benefits of the pacing itself and it should be adopted with extreme caution. Guidelines vary and, in general, local practice should be followed; however, carefully titrated IV ketamine boluses are an appealing option for both sedation and analgesia for transcutaneous pacing. Ketamine potentially avoids the hypotension and respiratory depression associated with midazolam and fentanyl, which is another common sedation regimen.

As with many prehospital therapies, transcutaneous pacing can provide several challenges that may not be encountered in the hospital setting. As the critical care clinician, you are likely to be the only member of the team who can deliver the procedure and associated therapies, such as sedation and airway support. Your access to the patient and monitoring equipment must always be considered and it may, on occasions, be of benefit to withhold pacing until the patient has been extricated from their environment, depending on how imminent the need to deliver the therapy is deemed.

> **PRACTICE TIP**
>
> When handing over the patient, establish clear responsibilities and a timeline to swap monitoring; take the lead in ensuring the continuation of pacing.

Key Evidence

Mangrum JM, DiMarco JP. The evaluation and management of bradycardia. *New England Journal of Medicine*. 2000;342(10):703–709. Available at: https://pubmed.ncbi.nlm.nih.gov/10706901/

Kusumoto FM, Schoenfeld MH, Barrett C et al. 2018 ACC/AHA/HRS guideline on the evaluation and management of patients with bradycardia and cardiac conduction delay: a report of the American College of Cardiology/American Heart Association Task Force on Clinical Practice Guidelines and the Heart Rhythm Society. *Journal of the American College of Cardiology*. 2019;74(7):e51–156. Available at: https://www.jacc.org/doi/10.1016/j.jacc.2018.10.044

Self-Reflection Questions

1. What are some of the logistical challenges of prehospital pacing?
2. What would be your choice of medication for the bradycardic patient?
3. What sedation agents and strategy would you use to optimise patient comfort during pacing?
4. Patients with profound bradycardia are often complex in terms of pre-morbid state and frailty. How would this impact your treatment choice?
5. Handover and changeover from the prehospital monitor to the hospital monitor is a complex and high-risk process. How would you ensure that pacing is not interrupted in this phase?

CHAPTER 9 The Management of Unstable Bradycardia

References

1. Wung SF. Bradyarrhythmias: clinical presentation, diagnosis, and management. *Critical Care Nursing Clinics of North America*. 2016;28(3):297–308. Available at: https://pubmed.ncbi.nlm.nih.gov/27484658/
2. Kusumoto FM, Schoenfeld MH, Barrett C et al. 2018 ACC/AHA/HRS guideline on the evaluation and management of patients with bradycardia and cardiac conduction delay: a report of the American College of Cardiology/American Heart Association Task Force on Clinical Practice Guidelines and the Heart Rhythm Society. *Journal of the American College of Cardiology*. 2019;74(7):e51–156. Available at: https://www.jacc.org/doi/10.1016/j.jacc.2018.10.044
3. Mangrum JM, DiMarco JP. The evaluation and management of bradycardia. *New England Journal of Medicine*. 2000;342(10):703–709.
4. Sidhu S, Marine JE. Evaluating and managing bradycardia. *Trends in Cardiovascular Medicine*. 2020;30(5):265–272. Available at: https://pubmed.ncbi.nlm.nih.gov/31311698/
5. Stahmer SA. Bradyarrhythmias. In: Adams JG (ed.) *Emergency Medicine: Clinical Essentials*, 2nd edn. Philadelphia, PA: Elsevier; 2013.
6. Bernheim A, Fatio R, Kiowski W et al. Atropine often results in complete atrioventricular block or sinus arrest after cardiac transplantation: an unpredictable and dose-independent phenomenon. *Transplantation*. 2004;77(8):1181–1185. Available at: https://pubmed.ncbi.nlm.nih.gov/15114081/
7. Brady WJ, Swart G, DeBehnke DJ et al. The efficacy of atropine in the treatment of hemodynamically unstable bradycardia and atrioventricular block: prehospital and emergency department considerations. *Resuscitation*. 1999;41:47–55.
8. Burri H, Dayal N. Acute management of bradycardia in the emergency setting. *Cardiovascular Medicine*. 2018;21(04):98–104. Available at: https://doi.org/10.4414/cvm.2018.00554
9. Soar J, Nolan JP, Bottiger BW et al. European Resuscitation Council Guidelines for Resuscitation 2015: Section 3. Adult advanced life support. *Resuscitation*. 2015;95:100–147.
10. Lim S, Teo W, Anantharaman V. Cardiac pacing and Implanted defibrillation. In: Tintinalli JE, et al. (eds) *Tintinalli's Emergency Medicine: A Comprehensive Study Guide*, 9th edn. New York: McGraw-Hill Education; 2020.

10

Palpitations and Chest Pain: Paramedic Management of Narrow Complex Tachycardias

Andrew Bishop

In this chapter you will learn:

- The differential diagnosis for narrow complex tachycardias
- What management options are available to paramedics to manage narrow complex tachycardias
- Whether paramedics can safely manage narrow complex tachycardias
- The post-reversion management of supraventricular tachycardias (SVT).

Case Details

Dispatch

26-year-old female, chest pain, palpitations.

History

A 26-year-old female started experiencing palpitations and mild chest pain 30 minutes ago after an argument with her partner. Her partner called an ambulance when the symptoms did not resolve. A double-crewed ambulance and a single responder critical care paramedic are dispatched.

On Arrival of the First Crew

The scene is safe, with both parties no longer arguing. The patient is sitting on a couch, calm, but appears anxious. Her primary survey findings and initial vital signs are:

Airway	Patent
Breathing	RR 20, SpO$_2$ 99% on room air
Circulation	Peripheral pulses weak, HR 190, BP 102/64, cool peripheries
Disability	GCS E4, V5, M6 (15), BGL 5.5 mmol/L
Environmental	Temp 36.8 °C

The first paramedics arrive to find the patient sitting up, complaining of mild, central chest pain and feeling anxious about her palpitations. The patient's pain is 2/10, described as an 'ache'; she has never experienced this pain before. There is no radiation and no change

CHAPTER 10 Palpitations and Chest Pain

on movement, inspiration or palpation. The secondary survey is otherwise unremarkable. A 12-lead ECG is placed and shows a regular, narrow complex tachycardia (**Figure 10.1**).

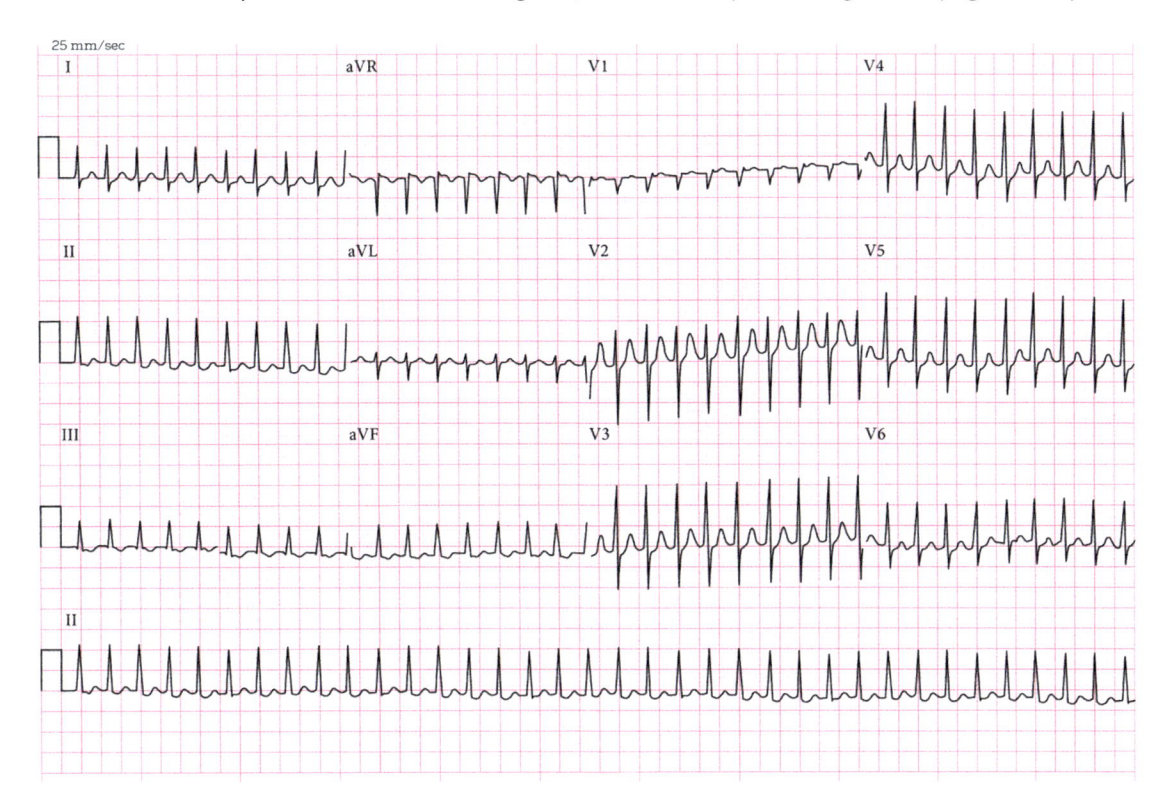

Figure 10.1 ECG showing a regular, narrow complex tachycardia.
Source: Adobe stock by alfa md.

The initial paramedics place an 18-gauge IV in the right cubital fossa and request that the critical care paramedic continues with this.

On Your Arrival as the Critical Care Paramedic

On your arrival you find no change in the patient's status. The chest pain and palpitations are still present.

AMPLE

Allergies	NKDA
Medications	Nil
Past history	Nil
Last ins and outs	Normal
Events	Chest pain and palpitations after an argument

SECTION 3   Circulation

Decision Point
What is the best management strategy for treating narrow complex tachycardias in this patient?

Question 1: What Is the Differential Diagnosis for a Narrow Complex Tachycardia?

Narrow complex tachycardia is defined as a tachycardia with a QRS duration of <120 msec and supraventricular the vast majority of the time, with the exception being high septal or fascicular ventricular tachycardia.

The most common cause of narrow complex tachycardia, typically placed under the umbrella of supraventricular tachycardia (SVT), is atrioventricular nodal re-entrant tachycardia (AVNRT) (56%), followed by atrioventricular re-entrant tachycardia (AVRT) (27%).[1] The mechanism by which AVNRT and AVRT occur is by the function of a re-entry circuit occurring, either around or within the AV node in the case of AVNRT, or via an atrioventricular accessory pathway in the case of AVRT. Wolff–Parkinson–White (WPW) syndrome is the most well-recognised disease process in which a tachyarrhythmia is associated with an accessory pathway.

Other potential causes of narrow complex tachycardia include atrial flutter, atrial fibrillation (AF) with rapid ventricular response (RVR) and multifocal atrial tachycardia (MAT). Both AF and MAT are irregularly irregular rhythms, while atrial flutter can be either regular or irregular. Atrial flutter is often diagnosed by the typical sawtooth pattern, most visually striking in the inferior leads, but can also be diagnosed by distinctive flutter waves in lead V1.

In case of the paramedic being unsure of whether there are underlying flutter waves, the use of the 'Lewis lead' electrode configuration can also be beneficial in revealing hidden atrial activity (**Figure 10.2**).[2] When using the Lewis lead configuration, increasing the calibration from 10 to 20 mm/mV and the paper speed from 25 to 50 mm/second can further amplify the atrial activity.

Prior to initiating management for SVT, one must ensure that sinus tachycardia is also excluded.

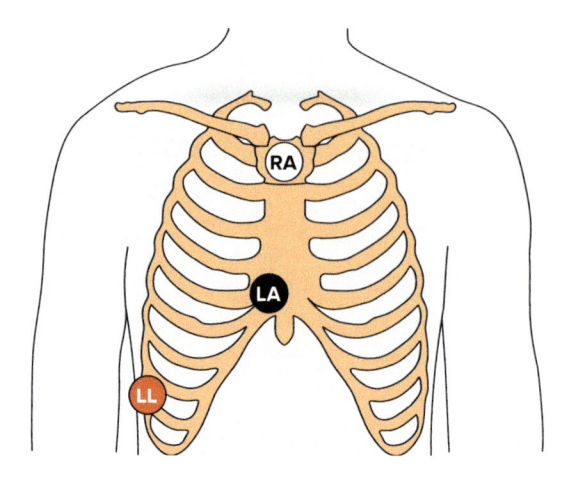

Figure 10.2   Lewis lead placement. Monitor lead I or II.

CHAPTER 10 Palpitations and Chest Pain

Question 2: What Management Options Are Available to Paramedics to Manage Supraventricular Tachycardia?

The management options for managing narrow complex tachycardia in the prehospital environment are focused on the tachycardias that come under the SVT banner, rather than treating AF or atrial flutter, for example. When it comes to these rhythms, AF with RVR in particular, the focus should be on treating the underlying cause of the tachycardia, rather than trying to revert the patient out of the rhythm. Reverting AF is a procedure that ideally should be done once the patient's coagulation status, length of time in AF and underlying cause of the tachycardia have all been assessed.

When considering what management options are available to the paramedic and what is best for the patient in front of them, a prudent first step is to assess the haemodynamic stability of the patient. The haemodynamics of the patient will help guide you to which management pathway is most appropriate for your patient; that is, how quickly you need to revert the patient.

Signs that the patient is unstable include, but are not limited to:

- Hypotension
- Altered conscious state
- Poor perfusion
- Ischaemic chest pain
- Dyspnoea.

If the patient is stable, then a prudent approach would be to attempt a Valsalva manoeuvre, followed by pharmacological management. In contrast, if the patient is unstable, adenosine or synchronised cardioversion are appropriate options.

PRACTICE TIP

Decision making to determine treatment pathways:

IS THE PATIENT HAEMODYNAMICALLY STABLE OR UNSTABLE?

Valsalva Manoeuvres

Valsalva manoeuvres are a common, safe way to manage supraventricular tachycardias in both prehospital and in-hospital environments. Unfortunately, the efficacy of these manoeuvres has been reported to be low, with rates of successful reversion of 19–55% recently being cited.[3]

The Valsalva is a breathing manoeuvre where the patient forcefully exhales against a closed glottis. There are different ways this can be employed, but blowing into a syringe with enough force to move the plunger is used most often. Other mechanisms such as carotid sinus massage or employing the diving reflex are shown to be effective but are not typically used in the prehospital environment.

The Valsalva works by increasing vagal tone, which therefore slows conduction through the atrioventricular node, prolonging its refractory period.

SECTION 3 Circulation

The REVERT trial[4] suggested a modified approach to the Valsalva manoeuvre, which resulted in a greater reversion rate with no serious adverse effects being reported.

In contrast to the 'standard' approach, where the patient will typically stay in the same position during the Valsalva, the modified approach had the patient stay semi-recumbent, but at the end of the strain, the patient was laid flat with their legs raised. Using this approach, the rates of successful reversion were greater than 40%.

If the patient shows signs of haemodynamic instability, other methods of reversion should be employed, rather than the Valsalva manoeuvre.

Adenosine

Adenosine is classified as a miscellaneous anti-arrhythmic drug outside the Vaughan Williams classifications. Adenosine works by activating specific potassium channels, which drives potassium outside the cell, while simultaneously inhibiting the influx of calcium. By moving the potassium out of the cell and inhibiting calcium influx, it causes a hyperpolarisation of the resting membrane potential and prolonged the time for depolarisation of the cell. This can terminate the SVT by breaking the re-entry circuit that occurs in AVNRT and AVRT.

The typical adult dose starts at 6 mg, increasing to 12 mg if unsuccessful. The 12 mg dose has been shown to effectively revert approximately 90% of SVTs. When administering adenosine, due to the short half-life of approximately 10 seconds, it is essential that it be given rapidly, through a large IV with a large, rapid flush after administration.

Some of the side-effects of adenosine include chest pain, dyspnoea and pre-syncope, often described as a 'sense of impending doom'. Indeed, this pre-syncopal experience can be so severe that patients may decline the use of adenosine due to previous experiences of this particular side-effect.

Calcium Channel Blockers

Calcium channel blockers have been used in SVT management for many years, and are often an option in the haemodynamically stable patient who does not wish to receive adenosine or where it has been ineffective.[5] Calcium channel blockers, typically verapamil, have been shown to have an equivalent efficacy to a graded dose approach of adenosine (65–95%),[6] without the aforementioned side-effect of a sense of impending doom.

Calcium channel blocker drugs in SVT work by closing conduction through the AV node, breaking the re-entry circuit. The dose of verapamil is 5–10 mg IV given over five minutes, with a repeat dose of another 5–10 mg IV if the initial dose is unsuccessful.

Typical side-effects include bradycardia, AV block and hypotension if given too quickly. The half-life of calcium channel blockers is also significantly longer than adenosine, so this must be taken into account when considering side-effects and their duration. Calcium channel blockers are contraindicated in ventricular tachycardia (VT), so extreme caution should be exercised if the differential is SVT with aberrancy.

Synchronised Cardioversion

Synchronised cardioversion is a well-established treatment of SVT and is recommended for any haemodynamically unstable SVT, or if the pharmacological options are ineffective or contraindicated.[7] Prehospital synchronised cardioversion of tachyarrhythmias has been shown to have successful reversion rates of approximately 96%.[8]

Typically, the pads are placed in an anterolateral position, similar to the normal placement that would occur for a patient in cardiac arrest; however, an anteroposterior placement can be used in patients where the initial cardioversion is ineffective, or there is increased chest wall size.

Synchronised cardioversion differs from defibrillation in that the delivery of energy is synchronised to the QRS complex, in contrast to the delivery of energy in ventricular fibrillation, where it is unsynchronised. In synchronised cardioversion, we are delivering energy during the relative refractory period, with the goal of interrupting the re-entry circuit of the SVT and allowing a sinus rhythm to take over.

Prior to synchronised cardioversion, procedural sedation and analgesia should be administered, with the aim of rousable drowsiness. Typically, small doses of midazolam, propofol or ketamine are used, titrating to effect. Typical side-effects are often associated with either the excessive use of procedural sedation or increased frequency of dosing. Recall that in patients who are hypoperfused, the onset time of medications is prolonged, resulting in a longer interval between dosing being required when compared to a patient with normal haemodynamics.

The starting joules typically recommended to manage SVTs are lower than those recommended for defibrillation of the ventricular fibrillation patient, and the widespread use of biphasic defibrillators has allowed lower joules to be used to achieve successful reversion. Usually, cardioversion at lower joules (50–100 joules) is attempted first, increasing up to 200 joules if unsuccessful.

> **PRACTICE TIP**
>
> When administering procedural sedation in the hypotensive patient, go slow and low. Use small doses and wait for effect prior to more medication.

Question 3: What Is the Post-Reversion Management of SVT?

Post-reversion management of SVTs is typically supportive in nature. For patients who have received procedural sedation for synchronised cardioversion, they may be drowsy for a period of time afterwards, potentially requiring oxygen and basic airway manoeuvres.

The post-reversion ECG should be scrutinised for any signs of acute coronary artery occlusion, and should be monitored for any return of the SVT. Depending on numerous factors, such as duration of the SVT or pre-existing cardiac disease, diffuse ST-segment depression suggestive of diffuse, subendocardial ischaemia may be present in the post-reversion period. This is usually self-limiting and will resolve with time once there is normal cardiac blood flow.

The patient may experience lingering pain in the post-reversion period, either due to persistent cardiac ischaemia or associated with synchronised cardioversion. This will often also resolve, though low-dose opiates may also be effective.

Ongoing anti-arrhythmic drugs after successful reversion of SVT are not typically required in the prehospital environment.

SECTION 3 Circulation

Question 4: Can Paramedics Safely Manage Narrow Complex Tachycardias?

Evidence has shown that paramedic management of SVT is both safe and efficacious.[9] The use of adenosine in both the prehospital and in-hospital setting is very effective at reverting SVT and even in the setting of inappropriate use of adenosine, it is not associated with adverse outcomes.[10] Evidence has shown that paramedic interpretation of SVT is good, with some studies citing up to 98% paramedic recognition rate,[9] and that, with appropriate training, the chance of inappropriate administration is minimal.

Synchronised cardioversion in the prehospital environment has also been shown to be a safe and effective tool for paramedics to manage tachycardias. A study published in 2021[8] showed that paramedics using synchronised cardioversion in patients presenting with unstable primary tachyarrhythmias (SVT and VT) had an efficacy of approximately 96%.

Key Evidence

Appelboam, A., Reuben, A., Mann, C. et al. (2014). Randomised evaluation of modified Valsalva effectiveness in re-entrant tachycardias (REVERT) study. *BMJ Open*, 4, p.e004525. Available at: https://pubmed.ncbi.nlm.nih.gov/24622951/

Honarbakhsh, S., Baker, V., Kirkby, C. et al. (2017). Safety and efficacy of paramedic treatment of regular supraventricular tachycardia: a randomised controlled trial. *Heart*, 103, pp. 1413–1418.

Page, R.L., Joglar, J.A., Caldwell, M.A. et al. (2016). 2015 ACC/AHA/HRS guideline for the management of adult patients with supraventricular tachycardia. *Circulation*, 133(14), pp.e506–574. Available at: https://pubmed.ncbi.nlm.nih.gov/26399663/

Self-Reflection Questions

1. What aspects of the ECG would you use to differentiate narrow complex tachycardias?
2. How would you manage a haemodynamically stable patient in SVT?
3. How would you manage the haemodynamically stable SVT patient who is refractory to pharmacological management?
4. What medication/s and doses would you use for procedural sedation prior to synchronised cardioversion?
5. How would you manage the patient who is refractory to synchronised cardioversion?

References

1. Katritsis, D.G. and Josephson, M.E. (2015). Differential diagnosis of regular, narrow-QRS tachycardias. *Heart Rhythm*, 12(7), pp. 1667–1676.
2. Mizuno, A., Masuda, K. and Niwa, K. (2014). Usefulness of Lewis lead for visualizing P-wave. *Circulation*, 78(11), pp. 2774–2775. Available at: https://pubmed.ncbi.nlm.nih.gov/25131523/
3. Smith, G.D., Fry, M.M., Taylor, D. et al. (2015). Effectiveness of the Valsalva manoeuvre for reversion of supraventricular tachycardia. *Cochrane Database of Systematic Reviews*, 2015(2):CD009502. Available at: https://pubmed.ncbi.nlm.nih.gov/25922864/
4. Appelboam, A., Reuben, A., Mann, C. et al. (2015). Postural modification to the standard Valsalva manoeuvre for emergency treatment of supraventricular tachycardias (REVERT): a randomised controlled trial. *Lancet*, 386(10005), pp. 1747–1753. Available at: https://pubmed.ncbi.nlm.nih.gov/26314489/
5. Page, R.L., Joglar, J.A., Caldwell, M.A. et al. (2016). 2015 ACC/AHA/HRS guideline for the management of adult patients with supraventricular tachycardia. *Circulation*, 133(14), pp. e506–574. Available at: https://pubmed.ncbi.nlm.nih.gov/26399663/

6. Kotadia, I.D., Williams, S.E. and O'Neill, M. (2020). Supraventricular tachycardia: an overview of diagnosis and management. *Clinical Medicine*, 20(1), pp. 43–47. Available at: https://pubmed.ncbi.nlm.nih.gov/31941731/
7. Roth, A., Elkayam, I., Shapira, I. et al. (2003). Effectiveness of prehospital synchronous direct-current cardioversion for supraventricular tachyarrhythmias causing unstable hemodynamic states. *American Journal of Cardiology*, 91(4), pp. 489–491. Available at: https://pubmed.ncbi.nlm.nih.gov/12586276/
8. Cowley, A., Cody, D. and Nelson, M. (2021). The epidemiology and effectiveness of synchronized cardioversion in a UK prehospital setting: a retrospective cross-sectional study. *Prehospital and Disaster Medicine*, 36(4), pp. 1–5. Available at: https://pubmed.ncbi.nlm.nih.gov/34127157/
9. Sharp, A. (2015). Pre-hospital treatment of supraventricular tachycardia: a literature review. *Journal of Paramedic Practice*, 7(12), pp. 618–628. Available at: https://www.magonlinelibrary.com/doi/abs/10.12968/jpar.2015.7.12.618
10. Rankin, A.C., Brooks, R., Ruskin, J.N. et al. (1992). Adenosine and the treatment of supraventricular tachycardia. *American Journal of Medicine*, 92(6), pp. 655–664. Available at: https://pubmed.ncbi.nlm.nih.gov/1605147/

11 Broad Complex Tachycardia

Tim Edwards and Kieren Pugh

In this chapter you will learn:

- The management of broad complex tachycardia in the prehospital setting
- The differences in management of narrow complex versus broad complex tachycardia
- Characteristics of the ECG in various forms of broad complex tachycardia
- Electrical versus chemical cardioversion
- When sedation is indicated and the choice of agent.

Case Details

Dispatch
60-year-old male, shortness of breath and palpitations.

History
A 60-year-old male has had a sudden onset of chest pain, shortness of breath and palpitations while at home. He has a history of acute ST segment elevation myocardial infarction (STEMI) during the preceding six months and has been experiencing a sensation of occasional 'flutters' in his chest during the past few days.

On Arrival of the First Crew
The patient is pale, diaphoretic and peripherally cyanosed. His primary survey findings and initial vital signs are listed below:

Airway	Patent
Breathing	RR 24, SpO$_2$ unable to read due to poor perfusion
Circulation	Peripheral pulses absent, central pulses present, HR 170, BP 60/20, cool, clammy peripheries
Disability	GCS E3, V4, M6 (13), BGL 6.6 mmol/L
Environmental	Temp 36.2 °C

CHAPTER 11 Broad Complex Tachycardia

On Your Arrival as the Critical Care Paramedic

The first paramedics to attend the scene have obtained intravenous access and commenced an infusion of normal saline. Oxygen therapy is being provided via a non-rebreather mask at 15 LPM. ECG monitoring is ongoing, and a broad complex tachycardia is present (**Figure 11.1**).

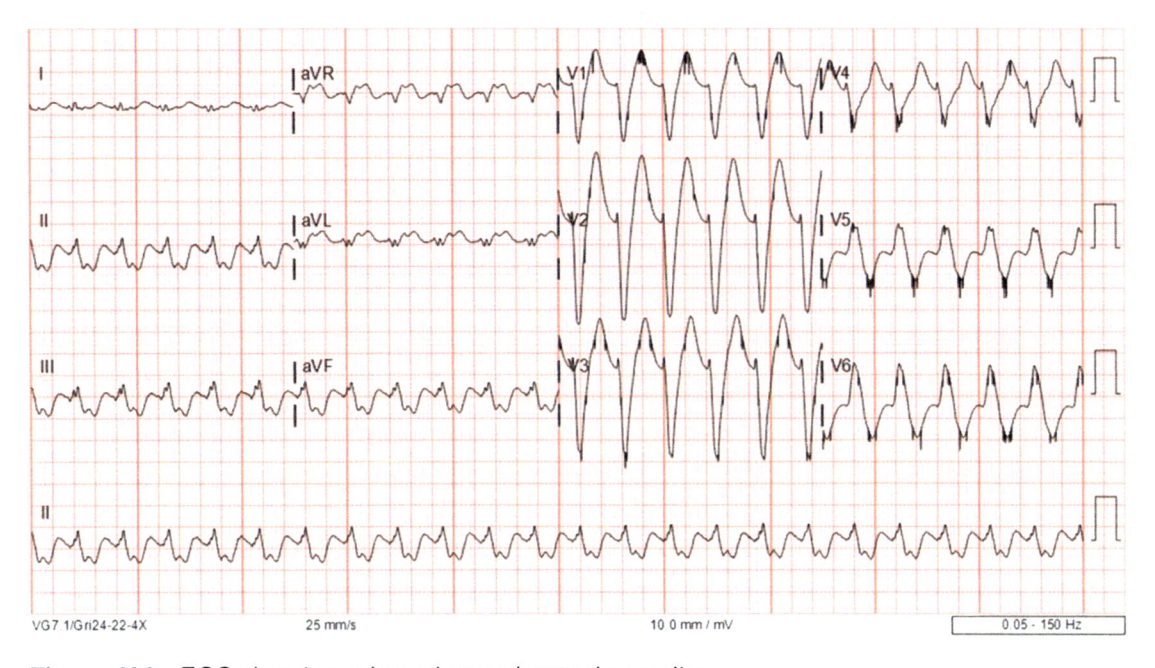

Figure 11.1 ECG showing a broad complex tachycardia.
Source: Regeer MV, Tops LF, de Riva Silva M. Broad complex tachycardia: never judge a book by its cover. *Netherlands Heart Journal*. 2021;29:168–171. Available at: https://link.springer.com/article/10.1007/s12471-020-01495-x (Creative Commons Attribution 4.0 International License).

AMPLE

The patient has had a previous myocardial infarction and takes anti-hypertensive medicine alongside anti-platelet drugs. He is otherwise well and lives a healthy lifestyle after giving up smoking 20 years ago. He has no allergies and has not eaten prior to your arrival.

Allergies	NKDA
Medications	Anti-hypertensive Anti-platelet
Past history	STEMI for past six months
Last ins and outs	Nil
Events prior	Sudden onset of chest pain, palpitations and SOB

SECTION 3 Circulation

Decision Point
What are your clinical priorities in this situation?
This patient is suffering from cardiogenic shock. He needs immediate management to prevent imminent cardiac arrest.

Question 1: What Is a Broad Complex Tachycardia?

Broad complex tachycardia is characterised by ventricular complexes with a duration greater than 120 msec. The term broad complex tachycardia refers to a range of tachyarrhythmias that may be ventricular or supraventricular in origin. Ventricular tachycardia (VT) is the most common form of broad complex tachycardia, and is defined as three or more ventricular extrasystoles at a rate in excess of 120/minute.[1] Other arrhythmias, such as atrioventricular re-entrant tachycardia (for example, Wolff–Parkinson–White syndrome), may present with a prolonged QRS morphology in certain circumstances but are in fact supraventricular in origin. Similarly, a broad complex tachycardia may be seen where a patient has a history of left bundle branch block, and supraventricular tachycardia ensues. Conversely, certain forms of VT, such as right ventricular outflow tract tachycardia (RVOT) or fascicular tachycardia, may be associated with relatively narrow complexes.[2]

Broad complex tachycardias are generally regular; however, an irregular appearance may be seen in scenarios such as polymorphic ventricular tachycardia and atrial fibrillation in combination with left bundle branch block. In some cases, there may be diagnostic uncertainty regarding the underlying cause; therefore, broad complex tachycardia is used as an umbrella term in resuscitation guidelines to simplify risk stratification and guide immediate management in the emergency setting. In prehospital care, the safest approach is to assume that a broad complex tachycardia is ventricular in origin until proven otherwise.

Question 2: What Are the ECG Characteristics of Broad Complex Tachycardia?

Broad complex tachycardia is associated with ventricular complexes greater than 120 msec at a rate exceeding 100/minute. VT is referred to as monomorphic where complexes have the same appearance and polymorphic where the morphology differs. The rate is generally 120–300/minute,[1] although broad complex tachycardias at the extreme end of this spectrum are less likely to be associated with VT and should prompt consideration of the potential for a supraventricular origin. A narrower QRS morphology is also less likely to be ventricular in origin; however, this is not always the case (see discussion of RVOT above).

Several different criteria for identification of VT based on 12-lead ECG findings have been developed with varying levels of sensitivity and specificity. Where the onset of broad complex tachycardia is witnessed in a monitored patient, VT is more likely where this is seen in association with significant axis deviation, particularly leftward deviation. The presence of concordance where ECG complexes share the same general direction is also indicative of VT as the underlying rhythm. Concordance may be associated with positive or negative deflection, with positive complexes more likely to be seen in VT.[1]

Table 11.1 outlines factors that can contribute to an increase in the likelihood of VT.

CHAPTER 11 Broad Complex Tachycardia

Table 11.1 Factors increasing the likelihood of ventricular tachycardia

Contributing factor	Characteristics
Concordance	All complexes have same axis, often extreme leftward or rightward axis.
QRS width	Typically >160 ms.
Atrioventricular dissociation	P-waves may be seen superimposed on QRS complexes.
Capture beats	Brief periods of normal morphology QRS complexes preceded by P-waves.
Fusion beats	Broad QRS superimposed on a normally transmitted narrow complex.

It should be noted that although broad complexes originating from the ventricles are the dominant ECG finding in VT, evidence of atrial activity may also be seen. Where these features are present, they provide further evidence that the underlying rhythm is ventricular as opposed to supraventricular in origin. Evidence of independent P-waves, which may be seen embedded in ventricular complexes, is strongly indicative of VT.[3] In this situation P-waves generally occur at regular intervals and measuring the P–P interval may assist in identifying this feature. At lower VT rates, occasional evidence of atrioventricular conduction may be seen in the form of capture and fusion beats. The term capture beat refers to an isolated narrow complex sinus beat conducted via the normal pathway in the midst of a broad complex tachycardia. Fusion beats are a hybrid of a normally conducted impulse and a ventricular impulse fused together and are characterised by abnormal but usually narrower complexes with a different morphology interspersed between broad complexes.[1]

As discussed, patients with supraventricular tachycardia in the presence of LBBB will, by definition, present with a broad complex tachycardia. Concordance is less likely in this situation and if previous ECG traces are available, it may be possible to compare the appearance of the QRS complexes. This is one of many good reasons to ensure that all patients are provided with a copy of their ECG by prehospital providers. Where the QRS morphology has the same appearance as previous ECG traces but at a more rapid rate, a supraventricular origin is more likely, especially if the arrhythmia appears reasonably well tolerated. The most common cause of an irregularly irregular broad complex tachycardia in these circumstances is acute onset atrial fibrillation, which may be caused by a range of underlying conditions including infection. Similarly, the presence of sinus tachycardia in response to common provoking factors, such as pain, infection, hypovolaemia, anxiety and hypoxia, will produce a broad complex tachycardia; however, the focus in these situations should be on recognising and managing the underlying cause.

As a general rule, supraventricular tachycardia is better tolerated and less likely to result in adverse features than VT. However, the extent to which any form of tachycardia results in haemodynamic compromise is at least in part dependent on the condition of the heart prior to the onset of the arrhythmia. Where pre-existing structural heart disease is present, any form of arrhythmia, including those of with a supraventricular origin, is likely to be poorly

SECTION 3   Circulation

tolerated, especially over a prolonged period. It is therefore vital that immediate management to prevent further deterioration is initiated in any form of broad complex tachycardia where adverse signs are seen.

Question 3: How Is a Broad Complex Tachycardia Managed Out of Hospital?

Treatment of tachyarrhythmias, including broad complex tachycardia, falls into two broad categories, regardless of whether the patient presents in a hospital or prehospital setting. These are electrical, where DC counter shocks are provided, and chemical, involving administration of medication with the intention of terminating the arrhythmia. It should be noted that these interventions are indicated where arrhythmia is known to be present, as opposed to other forms of non-arrhythmogenic broad complex tachycardia, where interventions should be targeted at the underlying cause, for example, management of infection, hypoxia or hypovolaemia. Where the decision is taken to attempt cardioversion in an irregular broad complex tachycardia, the potential for atrial fibrillation and associated risk of a thromboembolic event associated with restoration of sinus rhythm must be taken into consideration. In prehospital care it should be noted that immediate intervention will not always be required and therefore it is always an option to do nothing in favour of ongoing monitoring and a transfer to definitive care.

> **PRACTICE TIP**
>
> Always consider whether immediate cardioversion in the prehospital phase is required, taking into account availability of other services and transfer times and modes.

Broad complex tachycardia with adverse clinical features, such as hypotension, is generally managed via electrical cardioversion. Delivery of shocks to the patient may be uncomfortable or painful, and therefore consideration must be given to the requirement for analgesia and sedation, especially where the patient is conscious. As with all attempts at cardioversion, equipment and personnel to facilitate immediate cardiopulmonary resuscitation must be available at all times. With the exception of cardiac arrest, any shocks must be synchronised to ensure that they are delivered at the appropriate phase of the cardiac cycle.[3] Failure to do so may result in R-on-T phenomenon, whereby a shock delivered during ventricular repolarisation induces ventricular fibrillation. Guidelines for electrical cardioversion in broad complex tachycardia differ, with some recommending escalating energy levels and others advocating maximum energy levels for the first and subsequent shocks. As a general rule, higher energy levels are utilised in electrical cardioversion in broad versus narrow complex tachycardia.

Where adverse signs are not present or electrical cardioversion is not within the clinician's scope of practice, various medications may be used. Chemical cardioversion is usually slower than electrical cardioversion and all antiarrhythmic drugs are also potentially pro-arrhythmic, meaning they have the potential to generate as well as terminate arrhythmias.[3] Where a given agent fails to terminate a broad complex tachycardia, repeat doses are unlikely to change the situation, and an alternative is usually required. Administration of multiple drugs

CHAPTER 11 Broad Complex Tachycardia

further increases the potential for generation of arrhythmias, and therefore the requirement for expert advice should always be considered when contemplating further pharmacological intervention.

> **PRACTICE TIP**
>
> If the patient is shocked or haemodynamically unstable with adverse signs, electrical cardioversion is the treatment of choice.

The most common agents used in the management of broad complex tachycardia are amiodarone and lidocaine.[4] On the rare occasion that the specific form or polymorphic VT referred to as torsades de pointes occurs, magnesium is the antiarrhythmic of choice. Similarly, broad complex tachycardia occurring as a consequence of tricyclic antidepressant overdose should be managed with sodium bicarbonate.[4]

Question 4: When to Intervene?

Once an initial assessment is complete, the clinician should seek to identify the presence or otherwise of signs and symptoms indicative of haemodynamic compromise. These are referred to as adverse signs and include the presence of hypotension, heart failure, chest pain, confusion and other features of cardiogenic shock. When considering the need for intervention, the prehospital clinician will also need to take into consideration factors such as the proximity of appropriate receiving facilities and associated transfer times and modalities. For example, a conscious patient with broad complex tachycardia may not require immediate intervention where a short transfer by land ambulance to a specialist cardiac centre is available, but the same patient might well need to undergo cardioversion where aeromedical transfer over a longer distance is contemplated. Consideration should also be given to the scope of practice of the attending clinicians and the option to seek expert advice where this is available.

> **PRACTICE TIP**
>
> Remember that sedation and analgesia may be required when electrical cardioversion is contemplated.

Question 5: What Is the Evidence Base Surrounding Optimal Management Strategies?

There is a paucity of evidence relating to prehospital, and specifically paramedic, cardioversion of VT, especially in relation to chemical as opposed to electrical cardioversion. Historically, lidocaine and amiodarone have formed the mainstay of pharmacological interventions for VT in paramedic systems, with lidocaine largely falling out of favour as a first-line agent in recent years in favour of amiodarone.[5] A systematic review comparing the relative efficacy of various agents for the treatment of stable, monomorphic VT found that procainamide, ajmaline and sotalol were all superior to lidocaine and that amiodarone was not more effective than procainamide.[6] An Australian study investigating paramedic chemical cardioversion in 61 haemodynamically stable patients with pulsed VT found that 52% (n = 32) reverted successfully following administration of amiodarone while 48% (n = 29) did not. Two patients required cardioversion amiodarone administration and one suffered cardiac arrest from which they were successfully resuscitated.[7]

Findings from a small-scale study of 22 patients who underwent prehospital synchronised cardioversion by doctors reported a 100% reversion rate in five (22.7%) patients, with pulsed VT within three shocks.[8] A more recent UK study, investigating electrical cardioversion by paramedics of both narrow and broad complex tachycardia, found a synchronised cardioversion success rate of 96% with a mean of 1.33 attempts in 43 patients presenting with primary tachyarrhythmia, including 29 (64.4%) cases of pulsed VT.[9,10]

In summary, limited evidence exists in relation to prehospital management of broad complex tachycardia including pulse VT. In keeping with hospital data, electrical cardioversion is generally more efficacious than chemical cardioversion and is the treatment of choice in the unstable patient with adverse signs.[11] Chemical cardioversion by paramedics appears safe but is associated with lower reversion rates and a more limited range of available pharmacological interventions compared with the hospital setting. Given varying levels of efficacy of different anti-arrhythmic agents, future paramedic drug formularies may need to evolve and adapt to ensure that patients are offered the most appropriate and efficacious agents where prehospital chemical cardioversion is contemplated. Finally, it should be noted that the majority of studies utilised prehospital physicians or paramedics with specialist and advanced levels of training and, therefore, results may not be generalisable to the wider paramedic profession.

Question 6: How Should the Requirement for Sedation Be Managed?

Where electrical cardioversion is undertaken, the requirement for sedation and analgesia must be considered. The extent to which this is required will depend on the conscious level of the patient and in some cases level of haemodynamic stability. It should be noted that while sedation may reduce awareness, this may not provide adequate analgesia depending on the drug regime adopted. The ideal agent for sedation should be haemodynamically stable and provide a rapid onset of action. In practice, this may prove challenging to achieve given the variation in the characteristics of various different classes of drug used for this purpose. Whereas benzodiazepines such as midazolam may be familiar to paramedics and produce a relatively rapid onset of action, they offer no analgesic effect and may result in a precipitous drop in blood pressure. In contrast, ketamine may provide analgesic as well as sedating effects and is relatively cardiovascularly stable; however, side-effects include tachycardia and increased myocardial oxygen demand.

Key Evidence

Havakuk O, Viskin D, Viskin S et al. Clinical presentation of sustained monomorphic ventricular tachycardia without cardiac arrest. *Journal of the American Heart Association*. 2020;9(22):e016673.

Wesley K. *Huszar's ECG and 12-lead Interpretation*. Oxford: Elsevier Health Sciences; 2016.

Whitaker J, Wright MJ, Tedrow U. Diagnosis and management of ventricular tachycardia. *Clinical Medicine*. 2023;23(5):442.

CHAPTER 11 Broad Complex Tachycardia

Self-Reflection Questions

1. How does practice on cardioversion vary in prehospital services around the world? Can everyone perform this skill? And if not, would it be beneficial?
2. Have you ever experienced a time where cardioversion was unsuccessful, and what was the differing hospital management that successfully cardioverted that patient?
3. Have you considered the differing aetiologies of how a tachycardia starts and whether that would affect your management?
4. Is fluid therapy detrimental or useful in this patient group before and during cardioversion, and does the evidence support this?
5. Does your local guideline for pharmacological cardioversion and electrical cardioversion differ from international and national guidance?

References

1. Edhouse J. Broad complex tachycardia – part I. *BMJ*. 2002; 324 :719. Available at: https://www.bmj.com/content/324/7339/719.1.full.
2. Ramrakha P, Hill J. Arrhythmias. In Ramrakha P and Hill J. *Oxford Handbook of Cardiology*. OUP. 2006; 404-453.
3. Soar J, Böttiger BW, Carli P et al. European Resuscitation Council Guidelines 2021: Adult advanced life support. *Resuscitation*. 2021;161:115–151. Available at: https://pubmed.ncbi.nlm.nih.gov/33773825/. Erratum in: *Resuscitation*. 2021;167:105–106.
4. Lott C, Truhlář A, Alfonzo A et al. European Resuscitation Council Guidelines 2021: Cardiac arrest in special circumstances. *Resuscitation*. 2021;161:152–219. https://pubmed.ncbi.nlm.nih.gov/33773826/. Erratum in: *Resuscitation*. 2021;167:91–92.
5. Corey M, Slovis PJ, Kudenchuk MA et al. Prehospital management of acute tachyarrhythmias. *Prehospital Emergency Care*. 2003;7(1):2–12. Available at: https://pubmed.ncbi.nlm.nih.gov/12540138/
6. deSouza IS, Martindale JL, Sinert R. Antidysrhythmic drug therapy for the termination of stable, monomorphic ventricular tachycardia: a systematic review. *Emergency Medicine Journal*. 2015;32(2):161–167. Available at: https://pubmed.ncbi.nlm.nih.gov/24042252/
7. Foerster CR, Andrew E, Smith K et al. Amiodarone for sustained stable ventricular tachycardia in the prehospital setting. *Emergency Medicine Australasia*. 2018;30(5):694–698. Available at: https://onlinelibrary.wiley.com/doi/abs/10.1111/1742-6723.13146
8. Jelatancev A, Grmec S, Klemen P et al. Synchronized cardioversion in a prehospital setting: a safe and reliable method for urgent treatment of tachyarrhythmias. *Critical Care*. 2005;9(1):307. Available at: https://ccforum.biomedcentral.com/articles/10.1186/cc3370
9. Cowley A, Cody D, Nelson M. The epidemiology and effectiveness of synchronized cardioversion in a UK prehospital setting: a retrospective cross-sectional study. *Prehospital and Disaster Medicine*. 2021;36(4):440–444. Available at: https://pubmed.ncbi.nlm.nih.gov/34127157/
10. Docherty E, Morris FP. Broad complex tachycardias [online]. Available at: https://www.rcemlearning.co.uk/reference/broad-complex-tachycardias/#1568295536268-4363201a-5ee5
11. Long B, Koyfman A. Best clinical practice: emergency medicine management of stable monomorphic ventricular tachycardia. *Journal of Emergency Medicine*. 2017;52(4):484–492. Available at: https://pubmed.ncbi.nlm.nih.gov/27751700/

12

Acute Chest Pain and Shortness of Breath: Cardiogenic Shock Complicating Acute Myocardial Infarction

Jason Bloom and Dave Hawkins

In this chapter you will learn:

- How to define hypoperfusion
- The common causes of cardiogenic shock
- Commonly used medications to support perfusion: pharmacology and clinical evidence
- How to select the appropriate disposition for patients with cardiogenic shock.

Case Details

Dispatch

54-year-old male, acute chest pain, shortness of breath, agitated.

History

A 54-year-old man developed acute onset chest pain at work. There is associated nausea, shortness of breath and agitation. A colleague called for an ambulance. A double-crewed advanced life support ambulance and a single unit critical care paramedic are dispatched.

On Arrival of the First Crew

The crew arrive and find the scene to be safe and the call as given. On taking a patient history, they identify that the patient has experienced a previous STEMI, which was treated by stenting the left anterior descending coronary artery. Prior to this acute episode, the patient had been experiencing increasing shortness of breath on exertion, causing him to have to stop to recover after climbing a single staircase.

Airway	Patent
Breathing	RR 26, SpO$_2$ 89% on air
Circulation	Peripheral pulses weak, HR 50, BP 79/32, cool peripheries
Disability	GCS E3, V5, M6 (14), BGL 7.1 mmol/L
Environmental	Temp 36.6 °C

CHAPTER 12 Acute Chest Pain and Shortness of Breath

On Your Arrival as the Critical Care Paramedic

You arrive to find the crew attending to the agitated patient. They have administered high-flow oxygen therapy and are busy setting up an IV and preparing to give a Hartmann's infusion. They hand over that the patient is hypotensive and confused. They feel that the infusion is what the patient requires.

AMPLE

Allergies	Penicillin
Medications	Furosemide
	Ramipril
	Candesartan
Past history	Hypertension
	STEMI
	Angina
	Smoker 20 per day for 40 years
Last ins and outs	Lunch just before the call; normal outputs
Events prior	Acute onset chest pain

Decision Point

What are your clinical priorities in this situation?

The patient is complaining of chest pain and, from the initial assessment, appears to be in extremis. The crew have obtained a 12-lead ECG, which does not show evidence of a new STEMI. The patient's BP and heart rate are low, and you are considering your next actions.

Question 1: What Is Cardiogenic Shock and How Is It Defined?

Cardiogenic shock (CS) is a complex clinical syndrome that is characterised by insufficient cardiac output to meet basal metabolic requirements.[1,2] The development of CS has downstream effects on the entire circulation, leading to tissue hypoxia, injury and inflammation. Prompt identification of CS, treatment of the underlying disease process and haemodynamic support is essential to restore cellular metabolism and prevent worsening systemic perfusion that drives the 'shock spiral' that in many cases leads to circulatory collapse and death.

Defining CS has traditionally been challenging, owing to the numerous and varied definitions used in key clinical trials and major cardiac societal guidelines.[3] In 2019, the Society for Cardiovascular Angiography and Interventions (SCAI) published a seminal CS classification scheme to assist with the diagnosis and staging of the condition. This unique classification system can be applied to a range of clinical settings that include acute myocardial infarction, cardiac arrest and decompensated cardiomyopathy. Furthermore, it provides clinicians with the capacity to stage disease severity, ranging from stage A – 'at risk' – to fulminant circulatory collapse with stage E – 'extremis'.[4] A summary of the scoring system is provided in **Table 12.1**. Despite the use of invasive haemodynamics

SECTION 3 Circulation

and biochemical markers of hypoperfusion in the published classification system, the overarching description, clinical findings and basic non-invasive haemodynamic features can readily be applied to the prehospital setting.

> **PRACTICE TIP**
>
> The presence of hypotension (systolic blood pressure <90 mmHg or MAP <65 mmHg), tachycardia (heart rate >100 beats/minute), cool or mottled skin, delayed capillary refill and altered mentation are all easily identified bedside features of hypoperfusion.

Table 12.1 SCAI shock classification adapted for prehospital practice

Stage	Description	Clinical	Haemodynamic
A: 'At risk'	No signs or symptoms of CS	Warm, well-perfused, normal JVP, clear lungs and mentation	Normotensive, no tachycardia
B: 'Beginning'	Evidence of relative hypotension or tachycardia, without hypoperfusion	Warm, well-perfused, elevated JVP, rales in lungs	SBP <90 mmHg or MAP <60 mmHg or >30 mmHg drop from baseline, HR >100 BPM
C: 'Classic'	Hypoperfusion requiring intervention beyond volume resuscitation to restore perfusion	Unwell, ashen, mottled extremities, cold, clammy, volume overloaded	Any of SBP <90 or MAP <60 or >30 mmHg drop from baseline and drugs/devices used to maintain BP
D: 'Deteriorating'	Similar to C, but worse, fails to respond to initial interventions	Any of stage C above	Any of stage C above, and requiring multiple vasopressors or addition of MCS to maintain perfusion
E: 'Extremis'	Cardiac arrest with ongoing CPR and/or ECMO, supported by multiple interventions	Cardiac collapse, use of defibrillator, near pulselessness, need for mechanical ventilation	No SBP without resuscitation; PEA or refractory VT/VF; hypotension despite maximal support

Abbreviations: CS, cardiogenic shock; CPR, cardiopulmonary resuscitation; ECMO, extracorporeal membrane oxygenation; JVP, jugular venous pressure; SBP, systolic blood pressure; BP, blood pressure; VT, ventricular tachycardia; VF, ventricular fibrillation; MCS, mechanical circulatory support; PEA, pulseless electrical activity.

Source: Adapted from Naidu SS, Baran DA, Jentzer JC et al. SCAI SHOCK stage classification expert consensus update: a review and incorporation of validation studies. *Journal of the American College of Cardiology*. 2022;79(9):933–946.

CHAPTER 12 Acute Chest Pain and Shortness of Breath

Question 2: How Common Is Cardiogenic Shock and What Are Its Common Causes?

The epidemiology and outcomes of in-hospital CS have been well described; however, there remains a paucity of data in relation to the incidence and outcomes of CS in the prehospital environment. A recent population-based cohort study of a large Australian provincial ambulance service has shown that CS is a relatively common condition, with an overall incidence of paramedic-treated CS of 14.5 per 100,000 person-years and an overall 30-day all-cause mortality of 43.9%.[2,5]

Acute coronary syndromes (ACS) are the most common cause of CS.[1] Approximately one in ten ST-elevation myocardial infarction (STEMI) cases are complicated by the development of CS, having a two- to four-fold greater risk compared with non-ST-elevation myocardial infarction (NSTEMI) cases.[6] Risk factors for ACS cases developing CS include advanced age, anterior or left main culprit lesion, delayed revascularisation therapy and the presence of cardiac arrest on admission.[6]

A decade ago, 81% of CS was caused by ACS.[7] However, there has been a progressive decline in the contribution of ACS, due in part to reduced smoking rates and improved revascularisation therapies, with a resultant increase in ischaemic cardiomyopathy without ACS, non-ischaemic cardiomyopathy and other causes, including valvular heart disease.[8]

Question 3: How Is Perfusion Supported in the Prehospital Setting?

Initial Assessment for Hypoperfusion and Congestion

Assessing the adequacy of the patient's perfusion status will dictate whether therapy is required. The basic physical examination, which can readily be performed at the scene or during transfer, can provide a 'window' into the patient's perfusion and filling state (**Table 12.2**). The presence of hypotension (systolic blood pressure <90 mmHg or MAP <65 mmHg), tachycardia (heart rate >100 beats/minute), cool or mottled skin, delayed capillary refill and altered mentation are all easily identified bedside features of hypoperfusion. Elevated filling

Table 12.2 Summary of basic examination findings suggesting hypoperfusion and congestion

Features of hypoperfusion	Features of congestion

• Observations:
  ○ Systolic blood pressure <90 mmHg or mean arterial pressure <65 mmHg
  ○ Heart rate >100 beats per minute
• Peripheral findings:
  ○ Cool to touch
  ○ Mottled skin
  ○ Cyanosis
  ○ Capillary refill >3 seconds
• Altered mentation
  ○ Confused, drowsy or obtunded
	• Observations:
	  ○ Hypoxia
	• Pulmonary findings:
	  ○ Rales consistent with pulmonary oedema
	• Peripheral findings:
	  ○ Lower limb oedema
	  ○ Elevated jugular venous pressure

SECTION 3 Circulation

pressures can also be identified by the presence of pulmonary oedema, peripheral oedema and jugular venous pressure elevation.

> **PRACTICE TIP**
>
> For patients with hypoperfusion but no pulmonary oedema (rales on auscultation of the lungs or significant hypoxia), a trial of 250–500 mL of normal saline 0.9% should be considered.

Prehospital Therapies to Improve Perfusion

Having completed a primary assessment and identifying hypoperfusion in the presence or absence of congestion, there are two key therapeutic interventions that can be used in an attempt to improve perfusion: intravenous fluid therapy and/or vasoactive medication administration. A summary of a proposed treatment algorithm is presented in **Figure 12.1**.

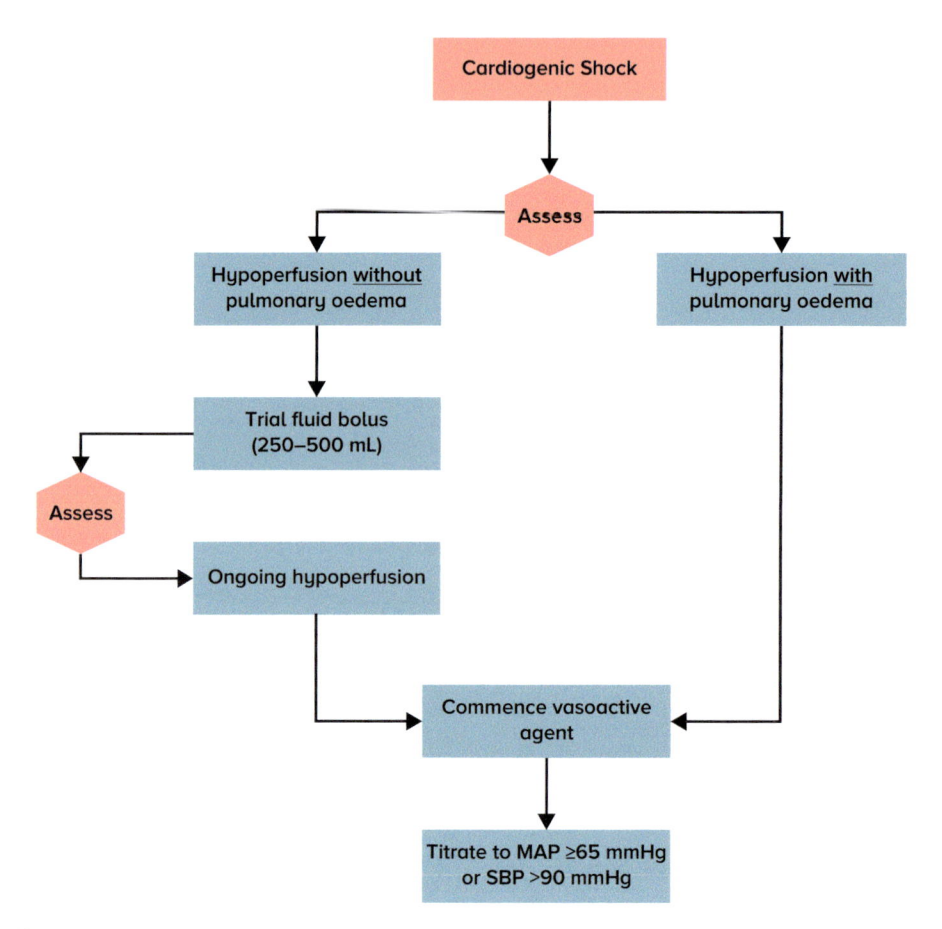

Figure 12.1 Proposed treatment pathway to support perfusion in patients with cardiogenic shock managed in the prehospital setting.
Source: © Image by Jason Bloom.

Fluid Administration

Determining the need for intravenous fluid therapy in CS is a clinical challenge, as it is often difficult to accurately assess for evidence of congestion. In right-sided heart failure, for example an acute inferior STEMI, a trial of a fluid bolus (for example, 500 mL of normal saline 0.9%) is a reasonable intervention. For patients with hypoperfusion but no pulmonary oedema (rales on auscultation of the lungs or significant hypoxia), a trial of 250–500 mL of normal saline 0.9% should be considered, followed by repeat clinical assessment of perfusion status. In the event of ongoing clinical features of hypoperfusion, commencement of a vasoactive infusion should be considered.

Vasoactive Agents

The use of vasoactive medications in CS constitutes a central component of the haemodynamic support. Within the intensive care setting, approximately 25% of patients admitted receive a vasoactive medication, which increases to over 90% in those with a diagnosis of CS.[9–11] Within the prehospital arena, in a single Australian EMS service, 54% of patients with CS were treated with adrenaline at the scene and during transport to hospital.[5] To date, there have been no further studies characterising the use of these agents for CS in the prehospital environment.

Vasoactive medications are broadly divided into three categories in accordance with their predominant haemodynamic effects: vasopressors, inotropes and inodilators. Vasopressors improve systemic perfusion through vasoconstriction, therefore increasing mean arterial pressure (MAP).[12] Inotropes augment cardiac output by increasing myocardial contractility and in many instances heart rate. Inodilators have the mixed effects of exerting inotropic effects on cardiac tissue and peripheral arterial vasodilation.

The most commonly administered class of vasopressors and inotropic medications is catecholamines. These agents act on alpha and beta adrenoreceptors, and act on the heart to increase heart rate and myocardial contractility and on the blood vessels to cause vasoconstriction in most vascular beds (beta-agonists will cause vasodilation in some vascular beds, for example, skeletal muscle). Traditionally, adrenaline is the most commonly used catecholamine in prehospital care, as well as in CS. Adrenaline is an inotrope and vasopressor with pronounced effects on all adrenoreceptors. It is typically administered as an infusion (ideally through a central line, although in the prehospital environment, administration through a large-bore peripheral IV line or IO administration is acceptable) but may also be administered as a bolus.[13] The haemodynamic effect of an adrenaline bolus can be unpredictable, so smaller boluses (for example, 10–20 mcg) should be used initially (this will usually require a double dilution so great care must be taken with medication identification and safety).

> **PRACTICE TIP**
>
> Two concentrations of bolus dose adrenaline may be required. To make up dilute (10 mcg/mL) adrenaline, draw up 1 mL of 100 mcg/ml (or 1:10,000) adrenaline into a 10 mL syringe and dilute with 9 mL of 0.9% saline. Ensure that both syringes are very carefully labelled and that other clinicians are aware that there are two different adrenaline concentrations.

SECTION 3 Circulation

Other vasoactive agents used in CS include noradrenaline, dobutamine, milrinone and levosimendan. These are not commonly used in the prehospital environment but may be encountered by critical care paramedics on interhospital critical care transfers. **Table 12.3** outlines the key properties of each agent. There is emerging interest in the use of noradrenaline in prehospital critical care.

Table 12.3 Comparison of commonly used vasopressors and inotropes

Agent	Mechanism of action	Infusion rate	Bolus dose	Adverse effects
Adrenaline	Vasopressor and inotrope – alpha and beta effects	1–30 mcg/min (no real upper limit but more limited effect at higher doses)	10–20 mcg (low dose), 100–200 mcg (high dose)	Hypertension, increased myocardial oxygen demand, tremor, elevated lactate
Noradrenaline	Vasopressor – predominant alpha 1 effects	1–30 mcg/min (no real upper limit but more limited effect at higher doses)	N/A	Hypertension, skin necrosis if extravasated
Dobutamine	Inotrope – predominant beta 1 effects	2.5–20 mcg/kg/min	N/A	Tachycardia, arrhythmias
Milrinone	Inodilator – phosphodiesterase inhibitor	0.375–0.75 mcg/kg/min	N/A	Hypotension (often co-infused with noradrenaline)
Levosimendan	Inodilator – calcium sensitiser	2.5 mg single dose, infused over 24 hours	N/A	Hypotension

Key Evidence

Bloom JE, Andrew E, Dawson LP et al. Incidence and outcomes of nontraumatic shock in adults using emergency medical services in Victoria, Australia. *JAMA Network Open*. 2022;5(1):e2145179.

van Diepen S, Katz JN, Albert NM et al. Contemporary management of cardiogenic shock: a scientific statement from the American Heart Association. *Circulation*. 2017;136(16):e232–e268. Available at: https://www.ahajournals.org/doi/10.1161/CIR.0000000000000525

Self-Reflection Questions

1. How do you define and classify cardiogenic shock?
2. What are currently the key causes of cardiogenic shock and how does this compare with previous key causes?

3. How would you clinically balance the concerns of hypoperfusion with features of congestion?
4. What are the challenges with assessing for congestion in the setting of hypoperfusion?
5. What are the pros and cons of different vasopressors and inotropes in your setting?

References

1. van Diepen S, Katz JN, Albert NM et al. Contemporary management of cardiogenic shock: a scientific statement from the American Heart Association. *Circulation*. 2017;136(16):e232–e268. Available at: https://www.ahajournals.org/doi/10.1161/CIR.0000000000000525
2. Bloom JE, Andrew E, Nehme Z et al. Gender disparities in cardiogenic shock treatment and outcomes. *American Journal of Cardiology*. 2022;177:14–21. Available at: https://pubmed.ncbi.nlm.nih.gov/35773044/
3. Baran DA, Grines CL, Bailey S et al. SCAI clinical expert consensus statement on the classification of cardiogenic shock. *Catheterization and Cardiovascular Interventions*. 2019;94(1):29–37. Available at: https://pubmed.ncbi.nlm.nih.gov/31104355/
4. Naidu SS, Baran DA, Jentzer JC et al. SCAI SHOCK stage classification expert consensus update: a review and incorporation of validation studies. *Journal of the American College of Cardiology*. 2022;79(9): 933–946. Available at: https://pubmed.ncbi.nlm.nih.gov/35115207/
5. Bloom JE, Andrew E, Dawson LP et al. Incidence and outcomes of nontraumatic shock in adults using emergency medical services in Victoria, Australia. *JAMA Network Open*. 2022;5(1):e2145179.
6. Berg DD, Bohula EA, Morrow DA. Epidemiology and causes of cardiogenic shock. *Current Opinion in Critical Care*. 2021;27(4):401. Available at: https://pubmed.ncbi.nlm.nih.gov/34010224/
7. Harjola VP, Lassus J, Sionis A et al. Clinical picture and risk prediction of short-term mortality in cardiogenic shock: clinical picture and outcome of cardiogenic shock. *European Journal of Heart Failure*. 2015;17(5):501–509. Available at: https://pubmed.ncbi.nlm.nih.gov/25820680/
8. Chioncel O, Parissis J, Mebazaa A et al. Epidemiology, pathophysiology and contemporary management of cardiogenic shock – a position statement from the Heart Failure Association of the European Society of Cardiology. *European Journal of Heart Failure*. 2020;22(8):1315–1341. Available at: https://pubmed.ncbi.nlm.nih.gov/32469155/
9. Berg D, Bohula E, van Diepen S et al. Epidemiology of shock in contemporary cardiac intensive care units. *Circulation. Cardiovascular Quality and Outcomes*. 2019;12(3):e005618. Available at: https://pubmed.ncbi.nlm.nih.gov/30879324/
10. Jentzer JC, Wiley B, Bennett C et al. Temporal trends and clinical outcomes associated with vasopressor and inotrope use in the cardiac intensive care unit. *Shock*. 2020;53(4):452–459. Available at: https://pubmed.ncbi.nlm.nih.gov/31169766/
11. Tarvasmäki T, Lassus J, Varpula M et al. Current real-life use of vasopressors and inotropes in cardiogenic shock – adrenaline use is associated with excess organ injury and mortality. *Critical Care*. 2016;20(1). Available at: https://pubmed.ncbi.nlm.nih.gov/27374027/#:~:text=Among%20vasopressors%20and%20inotropes%2C%20adrenaline%20was%20independently%20associated,with%20marked%20worsening%20in%20cardiac%20and%20renal%20biomarkers
12. Squara P, Hollenberg S, Payen D. Reconsidering vasopressors for cardiogenic shock: everything should be made as simple as possible, but not simpler. *Chest*. 2019;156(2):392–401. Available at: https://pubmed.ncbi.nlm.nih.gov/30935893/
13. Levy B, Bastien O, Bendjelid K et al. Experts' recommendations for the management of adult patients with cardiogenic shock. *Annals of Intensive Care*. 2015;5(1):17. Available at: https://www.ncbi.nlm.nih.gov/pmc/articles/PMC4495097/

13 Massive Upper Gastrointestinal Bleed (UGIB)

Sarah Yong and Michelle Murphy

In this chapter you will learn:

- Major differential diagnoses for acute upper gastrointestinal bleeding (UGIB)
- Early resuscitation priorities in acute UGIB, including massive UGIB
- Principles and evidence base for transfusion and coagulopathy management in GI haemorrhage
- The role of endoscopy in managing UGIB and the associated paramedic considerations with respect to disposition
- The evidence base for adjunct pharmacotherapy.

Case Details

Dispatch

52-year-old male, acute haematemesis.

History

A 52-year-old indigenous Australian man, living in a rural community, has had multiple episodes of frank haematemesis over the course of the day. His brother calls for an ambulance late in the day when he thinks the patient is 'not looking too well'. He tells the call-taker that 'the vomit is bright red and half filled a bucket'. A double-crewed ambulance with a qualified paramedic and yourself (a critical care paramedic) are dispatched.

On Your Arrival as the Critical Care Paramedic

The scene is safe and the patient is found on the porch of the house, located at the end of a dirt road. He is semi-recumbent in an old rattan chair. His primary survey findings and initial vital signs are:

Airway	Patent
Breathing	RR 26, SpO_2 86% on air
Circulation	Peripheral pulses weak, HR 118, BP 95/70, cool peripheries
Disability	GCS E3, V5, M6 (14), BGL 4.1 mmol/L
Environmental	Temp 36.3 °C

CHAPTER 13   Massive Upper Gastrointestinal Bleed (UGIB)

The patient is lethargic but compliant. His skin is jaundiced with pale dry mucosa and he complains of thirst. He has no obvious injuries and there is approximately 1500 ml of frank haematemesis in a bucket beside the chair. You ask your partner to administer oxygen via nasal prongs at 4 l/min and you gather a history.

AMPLE

The patient smokes 20 cigarettes a day and is moderately obese, with chronic health issues complicated by poor compliance with lifestyle behaviours and medication regime. He rarely attends a GP, as it is too far to travel to the nearest town, and occasionally a community healthcare worker visits him at home.

Allergies	NKDA
Medications	Esomeprazole, ipratropium, salbutamol
Past history	Hepatitis C, alcoholic cirrhosis, GORD, COPD
Last ins and outs	Breakfast ~7 hours ago and coffee ~2 hours ago
Events	After breakfast, the patient began to feel bloated (more than usual) and nauseated. He experienced his first vomit of bright red blood mixed with breakfast about 10am and told his brother he has had a few more episodes since then. When he started feeling dizzy, he called his brother. He has had burning upper chest/throat pain during the past hour

Decision Point 1
What are your clinical priorities in this situation?

With altered mentation (or decreased GCS) most likely due to uncontrolled haemorrhage, control of the haemorrhage is the priority. This requires expedited transport to surgical intervention. However, due to uncontrolled co-morbidities and hypoperfusion in a semi-recumbent position, this patient is at high risk of rapid deterioration on movement.

The safest plan would be to oxygenate the patient and prepare for rapid deterioration on movement, prior to transport.

Decision Point 2
Where is your destination?

This patient requires definitive surgical intervention, most likely at a specialist tertiary hospital, but there are blood products, pharmacological interventions and procedures (for example, a balloon tamponade device such as a Sengstaken–Blakemore tube) that could support perfusion and slow haemorrhage until arrival at definitive care (operating theatre or endoscopy suite). Consideration could be given to bringing these to the patient or stopping at an intermediate facility on route to definitive treatment.

SECTION 3 Circulation

Question 1: What Are the Common Presentations and Major Differentials for Upper Gastrointestinal Bleeding?

Upper gastrointestinal bleeding (UGIB) is defined as bleeding that originates proximal to the ligament of Treitz, the suspensory ligament of the duodenum located at the duodenojejunal flexure.

Upper GI bleeding commonly presents with haematemesis (vomiting of blood or coffee ground-like material) with or without melaena (black, tarry stools due to altered blood having passed through the GI tract). In a minority of patients (5–10%), it may present as haematochezia (bright, bloody stools) due to massive or brisk UGIB. Abdominal pain may be associated but is usually not present. History may reveal risk factors suggestive of aetiology of the UGIB, such as use of NSAIDS, anticoagulants or antiplatelet agents, alcohol abuse, liver disease, previous GI bleed or coagulopathy.

Examination findings include haemodynamic instability suggestive of life-threatening blood loss (tachycardia, orthostatic hypotension or hypotension), abdominal tenderness with possible signs of peritoneal irritation (for example, involuntary guarding, suggestive of perforation).

PRACTICE TIP

UGIB can be life threatening and the volume of haematemesis may not reflect the severity of the bleeding.

Gastric or duodenal ulcers are the most common cause of major UGIB. Other differentials (see **Figure 13.1**) for major upper GI bleeding include, in descending order of frequency:[1]

- Severe or erosive gastritis/duodenitis
- Severe or erosive oesophagitis
- Oesophagogastric varices
- Portal hypertensive gastropathy
- Angiodysplasia (vascular ectasia)
- Mallory–Weiss syndrome
- Mass lesions (polyps/cancers).

In up to 18% of patients presenting with an apparent upper GI bleed, endoscopy does not reveal a cause.[1,2]

It is not possible to differentiate between bleeding caused by ulcers, gastritis/oesophagitis/duodenitis or varices in the prehospital setting. Variceal bleeding is more likely in patients with a history of cirrhosis and, wherever possible, patients with such a history should be transported to a tertiary hospital.

Question 2: What Are the Early Management Priorities in Severe UGIB?

Rapid identification of the haemodynamically unstable patient with severe UGIB, with consideration of high-risk co-morbidities, along with simultaneous assessment and resuscitation, is essential. Ensure the patient remains nil orally as resuscitation proceeds.

CHAPTER 13 Massive Upper Gastrointestinal Bleed (UGIB)

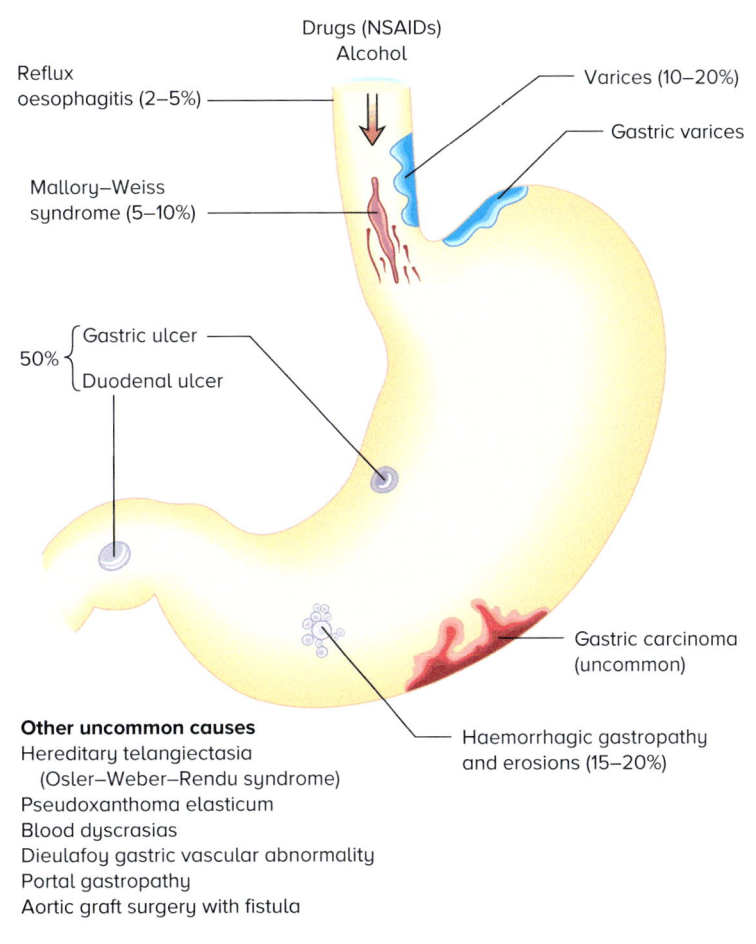

Figure 13.1 Causes of upper gastrointestinal bleeding.

Labels on figure:
- Drugs (NSAIDs) / Alcohol
- Reflux oesophagitis (2–5%)
- Varices (10–20%)
- Gastric varices
- Mallory–Weiss syndrome (5–10%)
- 50% {Gastric ulcer, Duodenal ulcer}
- Gastric carcinoma (uncommon)
- Haemorrhagic gastropathy and erosions (15–20%)

Other uncommon causes
Hereditary telangiectasia (Osler–Weber–Rendu syndrome)
Pseudoxanthoma elasticum
Blood dyscrasias
Dieulafoy gastric vascular abnormality
Portal gastropathy
Aortic graft surgery with fistula

Intravenous or intraosseous access with two large-bore cannulae (18 gauge or larger) should be obtained, while closely monitoring the airway, vital signs, cardiac rhythm, level of consciousness and overall clinical status. In haemodynamically unstable patients, treat initial hypotension with rapid bolus infusions of isotonic crystalloid (for example, 500–1000 mL per bolus, smaller boluses if there is a history of cardiac dysfunction). This should not be delayed pending transfer of the patient to an emergency department. Supplemental oxygen should be administered aiming for SpO_2 ≥94% (88–92% if there is a history of COPD).[3]

Principles of management thereafter include:

- Haemostatic resuscitation with packed red blood cells and also plasma if available
- If point-of-care blood testing is available, aiming for Hb >70 (or >80 if the patient is high risk)

SECTION 3 Circulation

- Avoidance of over-transfusion if variceal bleeding is a possibility
- Rapid transport to hospital, ideally with a gastroenterologist and also surgical and interventional radiology facilities for definitive management of UGIB
- Pharmacotherapy with PPI or somatostatin analogue may be appropriate in some environments (for example, interhospital transfers or remote areas).

These will be discussed in further detail below.

Patients who are haemodynamically unstable or have clear evidence of active bleeding (haematemesis or haematochezia) should be transported to a hospital with ICU facilities, as they will almost certainly require ongoing resuscitation and close observation. When transfer decisions are being considered, it is essential to be aware of specific hospital capability with respect to the trajectory of the individual patient's clinical picture. In addition, consideration should be given to transportation for initial resuscitation/stabilisation and then ongoing transport for definitive treatment or rendezvous with an experienced retrieval team for additional management, such as a Sengstaken–Blakemore tube.

Question 3: What Considerations Are Important for Prehospital Blood Administration in Acute Upper GI Bleeding?

Increasingly, transfusion of blood products such as packed red blood cells (PRBC) or plasma (thawed or freeze dried) is being adopted as a treatment for major bleeding in the prehospital setting. The evidence base for prehospital transfusion largely comes from the trauma setting, but other bleeding patients, such as those with UGIB, obstetric haemorrhage or a leaking abdominal aortic aneurysm, will also likely benefit from prehospital transfusion.

Ideally, patients with massive UGIB should be transfused with PRBC, platelets and plasma in a 1:1:1 ratio. In the prehospital setting it is likely that only PRBC (and possibly freeze-dried plasma) will be available. Decisions on blood transfusion should be based on a comprehensive patient assessment and possibly consultation with a critical care doctor or another CCP, recognising that over-transfusion may also have associated adverse effects.[3–5]

If point-of-care testing is available, the evidence supports the use of a restrictive transfusion strategy defending a haemoglobin of >70 g/L in most haemodynamically stable patients with UGIB.[3–7] A haemoglobin target of >80 g/L can be considered in patients at higher risk of adverse events in the setting of significant anaemia, such as those with cardiovascular disease or evidence of ongoing active bleeding.[3,8] In the prehospital setting, transfusion will likely be guided largely by shock state; however, Hb measurement may be relevant in the setting of an interhospital transfer.

A very high index of suspicion must be maintained in patients who are taking anticoagulants (such as warfarin or apixaban) or antiplatelets (such as aspirin or clopidogrel).

PRACTICE TIP

Beware patients who are taking anticoagulant or antiplatelet medications.

CHAPTER 13 Massive Upper Gastrointestinal Bleed (UGIB)

Question 4: What Are the Options for Managing UGIB in Hospital?

Endoscopy is the cornerstone of acute UBIG management, with high sensitivity and specificity for locating and identifying bleeding lesions in the upper GI tract, while providing prognostic information (**Figure 13.2**). Additionally, once the culprit lesion is identified, therapeutic endoscopy achieves acute haemostasis and prevents recurrent bleeding in most patients.[4]

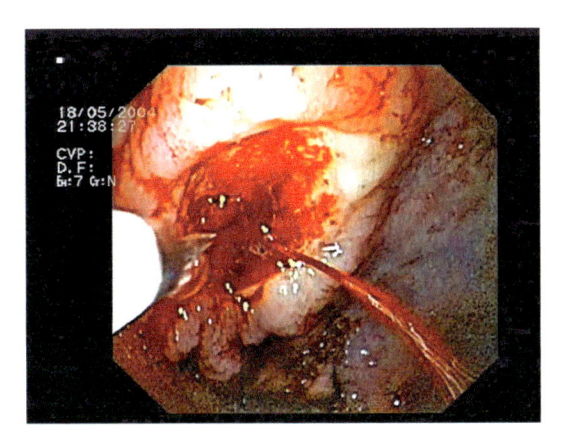

Figure 13.2 Endoscopic view of actively bleeding gastric ulcer.

Source: Jeremias, CC BY-SA 3.0 via Wikimedia Commons: https://commons.wikimedia.org/wiki/File:Bleeding_gastric_ulcer.png

Endoscopy is associated with complications, which may be life threatening in patients who are actively bleeding, physiologically unstable or with medical co-morbidities. It is crucial that patients are optimally resuscitated before endoscopy, to minimise the risk of complications. However, endoscopy should not be delayed because of anticoagulant or antiplatelet use,[8] and provided the patient is haemodynamically stable, urgent endoscopy can usually be carried out simultaneously with ongoing management of antithrombotic medications.[9]

Acid-suppressive therapies, somatostatin analogues and antibiotics have a role to play in acute UGIB. Acid-suppressing drugs such as PPIs are thought to reduce the risk of ongoing bleeding and re-bleeding by achieving an intragastric pH of at least 6.5, which stabilises blood clot formation within the bleeding ulcer crater, optimises platelet function, inhibits fibrinolysis and minimises peptic activity.[10] Infusions of PPI are often used and may be continued on an interhospital transfer.

Somatostatin analogues, such as octreotide, and vasopressin analogues, such as terlipressin, are used in the management of variceal bleeding. Both are thought to reduce portal pressure by reducing splanchnic flow to therefore reduce severity of variceal bleeding.[4] CCPs may also be requested to supervise infusions of these drugs on interhospital transfers.

Tranexamic acid is not routinely used in the management of acute UGIB. Its use has been studied in patients with acute UGIB, with randomised trials and meta-analyses concluding that there is no role for it, as its use was associated with an increase in venous thromboembolic events and seizures compared with placebo, with no improvement in bleeding risk.[11]

SECTION 3 Circulation

> **PRACTICE TIP**
>
> Packed red bloods cells are the ideal resuscitation fluid for patients with severe UGIB.

In patients with life-threatening variceal haemorrhage, a balloon tamponade device, such as a Sengstaken–Blakemore or a Minnesota tube, can help to temporise bleeding while a patient is transported to a facility capable of definitive endoscopic management of the varices. These devices are usually large-bore orogastric tubes with one or more balloons at the distal end. The balloons are inflated after insertion to tamponade bleeding from the varices (**Figure 13.3**). Traction is also used, with the device usually secured to an IV pole at the foot end of the stretcher. Complications include pressure necrosis and oesophageal rupture. Critical care paramedics may be called on to transport patients with a Sengstaken–Blakemore or Minnesota tube in place. Care should be taken to ensure that it is well secured, and the balloon pressure should be checked periodically with an ETT cuff manometer if available.

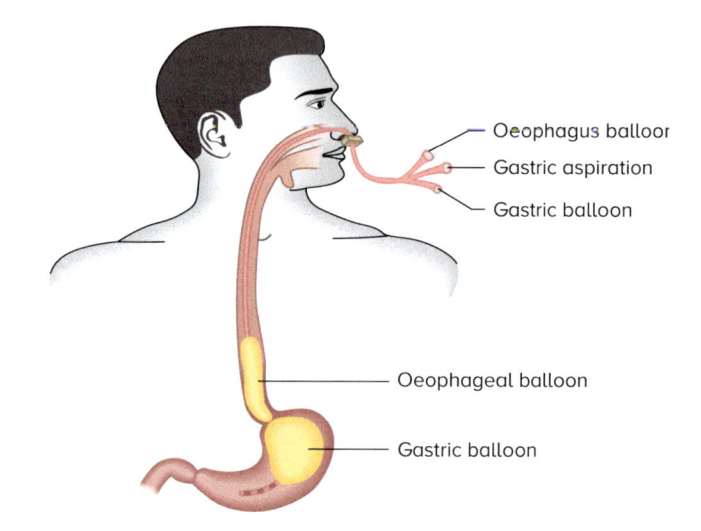

Figure 13.3 Sengstaken–Blakemore tube for balloon tamponade of variceal bleeding.

> **PRACTICE TIP**
>
> Balloon tamponade can be life-saving and may be available at district hospitals or with interhospital retrieval teams.

Key Evidence

Barkun AN, Almadi M, Kuipers EJ et al. Management of nonvariceal upper gastrointestinal bleeding: guideline recommendations from the international consensus group. *Annals of Internal Medicine*. 2019;171(11): 805–822. Available at: https://pubmed.ncbi.nlm.nih.gov/31634917/

National Institute for Health and Care Excellence. Acute upper gastrointestinal bleeding in over 16s: management. Clinical guideline [CG141]. 2012. Available at: https://www.nice.org.uk/guidance/cg141

Odutayo A, Desborough MJR, Trivella M et al. Restrictive versus liberal blood transfusion for gastrointestinal bleeding: systematic review and meta-analyses of randomised controlled trials. *Lancet. Gastroenterology and Hepatology*. 2017;2(5):354–360. Available at: https://pubmed.ncbi.nlm.nih.gov/28397699/

Self-Reflection Questions

1. What do you think is the most likely trajectory for this patient's illness if you are >90 minutes from hospital, and what are five contributing factors based on the information and knowledge you now have?
2. What are your considerations for fluid resuscitation, at what point physiologically would you start, and how much would you administer? What's your target?
3. If available in your region, how would you facilitate administration of PRBC to this patient?
4. What indications would you look for to intubate this person, and what medications would you choose for induction of anaesthesia, paralysis to achieve intubation, post-intubation sedation and analgesia?
5. Given this patient is likely to deteriorate on transfer, what other actions would you consider? Is there any consideration for bringing the treatment to the patient prior to transfer?
6. What are your priorities for 'goals' of care for this patient, and what is the role that this patient and his family will play in that decision making?

References

1. Rockey DC. Causes of upper gastrointestinal bleeding in adults [online]. UpToDate. 2022. Available at: https://www.uptodate.com/contents/causes-of-upper-gastrointestinal-bleeding-in-adults?search=upper%20gi%20bleeding&topicRef=2548&source=see_link
2. Papadinas A, Butt J. Outcomes in patients with acute upper gastrointestinal bleeding following changes to management protocols at an Australian hospital. *Journal of Gastroenterology and Hepatology Open*. 2020;4(4):617–623. Available at: https://www.ncbi.nlm.nih.gov/pmc/articles/PMC7411648/
3. Saltzman JR. Approach to acute upper gastrointestinal bleeding in adults [online]. UpToDate. 2024. Available at: https://www.uptodate.com/contents/approach-to-acute-upper-gastrointestinal-bleeding-in-adults?search=upper%20gi%20bleeding&source=search_result&selectedTitle=1~150&usage_type=default&display_rank=1#H1
4. National Institute for Health and Care Excellence. Acute upper gastrointestinal bleeding in over 16s: management. Clinical guideline [CG141]. 2012. Available at: https://www.nice.org.uk/guidance/cg141
5. National Blood Authority. *Patient Blood Management Guidelines: Module 1 Critical Bleeding Massive Transfusion*. 2012. Available at: https://www.blood.gov.au/system/files/documents/20140904-pbm-mod1-qrg.pdf
6. Jairath V, Kahan BC, Gray A et al. Restrictive versus liberal blood transfusion for acute upper gastrointestinal bleeding (TRIGGER): a pragmatic, open-label, cluster randomised feasibility trial. *Lancet*. 2015;386:137–144. Available at: https://pubmed.ncbi.nlm.nih.gov/25956718/
7. Odutayo A, Desborough MJR, Trivella M et al. Restrictive versus liberal blood transfusion for gastrointestinal bleeding: systematic review and meta-analyses of randomised controlled trials. *Lancet. Gastroenterology and Hepatology*. 2017;2(5):354–360. Available at: https://pubmed.ncbi.nlm.nih.gov/28397699/
8. Barkun AN, Almadi M, Kuipers EJ et al. Management of nonvariceal upper gastrointestinal bleeding: guideline recommendations from the international consensus group. *Annals of Internal Medicine*. 2019;171(11):805–822. Available at: https://pubmed.ncbi.nlm.nih.gov/31634917/
9. ASGE Standards of Practice Committee, Acosta RD, Abraham NS et al. The management of antithrombotic agents for patients undergoing GI endoscopy. *Gastrointestinal Endoscopy*. 2016;83(1):3–16. Available at: https://pubmed.ncbi.nlm.nih.gov/26621548/

10. Leontiadis GI, Sharma VK, Howden CW. Systematic review and meta-analysis of proton pump inhibitor therapy in peptic ulcer bleeding. *British Medical Journal*. 2005;330(7491):568. Available at: https://pubmed.ncbi.nlm.nih.gov/15684023/
11. HALT-IT Trial Collaborators. Effects of a high-dose 24-h infusion of tranexamic acid on death and thromboembolic events in patients with acute gastrointestinal bleeding (HALT-IT): an international randomised, double-blind, placebo-controlled trial. *Lancet*. 2020;395(10241):1927–1936. Available at: https://pubmed.ncbi.nlm.nih.gov/32563378/

Acute Pulmonary Oedema

14

Nick Trestrail and Luke Hamilton

> **In this chapter you will learn:**
> - The role of ultrasound in assisting with the diagnosis of acute pulmonary oedema (APO) in the prehospital environment
> - The benefits of continuous pulmonary airway pressure (CPAP) for patients suffering APO
> - The potential complications and restrictions of CPAP
> - The potential future treatments alongside CPAP in the prehospital phase.

Case Details

Dispatch
74-year-old woman, dyspnoea, difficulty speaking between breaths.

History
A 74-year-old woman with a history of hypertension and aortic stenosis reported becoming increasingly short of breath and dizzy over several hours one evening. Her wife phoned for an ambulance to help when she could no longer speak in sentences and her breathing was audibly laboured. A paramedic double-crewed ambulance was dispatched.

On Arrival of the First Crew
The scene is safe. The patient is half slumped in bed, attempting to keep herself upright. Her primary survey findings and initial vital signs are:

Airway	Patent
Breathing	RR 32, SpO$_2$ 82% on room air
Circulation	Peripheral pulses strong, HR 130 irregular, BP 170/110, cool peripheries
Disability	GCS E4, V5, M6 (15), BGL 7.2 mmol/L
Environmental	Temp 36.1 °C

The paramedic crew sit the patient up, apply high-flow oxygen therapy and nasal end-tidal carbon dioxide monitoring, revealing a non-bronchospastic waveform. They note global coarse crackles on auscultation, an elevated respiratory rate and an increased work of

SECTION 3   Circulation

breathing. The patient feels cool to the touch peripherally. The crew have administered a single 400 mcg dose of sublingual glyceryl trinitrate (GTN).

On Your Arrival as the Critical Care Paramedic

Patient positioning and oxygen therapy have increased oxygen saturations to 89% on 15 lpm. The patient no longer appears as cyanosed. However, her work of breathing is high. The paramedic is gaining intravenous access while handing over to you, and wonders if this APO was caused by left ventricular failure, asking if this patient would benefit from CPAP.

AMPLE

Allergies	NKDA
Medications	Amlodipine 5 mg Lisinopril 20 mg Spironolactone 25 mg Salbutamol PRN
Past history	Hypertension Aortic stenosis Gout Smoker
Last ins and outs	Small evening meal at approximately 1900
Events prior	Increasingly breathless before becoming tight-chested, developing palpitations and becoming significantly breathless

Decision Point
What are your clinical priorities in this situation?

You suspect that this patient has APO and would benefit from non-invasive ventilation, but you are not certain. You think point-of-care ultrasonography (POCUS) may add diagnostic benefit while your ventilator and CPAP device are retrieved from the car.

Question 1: How Is APO Diagnosed in the Prehospital Setting?

Heart failure can be chronic, acute on chronic (acutely decompensated), or *de novo* – normally as a serious complication of acute coronary syndrome.[1]

The patient in this case study has a past medical history that indicates established cardiovascular disease. The chain of events preceding the emergency call indicates a potentially cardiovascular and/or respiratory component. The patient's observations and physical signs indicate a congested circulation with a deteriorating picture of gas exchange reflected in poor oxygen saturations and increased work of breathing.

Early prehospital identification of APO and heart failure can initiate rapid and decisive treatment. However, identification of APO in the prehospital setting is notoriously difficult. Physical examination findings may be limited and inconsistent, and reported symptoms can

CHAPTER 14 Acute Pulmonary Oedema

potentially be non-specific and common in many disease states. Often examination findings and symptoms have a low sensitivity and poor predictive value (**Table 14.1**).

Table 14.1 Clinical features and examination sensitivity, specificity and predictive value

Clinical features	Sensitivity %	Specificity %	Predictive value %
Dyspnoea	66	52	23
Paroxysmal nocturnal dyspnoea	33	76	26
Examination			
Tachycardia	7	99	6
Crepitations	13	91	27
Oedema	10	93	3
Neck vein distention	10	97	2

Source: Watson, R.D.S., Gibbs, C.R. and Lip, G.Y.H. (2000). Clinical features and complications. ABC of heart failure. *British Medical Journal*, 320 (7229). Available at: https://www.ncbi.nlm.nih.gov/pmc/articles/PMC1117436/

The classic presenting symptoms include dyspnoea, hypoxia and fatigue. The patient may also complain of shortness of breath on bending over (bendopnoea).[2]

> **PRACTICE TIP**
>
> APO can be difficult to diagnose; point-of-care ultrasound (POCUS) can help differentiate respiratory failure secondary to APO from that with a respiratory cause.

The accuracy of auscultation to differentiate lung sounds when performed on a patient *in extremis* is inconsistent.[3] As such, diagnosing pulmonary oedema as a result of heart failure can be challenging prehospitally. However, with ultrasound technology in addition to signs, symptoms and history indicative of heart failure, that has changed. A systematic review and meta-analysis by Maw et al. in 2019[4] have shown that the presence of B-lines or comet tails (**see Figure 5.2** on p. 53) bilaterally on lung ultrasound (LUS) assessment is more sensitive, and as specific as chest x-ray in detecting pulmonary oedema. The 2021 guidelines for the diagnosis and treatment of acute and chronic heart failure highlight the utility of LUS alongside clinical signs in the diagnosis of APO.[5] It has been shown that, even after a relatively brief course, critical care paramedics can perform LUS with reasonable accuracy.[6] The presence of B-lines is directly proportional to the amount of congestion from a cardiac origin.[7] Schoeneck et al. have completed a pilot study of paramedic usage of ultrasound prehospitally, specifically for the detection of B-lines in the presence of congestive heart failure, with promising results.[8] Donovan et al. conducted a scoping review of respiratory distress assessment utilising ultrasound technology in the prehospital field, concluding that further robust research is required with an emphasis on a more standardised training and assessment protocol, but that the potential feasibility has been demonstrated.[6] Clearly, the adoption of ultrasound for

SECTION 3 Circulation

the wider prehospital workforce has investment, training and governance considerations, but enhanced care teams have already adopted its use with evident benefits for diagnosing the absence or presence of pulmonary oedema in the acute heart failure patient.

Source: https://www.researchgate.net/figure/Lung-ultrasound-scan-showing-multiple-B-lines-from-a-case-of-cardiogenic-pulmonary_fig1_280107036

Question 2: What Is the Role of Non-Invasive Ventilation (NIV) in the Paramedic Management of APO?

Continuous pulmonary airway pressure (CPAP) is a form of non-invasive ventilation (NIV) delivering positive pressure during both the inspiratory and expiratory phases of the respiratory cycle. CPAP is a widely recognised therapy and features in a variety of international guidelines for patients with respiratory failure.[9,10] CPAP generates positive end expiratory pressure (PEEP), which is delivered to the patient via a tight-fighting face mask or nasal cannula. Several CPAP devices lend themselves to their practical use in the prehospital setting by being simple to use, cheap, disposable and driven by oxygen, negating the need for a mechanical ventilator (**Figure 14.1**).

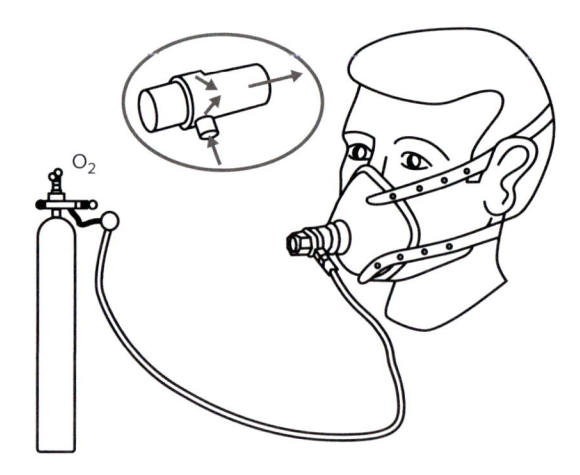

Figure 14.1 An example of a Boussignac CPAP mask.

Source: Spijker, E., de Bont, M., Bax, M. et al. (2013). Practical use, effects and complications of prehospital treatment of acute cardiogenic pulmonary edema using the Boussignac CPAP system. *International Journal of Emergency Medicine*, 6 (8). Available at: https://intjem.biomedcentral.com/articles/10.1186/1865-1380-6-8 (Creative Commons Attribution 2.0 International License).

CPAP and positive pressure ventilation affect both the respiratory and cardiovascular systems (**Figure 14.2**). Depending on the patient's physiology and disease processes, these treatments may be beneficial or detrimental.

In heart failure, CPAP and increases in PEEP prevent atelectasis at the end of expiration by improving the functional residual capacity (FRC) by splinting the smaller airways and preventing collapse. Increases in PEEP allow further recruitment of collapsed alveoli and alter hydrostatic pressure, inducing a shift of fluid or oedema from the alveoli to

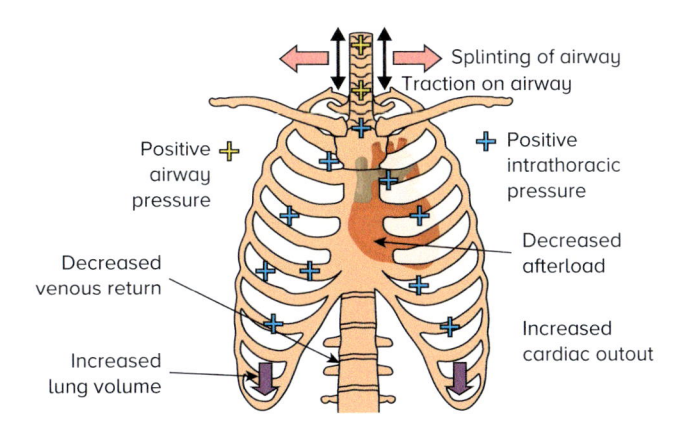

Figure 14.2 Effects of positive airway pressure on the respiratory and cardiovascular systems.

the pulmonary vasculature, helping to increase oxygenation and improving ventilation–perfusion ratios.[11–13] Furthermore, in those with hypoxic pulmonary vasoconstriction, the combined effects of the above mechanisms may relieve pulmonary vasoconstriction, further improving oxygenation.

CPAP and the provision of positive pressure cause both the mean airway and intrathoracic pressure to rise. Increased intrathoracic pressure diminishes systemic venous return, which alters the performance of the right and left sides of the heart.[14]

The right side of the heart operates under a low-pressure system, assisted by the negative pressure generated by spontaneous respiration, helping to augment venous return. As mean airway and intrathoracic pressure rise, the negative pressure gradient adding venous return reduces.[14] The reduction in preload can significantly affect the left ventricle, with reduced left ventricular filling decreasing the stroke volume and dependent mean arterial pressure (MAP). However, a protective mechanism may compensate for a reduction in MAP in the presence of left ventricular disease. Raised intrathoracic pressure creates a transaortic pressure gradient between higher pressures in the intrathoracic aorta and lower pressures in the extrathoracic aorta. The intrathoracic/extrathoracic aorta gradient reduces afterload, improves left ventricular ejection fraction and decreases the efficacy of its workload. This reduction in afterload can increase net cardiac output and reduce myocardial oxygen demands in a failing heart (**Figure 14.3**).[14]

Question 3: What Is the Evidence Supporting the Use of CPAP in Prehospital Care?

CPAP has been used in the management of APO over the past 40 years. The first randomised papers published in the 1980s and 1990s began to demonstrate physiological benefits and decreased incidence of tracheal intubation.[15,16] Several subsequent randomised studies and meta-analyses have replicated findings, demonstrating earlier resolution of respiratory failure, physiological improvement and decreased incidences of tracheal intubation.[17] Benefits have

SECTION 3   Circulation

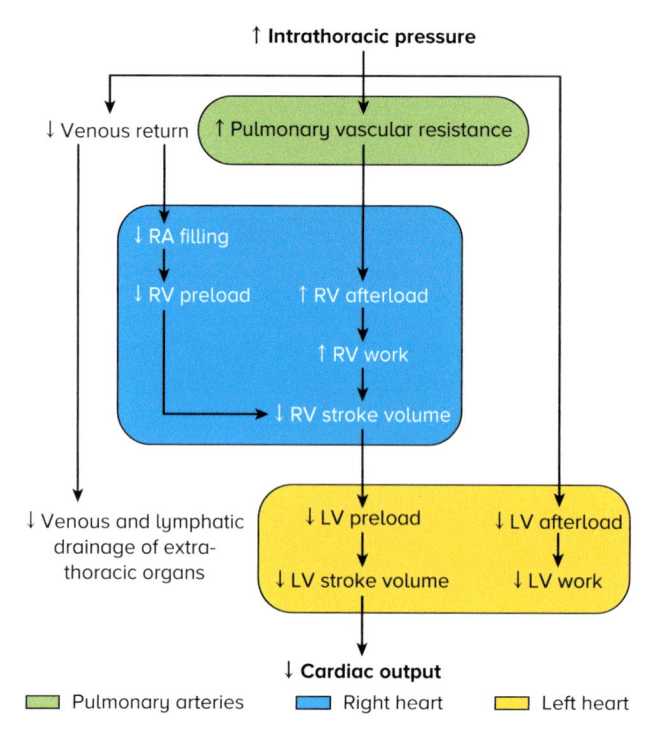

Figure 14.3   The cardiovascular effects of positive pressure ventilation.

Source: Class Professional Publishing. Based on Corp, A., Thomas, C. and Adlam M. 2021. The cardiovascular effects of positive pressure ventilation. *British Journal of Anaesthesia Education*, 21(6), pp. 202–209. Available at: https://www.bjaed.org/article/S2058-5349(21)00005-6/fulltext

been demonstrated in many hospital settings, including emergency, coronary and intensive care settings.[17]

Following the publication of several single-centre, low-powered studies, a trend of statistically significant data demonstrating a mortality benefit favouring the use of CPAP in APO was forming.[16] However, a later large randomised trial, 3CPO, showed no difference in mortality when comparing CPAP to standard therapies.[18] Several reasons may exist why 3CPO did not reproduce the expected trends, including enrolment of sicker patients with higher incidences of tracheal intubation, higher incidences of mortality than other studies and patients with lower levels of hypoxia potentially negating some benefits of CPAP and NIV.[16,18] Despite this, a 2019 Cochrane review analysing and undertaking power calculation from 21 studies examining CPAP and bi-level positive pressure ventilation in the treatment of APO concluded that NIV might reduce hospital mortality compared to standard medical therapies.

> **PRACTICE TIP**
>
> Early application of CPAP provides both symptomatic benefit and improved survival in APO.

CHAPTER 14 Acute Pulmonary Oedema

Paramedics in Europe and Australia have demonstrated safe and proficient use of CPAP.[19,20] Several studies show high sensitivity and specificity for paramedic ability to identify APO and respiratory failure, and additionally, safely and effectively apply CPAP in the prehospital setting.[19,20] Several studies demonstrate that prehospital CPAP may improve physiological parameters, decrease in-hospital tracheal intubation rates and improve patient comfort.[16,20,21] However, there appears to be an absence of high-quality empirical evidence supporting a mortality benefit or other patient-centred outcomes for early prehospital CPAP use.[20,22]

Question 4: What Are the Potential Risks, Complications and Contraindications of CPAP for APO?

Currently, two international guidelines recommend using CPAP to treat APO in the prehospital setting. The European Society of Cardiology (ERC) recommends the use of CPAP in the prehospital setting for patients identified as likely to have APO and respiratory distress (RR >25/min, SpO_2 <90%). The Joint ERC and ATS guideline recommends using CPAP in treating APO in the prehospital setting but without dictating physiological values to guide its use.[23]

PRACTICE TIP

Patient reassurance, and if required other means of anxiolysis, has an under-appreciated impact of the treatment of APO.

Contraindications associated with CPAP are connected mainly with the ability to ensure airway patency and minimise potential airway complications (**Table 14.2**). In some clinical settings, CPAP may be used in the presence of equivocal contraindications or cautions if contingency plans for rapid tracheal intubation have been made.[24] These may not be feasible or appropriate in the prehospital setting, so a more conservative approach may be required.

Table 14.2 British Thoracic Society/Intensive Care Society non-invasive ventilation contraindications and cautions

Absolute contraindications	Relative contraindications	Further cautions
• Severe facial deformity • Facial burns • Fixed upper airway obstruction	• GCS <8 • Confusion and agitation • Cognitive impairment	• Respiratory secretions • Vomiting • Recent facial surgery • Recent gastric surgery • Bowel obstructions

Source: British Thoracic Society: https://www.brit-thoracic.org.uk/quality-improvement/guidelines/niv/

Question 5: The Potential Future Treatments Alongside CPAP in the Prehospital Phase

The prehospital administration of furosemide, oxygen and glyceryl trinitrate have been utilised for patients suffering acute heart failure for a long time now.

Nitrates work by inducing changes at a cellular level that reduce intracellular calcium leading to venous vasodilation at low doses and arterial vasodilation at higher doses.

Administered to the patient with acute heart failure, the vasodilatory actions reduce end-diastolic filling pressures, while inducing a reduction in systemic and pulmonary vascular resistance, causing a systemic arterial blood pressure decrease. The result is a modest increase in stroke volume and cardiac output.[25]

However, with the increasing benefits that CPAP can contribute to the acute heart failure patient *in extremis*, it may be time to re-think how glyceryl trinitrate is delivered in the prehospital phase. If CPAP is fitted to the patient, breaking the seal on the tight-fitting mask to administer sublingual GTN has potentially deleterious consequences on the quality of care being delivered.

The use of intravenous nitrates has long been featured in guidelines for the management of acute decompensated heart failure.[26] Intravenous administration offers a potential solution to avoid delaying or interrupting the provision of CPAP, causing a potential loss of mask seal and a loss of PEEP and/or intrathoracic pressure. However, the benefit of using intravenous nitrates has been debated due to the small and limited evidence base.[27] More recently, the impact on mortality of prehospital intravenous nitrates has been explored by Miro et al.,[28] undertaking a large registry subanalysis examining the impact of intravenous nitroglycerin in heart failure given prehospitally, compared to within the emergency department or those who did not receive nitrate treatments. Within this study, 292 received prehospital intravenous nitrates, 1159 received intravenous nitrates in the ED setting, and 6973 did not receive them during their prehospital or ED phases. The authors identified that patients receiving intravenous nitrates appeared to be classified as sicker, with lower pulse oximetry values and greater degrees of hypertension, with patients who received prehospital intravenous nitrates having the worst prognostic scores when ranked. The authors found lower risks of one-year mortality in patients receiving prehospital intravenous nitrates, even after adjustments for differences in baseline characteristics and disease severity. However, the short-term 30-day survival or length of hospital admission did not appear to differ between groups. Although the favourable analysis supports the use of prehospital intravenous nitrates, consideration should be given to the limitations associated with retrospective, non-blinded registry analysis. In addition, the dosing strategy of prehospital nitrates was not recorded. Therefore, we are uncertain how generalisable or comparable these findings are to current practice.

Patrick et al. performed a retrospective chart review of all emergency medical services (EMS) and ED records of patients treated for presumed decompensated acute heart failure (AHF) and APO using bolus IV GTN +/- CPAP over a year-long period up to March 2019.[29] Paramedics were required to identify patients suffering AHF and APO and then had the option to administer GTN sublingually (400 mcg tablets) while intravenous or intraosseous access was gained. After access was gained, an initial dose of 1 mg IV GTN was slowly administered and repeated in five minutes if the systolic blood pressure remained greater than 160 mmHg. The maximum total dose was not to exceed 2 mg, CPAP was available and encouraged but not a requirement. A total of 250 EMS patients were identified and reviewed, as they satisfied the inclusion criteria. However, 162 patients were not included in the study, as an alternative diagnosis was more likely than AHF with APO. Of the 88 patients, 18 did not receive prehospital intravenous access and a further 22 patients did not receive IV GTN due to paramedic clinical decision making. Forty-eight (55%) patients received the treatment protocol. Prior to IV GTN, 16/48 received sublingual GTN, with 33/48 (69%) receiving a single 1 mg of IV GTN, compared with 15/48 (31%) receiving a second 1 mg dose. Supplemental oxygen was provided for patients in a variety of concentrations dependent on the patient presentation. Of the IV GTN group, 41/48 had an improvement in systolic blood pressure and 45/48 had an increase in oxygen saturation readings. There was one incident of a patient suffering hypotension after 1 mg of IV GTN, with a recorded drop from 203/88 to 71/38, which improved to 105/73 over four minutes without any treatment, and the patient arrived at ED with normotension, no chest pain and no syncope. The review did note that a further 40 patients could have potentially received IV GTN but did not, either due to cardiovascular access failure or paramedic decision making.

Other studies have examined the feasibility and efficacy of prehospital intravenous nitrate administration. One single-centre retrospective chart review by Patrick et al. examined 48 patients in a single centre who received one or two doses of 1 mg of nitroglycerin as a slow intravenous bolus in the setting of decompensated heart failure in addition to other standard therapies, including sublingual nitrates, supplemental oxygen and CPAP. The authors concluded that their care bundle, including the intravenous nitrates, improved median oxygen saturation while decreasing median blood pressure.[29] Only one adverse event of significant hypotension was reported in which a patient's blood pressure descended from 203/88 mmHg to 71/38 mmHg. However, this was reported to have self-normalised with no further interventions or adverse events. The authors found that their paramedics had a success rate of 94% at identifying heart failure. However, the authors identified that an additional 40 patients met the inclusion criteria for heart failure treatment, including intravenous nitrate therapies, who were not identified or treated with nitrates.

Comparisons between intravenous boluses and infusion of nitrates have been explored within the hospital setting. Although this research may not translate directly into prehospital practice, the findings of Abdelmoneum et al. may drive further research and guidelines offering a simpler alternative to the complexities that running infusions in the prehospital setting can bring.[30] Abdeloneum et al. undertook a randomised, single-centre, single-blinded study comparing intermittent boluses of GTN against continuous infusion to compare efficacy and safety within the ED. Intermittent boluses of GTN were found to be more effective at reducing hypertensive blood pressures and associated with fewer ICU admissions and shorter hospital lengths of stay than continuous infusions.[30] The safety and incidence of adverse events appear comparable between the two interventions.

The studies examined have indicated a potential for the benefits of early IV GTN administration on mortality after a year, and combined events after 90 days post discharge, especially for patients presenting with APO and AHF for the first time. The potential for a safe protocol to be adopted and enhanced with the use of prehospital ultrasound application to reinforce prehospital diagnosis of APO in AHF has been demonstrated, with only one patient suffering an episode of hypotension requiring no intervention. Also, bolus dosing of IV GTN for patients is as safe as a continuous infusion and is associated with fewer ICU admissions and shorter mean mechanical ventilation duration, with a similar safety and efficacy profile as current infusion strategies, potentially reducing the prehospital burden of preparing and commencing an infusion. AHF patients suffering APO would benefit from more definitive diagnostics provided by enhanced care teams that carry ultrasound technology.

SECTION 3 Circulation

In combination with an agreed protocol and inclusion criteria, including an IV GTN dosing strategy alongside standard care options and CPAP, the optimum prehospital care for this subset of critically ill medical patients could be achieved.

Key Evidence

Berbenetz, N., Wang, Y., Brown, J. et al. 2019. Non-invasive positive pressure ventilation (CPAP or bilevel NPPV) for cardiogenic pulmonary oedema. *Cochrane Database of Systematic Reviews*, *4*(4). Available at: https://pubmed.ncbi.nlm.nih.gov/30950507/

Finn, J.C., Brink, D., Mckenzie, N. et al. 2022. Prehospital continuous positive airway pressure (CPAP) for acute respiratory distress: a randomised controlled trial. *Emergency Medicine Journal*, *39*, pp. 37–44. Available at: https://emj.bmj.com/content/39/1/37.info

Gray, A., Goodacre, S., Newby, D.E. et al. 2008. Noninvasive ventilation in acute cardiogenic pulmonary edema. *New England Journal of Medicine*, *359*, pp. 142–151. Available at: https://www.nejm.org/doi/pdf/10.1056/nejmoa0707992

Schoeneck, J.H., Coughlin, R.F., Baloescu, C. et al. 2021. Paramedic-performed prehospital point-of-care ultrasound for patients with undifferentiated dyspnea: a pilot study. *Western Journal of Emergency Medicine*, *22*(3), pp. 750–755. Available at: https://pubmed.ncbi.nlm.nih.gov/34125056/

Self-Reflection Questions

1. What are the key clinical features of APO?
2. What are B-lines and how can they be used in diagnostic lung ultrasound?
3. What is the mechanism of action of CPAP in APO?
4. What are the contraindications for CPAP use in APO?
5. What is the role of IV GTN in critical care paramedic practice?

References

1. Kurmani, S. and Squire, I. 2017. Acute heart failure: definition, classification and epidemiology. *Current Heart Failure Reports*, *14*(5), pp. 385–392.
2. Thibodeau, J. T., Turer, A. T., Gualano, S. K. et al. 2014. characterization of a novel symptom of advanced heart failure: bendopnea. *JACC: Heart Failure*, *2*(1). Available at: https://pubmed.ncbi.nlm.nih.gov/24622115/
3. Arts, L., Lim, E.H.T., van de Ven, P.M. et al. 2020. The diagnostic accuracy of lung auscultation in adult patients with acute pulmonary pathologies: a meta-analysis. *Scientific Reports*, *10*(1), pp. 1–11.
4. Maw, A.M., Hassanin, A., Ho, P.M. et al. 2019. Diagnostic accuracy of point-of-care lung ultrasonography and chest radiography in adults with symptoms suggestive of acute decompensated heart failure: a systematic review and meta-analysis. *JAMA Network Open*, *2*(3). Available at: https://pubmed.ncbi.nlm.nih.gov/30874784/
5. McDonagh, T.A., Metra, M., Adamo, M. et al. 2021. 2021 ESC Guidelines for the diagnosis and treatment of acute and chronic heart failure: developed by the Task Force for the diagnosis and treatment of acute and chronic heart failure of the European Society of Cardiology (ESC) with the special contribution of the Heart Failure Association (HFA) of the ESC. *European Heart Journal*, *42*(36), pp. 3599–3726.
6. Donovan, J.K., Burton, S.O., Jones, S.L. et al. 2022. Use of point-of-care ultrasound by non-physicians to assess respiratory distress in the out-of-hospital environment: a scoping review. *Prehospital and Disaster Medicine*, *37*(4), pp. 520–528. Available at: https://pubmed.ncbi.nlm.nih.gov/35506171/
7. Mauro, C., Chianese, S., Cocchia, R. et al. 2023. Acute heart failure: diagnostic–therapeutic pathways and preventive strategies – a real-world clinician's guide. *Journal of Clinical Medicine*, *12*(3), p. 846.

CHAPTER 14 Acute Pulmonary Oedema

8. Schoeneck, J.H., Coughlin, R.F., Baloescu, C. et al. 2021. Paramedic-performed prehospital point-of-care ultrasound for patients with undifferentiated dyspnea: a pilot study. *Western Journal of Emergency Medicine*, *22*(3), pp. 750–755. Available at: https://pubmed.ncbi.nlm.nih.gov/34125056/
9. Ponikowski, P., Voors, A., A., Anker, D, S. et al. 2016. 2016 ESC Guidelines for the diagnosis and treatment of acute and chronic heart failure: The Task Force for the diagnosis and treatment of acute and chronic heart failure of the European Society of Cardiology (ESC). *European Heart Journal*, *37*(27). Available at: https://academic.oup.com/eurheartj/article/37/27/2129/1748921?login=false
10. Ezekowitz, J.A., O'Meara, E., McDonald, M.A. et al. 2017. Comprehensive update of the Canadian Cardiovascular Society Guidelines for the Management of Heart Failure. *Canadian Journal of Cardiology*, *33*(11), pp. 1342–1433. Available at: https://pubmed.ncbi.nlm.nih.gov/29111106/
11. Willams, A.T., Finn. J., Perkins, D.G. et al. 2012. Prehospital continuous positive airway pressure for acute respiratory failure: a systematic review and meta-analysis. *Prehospital Emergency Care*, *17*(2), pp. 261–273. Available at: https://www.tandfonline.com/doi/abs/10.3109/10903127.2012.749967
12. Kato, T., Suda, S. and Kasai, T. 2014. Positive airway pressure therapy for heart failure. *World Journal of Cardiology*, *6*(11), pp. 1175–1191. Available at: https://www.ncbi.nlm.nih.gov/pmc/articles/PMC4244615/
13. Santa Cruz, R., Villarejo, F., Irrazabal, C. et al. 2021. High versus low positive end-expiratory pressure (PEEP) levels for mechanically ventilated adult patients with acute lung injury and acute respiratory distress syndrome. *Cochrane Database of Systematic Reviews*, *3*(3). Available at: https://pubmed.ncbi.nlm.nih.gov/33784416/
14. Corp, A., Thomas, C. and Adlam M. 2021. The cardiovascular effects of positive pressure ventilation. *British Journal of Anaesthesia Education*, *21*(6), pp. 202–209. Available at: https://www.bjaed.org/article/S2058-5349(21)00005-6/fulltext
15. Kaminski J, Kaplan PD. The role of noninvasive positive pressure ventilation in the emergency department. *Advanced Emergency Nursing Journal*. 1999;21(4):68–73.
16. Masip, J., Peacock, W.F., Price, S. et al. 2018. Indications and practical approach to non-invasive ventilation in acute heart failure. *European Heart Journal*, *39*(1), pp. 17–25. Available at: https://academic.oup.com/eurheartj/article/39/1/17/4654494
17. Berbenetz, N., Wang, Y., Brown, J. et al. 2019. Non-invasive positive pressure ventilation (CPAP or bilevel NPPV) for cardiogenic pulmonary oedema. *Cochrane Database of Systematic Reviews*, *4*(4). Available at: https://pubmed.ncbi.nlm.nih.gov/30950507/
18. Gray, A., Goodacre, S., Newby, D.E. et al. 2008. Noninvasive ventilation in acute cardiogenic pulmonary edema. *New England Journal of Medicine*, *359*, pp. 142–151. Available at: https://www.nejm.org/doi/pdf/10.1056/nejmoa0707992
19. Spiker, E.E., Bont, D.M., Bax, M. et al. 2012. Practical use, effects and complications of prehospital treatment of acute cardiogenic pulmonary edema using the Boussignac CPAP system. *International Journal of Emergency Medicine*, *6*(8). Available at: https://intjem.biomedcentral.com/articles/10.1186/1865-1380-6-8
20. Finn, J.C., Brink, D., Mckenzie, N. et al. 2022. Prehospital continuous positive airway pressure (CPAP) for acute respiratory distress: a randomised controlled trial. *Emergency Medicine Journal*, *39*, pp. 37–44. Available at: https://emj.bmj.com/content/39/1/37.info
21. Plaisance, P., Pirracchio, R., Berton, C. et al. 2007. A randomized study of out-of-hospital continuous positive airway pressure for acute cardiogenic pulmonary oedema: physiological and clinical effects. *European Heart Journal*, *23*, pp. 2895–2901. Available at: https://pubmed.ncbi.nlm.nih.gov/17967821/
22. Fuller, G.W., Keating, S., Goodacre, S. et al. Prehospital continuous positive airway pressure for acute respiratory failure: the ACUTE feasibility RCT. *Health Technology Assessment*, 2021, *25*(7), 1.
23. Rochwerg, B., Brochard, L., Elliott, M.W. et al. 2017. Official ERS/ATS clinical practice guidelines: noninvasive ventilation for acute respiratory failure. *European Respiratory Journal*, *50*(2). Available at: https://pubmed.ncbi.nlm.nih.gov/28860265/
24. Kinnear, W. 2002. Non-invasive ventilation in acute respiratory failure. BTS Guidance. *Thorax*, *57*(3). Available at: https://thorax.bmj.com/content/57/3/192
25. Alzahri, M.S., Rohra, A. and Peacock, W.F., 2016. Nitrates as a treatment of acute heart failure. *Cardiac Failure Review*, *2*(1), p. 51.

26. DiDomenico, R.J., Park, H.Y., Southworth, M.R. et al. 2004. Guidelines for acute decompensated heart failure treatment. *Annals of Pharmacotherapy*, *38*(4). Available at: https://journals.sagepub.com/doi/abs/10.1345/aph.1D481
27. Wakai, A., Mccabe, A., Kidney, R. et al. 2013. Nitrates for acute heart failure syndromes. *Cochrane Database of Systematic Reviews*, *2013*(8). Available at: https://www.cochranelibrary.com/cdsr/doi/10.1002/14651858.CD005151.pub2/full
28. Miró, Ò., Llorens, P., Freund, Y. et al. 2021. Early intravenous nitroglycerin use in prehospital setting and in the emergency department to treat patients with acute heart failure: insights from the EAHFE Spanish registry. *International Journal of Cardiology*, *344*, pp. 127–134.
29. Patrick, C., Ward, B., Anderson, J. et al. 2020. Feasibility, effectiveness and safety of prehospital intravenous bolus dose nitroglycerin in patients with acute pulmonary edema. *Prehospital Emergency Care*, *24*(6), pp. 844–850.
30. Abdelmoneum, M.S., Eitta, M.I., Elrabat, K.A. et al. 2022. Bolus versus continuous infusion of nitroglycerin for the treatment of acute hypertensive heart failure. *International Journal of the Cardiovascular Academy*, *8*(1), p.14.

SECTION 4

Disability

Approach to an Altered Level of Consciousness

15

Luke De La Rue and Natalie Lavergne

In this chapter you will learn:
- Considerations to scene approach in patients with an altered level of consciousness
- An approach to undifferentiated altered level of consciousness
- General end points to consider when managing altered level of consciousness
- Best practice for the management of seizures and status epilepticus
- Other clinical syndromes to consider in seizure management.

Case Details

Dispatch
63-year-old male, found on the ground, altered conscious state, spontaneously breathing.

History
A 63-year-old man was found by his wife in the shed behind their house. She called an ambulance and reported that she last saw him well a few hours previously, then found him lying on the ground, making groaning noises. A double-crewed ambulance and a critical care paramedic are dispatched to the case.

On Arrival of the First Crew
The patient is lying on his side on the ground. His primary survey findings and initial vital signs are:

Airway	Requiring jaw thrust
Breathing	RR 28, SpO$_2$ 88% on air
Circulation	Peripheral pulses present, HR 130, regular, BP 165/90, warm peripheries
Disability	GCS E1, V2, M5 (8), pupils 5 mm and equally reactive, BGL 4.5 mmol/L
Environmental	Temp 36.5 °C

The crew that initially responds places the patient in a supine position and applies some jaw thrust, which overcomes the noisy breathing. A non-rebreather mask (NRB) is also applied at 15 L/min. Further assessment does not demonstrate any obvious signs of injury. The patient

SECTION 4 Disability

groans and localises only to pain but does not open his eyes. His pupils are 5 mm and equally reactive.

On Your Arrival as the Critical Care Paramedic

The initial crew have placed a nasopharyngeal airway (NPA) and with ongoing oxygen supplementation via a NRB, the oxygen saturations are now 98%. They have already obtained a single point of IV access in the patient's cubital fossa.

AMPLE

Allergies	NKDA
Medications	Perindopril 4 mg PO daily
	Metformin 1 g PO BD
	Thiamine 100 mg PO daily
Past history	Hypertension, T2DM (NIDDM), daily EtOH use, current smoker
Last ins and outs	Unknown
Events prior	Found ALOC on the ground without obvious signs of trauma, was well earlier in the day

Decision Point
What are your clinical priorities in this situation?

Question 1: Are There any Hazards at the Scene?

No matter the chief complaint, it is vital that every emergency call begins with an assessment for hazards. There are many causes of an altered level of consciousness (ALOC), including medical, traumatic, environmental and psychological.[1,2] Many of these causes of ALOC also have the potential to affect emergency responders and so careful consideration should be given to the call details for potential risks.

An infectious prodrome must prompt the paramedic to assess the need for contact or droplet personal protective equipment (PPE). Traumatic causes, such as assault, injury in a confined space or while on challenging terrain, or injury resulting from structure collapse or falling debris, may present an ongoing risk to the responding crew. Paramedics should consider the need for police response, assistance from a technical response team and additional PPE, such as helmets or stab vests as the case warrants. Additionally, possible chemical and biological exposures in the patient with an ALOC must be considered as this too can pose a risk to first responders.[3]

PRACTICE TIP

Don't become a patient yourself; always take a moment to evaluate for risk of exposure before entering a scene.

CHAPTER 15   Approach to an Altered Level of Consciousness

Question 2: What Initial Assessments and Investigations Should Occur in the Patient with an Altered Level of Consciousness?

Depending on the definition that is used, ALOC accounts for between 5% and 40% of emergency department visits.[1] As a priority, initial clinical assessment with all patient encounters should focus on the identification of any immediately life-threatening conditions. Is the airway patent and unobstructed? Is breathing inadequate to sustain life? Is there evidence of life-threatening bleeding? Is circulation sufficient to support vital organ function? What is the patient's response to stimulus?

Once immediate life threats have been identified and managed, cardiac monitoring and a complete set of vital signs, consisting of a Glasgow Coma Scale (GCS) assessment, heart rate and quality, respiratory rate and effort, oxygen saturation, blood pressure, pupil assessment, temperature and a blood glucose level should also be obtained. With any luck, clues identified in this initial assessment will assist in narrowing down the myriad possible differential diagnoses.

Having a structured approach to history gathering and physical assessment can aid in identifying signs and symptoms related to the patient's condition and assist in the formulation of a working diagnosis. Memory aids such as AEIOU-TIPS (**Figure 15.1**) can further assist in recalling the many potential causes of ALOC.

A	Alcohol
	Acidosis
	Ammonia
	Arrhythmias
E	Endocrine
	Electrolytes
	Encephalopathy
I	Infection
O	Oxygen
	Opiates
	Overdose
U	Uraemia
	Underdose
T	Trauma
	Temperature
	Thiamine
I	Insulin
P	Poisoning
	Psychiatric
S	Stroke
	Seizure
	Syncope
	Space-occupying lesions
	Shunt (VP) malfunction

Figure 15.1   AEIOU-TIPS mnemonic for altered mental status.

SECTION 4 Disability

History gathering, including recent events, past medical history, medications and family history, may also provide clues to the diagnosis.[4] Ideally, collateral information should also be obtained from family members or friends if available at the scene. It is important to identify if the patient was complaining of any symptoms prior to the decrease in consciousness. Did the episode occur suddenly or were the changes more gradual? Was there an illness or event that may have preceded or precipitated the current condition? Is there a possibility that this is a self-harm event? If stroke is suspected, the time the patient was last seen well is of critical importance, as this directs the care that the patient may receive in hospital.[5]

When obtaining the patient's past medical history, attention must be made to risk factors for the causes of ALOC.[6] Identify if there is a known neurological, endocrine, metabolic, cardiac or psychiatric disorder. Has the patient had any recent illness, trauma or significant life events? Have they had any recent surgical procedures or hospitalisations? What drugs have they been prescribed, are they taking them as indicated and have there been any recent additions or dosage changes? It is also important to enquire about any over-the-counter drugs use, as well as alcohol and other substance or recreational drug use.

Physical examination should include a detailed neurological assessment.[6] Does the patient respond to voice or painful stimulus? Are there any appreciable spontaneous movements? Are there focal findings, lateralisation or abnormal movements? Are there signs of meningeal irritation? Are the pupils equal and reactive or is there deconjugate gaze? When suspecting a stroke syndrome, physical assessment should also include a validated stroke scale where possible; however, this may be difficult or impossible in a patient with ALOC.[5]

Terminology such as 'coma' versus 'stupor' or 'unconscious' versus 'unresponsive' can be confusing, and so avoidance of global terms in favour of descriptions of the patient's specific responses can be more helpful. Re-assessment throughout the case is important, as changes in neurological status can be subtle and herald further deterioration. Other physical findings that may help differentiate causes include breath and body odours, skin discolouration, trauma and indwelling medical devices or catheters. The absence of any abnormal physical findings does not preclude an organic cause.[5]

Unfortunately, paramedics have limited tools for investigating illness in the field. In a patient with an ALOC, it is essential to check the patient's blood glucose and obtain a 12-lead ECG. If access to point-of-care labs is available, assessment of electrolytes, complete blood count and blood gas monitoring can be of significant benefit.[5] Other tools, such as point-of-care ultrasound or EEG monitoring, may be useful to critical care crews when transport times to hospital are delayed.

Treatment for the patient with an ALOC of undetermined cause is largely supportive. Intubation may be performed for airway protection in those patients at high risk of soiled airway or further deterioration.[6,7] Ventilatory support may be required in the patient with inadequate respiratory effort, elevated pCO_2, or in whom maintaining tight control over pCO_2 is desired, supplemental oxygen should be given to target SpO_2 >94%.[7]

If organ perfusion is insufficient to maintain vital function, cardiac output may be improved through the administration of crystalloid, vasopressors or through arrhythmia management.[7] Targeting a mean arterial pressure (MAP) of greater than 65 mmHg is generally considered ideal.[6,7] Conversely, correcting hypertension is a difficult decision to make in the prehospital environment. Hypertension may be the cause of the altered mentation, such as in posterior reversible encephalopathy syndrome (PRES), or it may be the result of physiological compensation for poor cerebral perfusion.[6] Given this, pain and agitation should first be addressed before any antihypertensive medication is administered.[8]

Additionally, hypoglycaemia should be corrected and normothermia maintained.[7] Consider thiamine if there is a risk of Wernicke's encephalopathy.[9] Administration of naloxone may be reasonable in a patient with suspected opioid overdose, but caution should be used in patients with chronic use as an acute withdrawal syndrome can be precipitated.[6] If a working diagnosis can be made, refer to the appropriate clinical practice guideline for additional interventions and treatment goals.

Question 3: The Patient is Showing Signs of a Brain Injury or Stroke. What Management Strategies and Interventions Should be Considered?

Stroke and stroke-like illnesses must be high on the list of differentials when faced with a patient with altered mentation. According to 2020 statistics, cerebrovascular disease is the third leading cause of death in women and the fourth leading cause of death in men in Australia.[10] In a study by Völk et al., of patients presenting to the emergency department in coma where a cause could be determined, cerebrovascular disease was the most common underlying cause (24%), followed by seizures (13%), psychiatric (8%), metabolic (7%) and intoxication (7%).[2]

Clinical evaluation may lead to suspicion of either ischaemic stroke or haemorrhagic stroke, but with limited diagnostics in the prehospital environment, it is difficult to achieve diagnostic certainty. Given this, emergency medical systems should have guidelines in place to transport patients with a suspected stroke to a hospital capable of definitive treatment, be that surgery, thrombolysis or endovascular clot retrieval (ECR).[5,11]

Hypoxia, hypotension and hypercarbia can significantly worsen patient outcomes, so it is essential to support ventilation and oxygenation to maintain pCO_2 at 35–45 mmHg and SpO_2 >94%.[7,11] Blood pressure should be optimised to maintain adequate organ perfusion (MAP >65 mmHg), and in the case of raised intracranial pressure (ICP), higher targets may be considered.[8,11] In patients with suspected intracranial haemorrhage and an initial SBP of 150–220 mmHg, cautiously lowering this to 130–150 mmHg may reduce haematoma expansion.[11] Transport with the head of the stretcher elevated to 30 degrees, the patient's head in a midline position and reduction in external stimulus where possible is also important.[8]

Both ischaemic and haemorrhagic stroke may lead to the development of raised ICP. It is vital to monitor closely for seizures, changes in respiratory pattern, pupillary response and for widening pulse pressure. ICP may be temporarily reduced through the administration of osmotic agents.[11] Intravenous mannitol 0.5–1.0 g/kg/dose and 3% hypertonic saline 3–5 mL/kg/dose have been shown to be equivalent at lowering ICP.[8,12] Hypertonic saline, however, may be more practical to administer in the prehospital environment, as it is not crystallised at room temperature and is a smaller volume to carry. Additionally, moderate hyperventilation targeting a pCO_2 of 30–35 mmHg can be attempted as a bridge to urgent definitive care if clinical signs of herniation occur.[8]

SECTION 4 Disability

Question 4: The Patient Subsequently has Multiple Seizures on Route to Hospital. What is Considered Current Best Practice for the Management of Refractory Seizures and Status Epilepticus?

While most seizures are brief, self-limiting and do not require treatment, prolonged or refractory seizures require immediate intervention to prevent neuronal injury and other respiratory, cardiovascular and metabolic complications. The provision of best supportive care using basic resuscitation concepts while attempting to identify possible precipitants, especially hypoglycaemia, is the priority in the prehospital setting, in addition to prompt termination of seizure activity.[13]

Status epilepticus is the persistence of seizure activity for more than five minutes without spontaneous resolution, or a recurrence of seizure activity without recovery between seizures.[14] This constitutes a medical emergency, and an escalation of therapeutic interventions up to and including intubation and administration of anaesthetic agents may be required.

The widely accepted first-line management of refractory seizures includes the administration of a benzodiazepine. The wide variety of drug administration routes and drug choices in this class makes it an effective and rapid treatment option. The suggested benzodiazepine of choice in Australia is midazolam at 5–10 mg intravenously (dose adjust if <60 kg or frail; paediatric dose 0.15 mg/kg IV, maximum 10 mg).[15] Alternatively, diazepam 10 mg intravenously can be given (paediatric dose 0.1–0.25 mg/kg IV). If intravenous access cannot be rapidly obtained, then midazolam can be given intramuscularly (5 mg IM if <40 kg, 10 mg IM if >40 kg; paediatric dose 0.15–0.2 mg/kg IM, maximum 10 mg), buccally or intranasally (5–10 mg; paediatric dose 0.2–0.3 mg/kg, maximum 10 mg).[16] In patients with severe and recalcitrant seizure disorders, it is common for patient-specific management plans to exist that utilise these non-standard administration routes which can be commenced early by parents and carers prior to first responder arrival. Administration of these first-line agents should be repeated if seizure activity fails to resolve within five minutes of treatment.[15,16]

If the seizure does not cease promptly and the cause cannot be identified or readily reversed, then further treatment with an anti-epileptic drug is required.[17] Practice in this area has changed over recent years, largely due to the Established Status Epilepticus Treatment Trial (ESETT) published in 2019.[18] This randomised, double-blinded, multicentre trial compared the efficacy of levetiracetam, fosphenytoin and valproic acid for the treatment of status epilepticus in both adults and children. It demonstrated that levetiracetam was non-inferior in the treatment of status epilepticus. These findings were further supported by the ConSEPT and EcLiPSE trials published in *The Lancet* in 2019, which compared levetiracetam to phenytoin in the paediatric population.[19,20] As such, the use of levetiracetam as the initial second-line agent is now preferred in the hospital setting, as well as in the prehospital and retrieval environment, due to its more favourable side-effect profile and ease of preparation and administration. The dose of levetiracetam is 60 mg/kg (maximum 4.5 g) given intravenously over five minutes.[17] Alternative second-line agents still include sodium valproate 40 mg/kg IV (maximum 3 g over 5–10 minutes) and phenytoin 20 mg/kg IV (given no faster than 50 mg/minute).[17] However, particularly in the retrieval setting, phenytoin is not preferred, due to its adverse risk profile, which includes arrhythmias and hypotension, in addition to the need for a slower infusion rate.[17]

CHAPTER 15 Approach to an Altered Level of Consciousness

In the absence of second-line agents, or if the status epilepticus remains refractory to the aforementioned treatments, progression to rapid-sequence induction (RSI) to facilitate general anaesthesia may be required to treat ongoing seizure activity. While there is no robust randomised controlled data available to guide anaesthetic agents for refractory status epilepticus, most clinical guidelines advocate the use of propofol for induction and to maintain anaesthesia, as well as continuous midazolam infusion for ongoing sedation and the treatment of seizures.[21] Alternatively, phenobarbitone or thiopentone still remain an option though are now rarely used for this purpose in Australia as a third-line agent. Fourth-line therapies, such as continuous ketamine infusion, can also be considered, as well as combining additional second-line therapies.[17] If safe to do so, the avoidance of long-acting neuromuscular blockade post RSI allows for monitoring of ongoing seizure activity and the need for further escalations in treatment.[17]

Question 5: What Other Clinical Syndromes Should be Considered when Managing Patients with Refractory Seizures?

It is important to consider various clinical syndromes that may require a non-standard approach to seizure management due to their underlying causes. Hypoglycaemia is a critical consideration as it can both cause seizures and be a result of prolonged seizure activity. Prompt treatment and exclusion of hypoglycaemia should be a priority in all seizure cases, particularly in diabetics taking insulin and sulfonylureas, as well as in those who are fasting, alcoholics and in critical illness where patients may have impaired hepatic function.[22] Electrolyte disturbances, such as severe hyponatraemia, hypocalcaemia, hypomagnesaemia, and extreme hypo- or hyperkalaemia, can also lead to seizures.[23] Although identifying this is challenging in prehospital settings without point-of-care testing, the speed of replacement of these electrolytes should be considered based on the patient's fluid state and the likely chronicity of the electrolyte abnormality.

Traumatic brain injury (TBI) often results in seizures, and although the use of seizure prophylaxis in patients with intracranial haemorrhage is controversial and at this stage not recommended, prompt termination of seizures if they occur and subsequent prevention with second-line agents are recommended as part of standard neuroprotective measures.[24] Infections, particularly involving the central nervous system (CNS), such as meningitis and encephalitis, can also cause seizures and it is crucial to initiate appropriate resuscitation and facilitate urgent transport to a hospital for administration of antivirals, antibiotics and steroids.[25] Prompt treatment of bacterial meningitis significantly improves morbidity and mortality outcomes, so in remote areas, where appropriate parenteral therapy may be substantially delayed, ceftriaxone 2 g IV or IM can be administered in the prehospital setting if the index of suspicion is high.[25]

Toxicological causes should always be considered in seizure cases. Tricyclic antidepressants in particular carry a significant risk of mortality. Screening patients with an ECG can provide a clue to potential deterioration in these cases, and prompt administration of sodium bicarbonate, along with RSI, hyperventilation and circulatory support for massive overdoses, is often required.[16,26] Additionally, certain medications, such as anti-psychotics and atypical opioid analgesics (for example, tramadol), may lower the seizure threshold, and illicit drugs, such as amphetamines, cocaine, synthetic cathinones and other novel

SECTION 4 Disability

psychoactive substances, can also induce seizures through their stimulatory effects on the central nervous system.[27]

> **PRACTICE TIP**
>
> If you don't think about toxicological causes, you won't find them; always consider toxicology in a patient with an altered level of consciousness.

Withdrawal syndromes, usually associated with alcohol but also with the reduction or abrupt cessation of benzodiazepines or barbiturates, can result in refractory seizures. Drug interactions leading to serotonin syndrome, as well as environmental hyperthermia, can also trigger seizure activity and active cooling measures are essential in such cases.[28]

Finally, eclampsia must be considered in pregnant patients presenting with seizures. Rapid administration of magnesium for seizure termination is crucial, in addition to blood pressure control and expedited delivery.[29]

Key Evidence

Randomised Controlled Trials

Chamberlain, J, Kapur, J, Shinnar, S et al. 2020. Efficacy of levetiracetam, fosphenytoin, and valproate for established status epilepticus by age group (ESETT): a double-blind, responsive adaptive, randomized controlled trial, *Lancet*, 395(10231), pp. 1217–1224. Available at: https://doi.org/10.1016/S0140-6736(20)30611-5

Dalziel, S, Borland, M, Furyk, J et al. 2019. Levetiracetam versus phenytoin for second-line treatment of convulsive status epilepticus in children (ConSEPT): an open-label, multicentre, randomised controlled trial, *Lancet*, 393(10186), pp. 2135–2145. Available at: https://doi.org/10.1016/S0140-6736(19)30722-6

Lyttle, M, Rainford, N, Gamble, C et al. 2019. Levetiracetam versus phenytoin for second-line treatment of paediatric convulsive status epilepticus (EcLiPSE): a multicentre, open-label, randomised trial, *Lancet*, 393(10186), pp. 2125–2134. Available at: https://doi.org/10.1016/S0140-6736(19)30724-X

Clinical Guidelines

Brophy, G, Bell, R, Claassen, J et al. 2012. Guidelines for the evaluation and management of status epilepticus, *Neurocritical Care*, 17, pp. 3–23. Available at: https://doi.org/10.1007/s12028-012-9695-z

Glauser, T, Shinnar, S, Gloss, D et al. 2016. Evidence-based guideline: treatment of convulsive status epilepticus in children and adults: report of the Guideline Committee of the American Epilepsy Society, *Epilepsy Currents*, 16(1), pp. 48–61. Available at: https://doi.org/10.5698/1535-7597-16.1.48

Powers, W, Rabinstein, A, Ackerson et al. 2019. Guidelines for the early management of patients with acute ischemic stroke: 2019 update to the 2018 guidelines for the early management of acute ischemic stroke: a guideline for healthcare professionals from the American Heart Association/American Stroke Association, *Stroke*, 50, pp. e344–e418. Available at: https://doi.org/10.1161/STR.0000000000000211

Stevens, RD, Shoykhet, M and Cadena, R. 2015. Emergency neurological life support: intracranial hypertension and herniation, *Neurocritical Care*, 23(suppl 2), pp. 76–82. Available at: https://doi.org/10.1007/s12028-015-0168-z

> **PRACTICE TIP**
>
> Know your Clinical Practice Guidelines and anticipate the need for escalating treatment options in status epilepticus.

CHAPTER 15 Approach to an Altered Level of Consciousness

Self-Reflection Questions

1. In your region of practice, are there particular industrial locations that pose a threat of exposure? What are the likely causative agents and how will you mitigate the risk?
2. Have you developed a structured approach to the assessment and management of a patient with ALOC, and how does it differ depending on your location of work?
3. Do you carry any point-of-care devices in your practice, and how do you apply them to patients with undifferentiated ALOC?
4. Do you carry second-line anti-epileptic drugs in your practice and, if not, what is your alternate management approach to refractory status epilepticus?
5. What are your thresholds for intubation in status epilepticus, and how do they change based on transport duration and platform used in your practice?

References

1. Jung, S, Jeon, J, Jung, C et al. 2020. The etiologies of altered level of consciousness in the emergency department, *Journal of Neurocritical Care*, 13(2), pp. 86–92. Available at: https://doi.org/10.18700/jnc.200010
2. Völk, S, Koedel, U, Pfister, H et al. 2019. Impaired consciousness in the emergency department, *European Neurology*, 80(3–4), pp. 179–186. Available at: https://doi.org/10.1159/000495363>
3. Domres, B, Taalab, Y and Hecker, N. 2021. CBRNE and decontamination, in Pikoulis, E and Doucet, J (eds), *Emergency Medicine, Trauma and Disaster Management. Hot Topics in Acute Care Surgery and Trauma*, Springer, Cham. Available at: https://doi.org/10.1007/978-3-030-34116-9_35
4. Wijdicks, E. 2010. The bare essentials: coma, *Practical Neurology*, 10(1), pp. 51–60. Available at: https://doi.org/10.1136/jnnp.2009.200097
5. Powers, W, Rabinstein, A, Ackerson, T et al. 2019. Guidelines for the early management of patients with acute ischemic stroke: 2019 update to the 2018 guidelines for the early management of acute ischemic stroke: a guideline for healthcare professionals from the American Heart Association/American Stroke Association, *Stroke*, 50, pp. e344–e418. Available at: https://doi.org/10.1161/STR.0000000000000211
6. Farkas, J, 2022. Approach to coma and stupor, Internet Book of Critical Care [online]. Available at: https://emcrit.org/ibcc/coma/
7. Traub, S and Wijdicks, E. 2016. Initial diagnosis and management of coma, *Emergency Medicine Clinics of North America*, 34(4), pp. 777–793. Available at: https://doi.org/10.1016/j.emc.2016.06.017
8. Stevens, R, Shoykhet, M and Cadena, R. 2015. Emergency neurological life support: intracranial hypertension and herniation, *Neurocritical Care*, 23(suppl 2), pp. 76–82. Available at: https://doi.org/10.1007/s12028-015-0168-z
9. Therapeutic Guidelines 2023, *Water-soluble Vitamin Deficiencies - Thiamine Supplementation in Adults*, eTG. Available at: https://tgldcdp.tg.org.au.acs.hcn.com.au/viewTopic?etgAccess=true&guidelinePage=Gastrointestinal&topicfile=c_GIG_Gastro-oesophageal-reflux-in-adultstopic_1&guidelinename=auto&sectionId=c_GIG_Water-soluble-vitamin-deficienciestopic_3#c_GIG_Water-soluble-vitamin-deficienciestopic_3
10. Australian Institute of Health and Welfare. 2022. *Deaths in Australia,* AIHW [online]. Available at: https://www.aihw.gov.au/reports-data/australias-health
11. Greenberg, S, Ziai, W, Cordonnier, C et al. 2022. 2022 Guideline for the management of patients with spontaneous intracerebral hemorrhage: a guideline from the American Heart Association/American Stroke Association, *Stroke*, 53, pp. e282–e361. Available at: https://doi.org/10.1161/STR.0000000000000407
12. Brophy, G and Human, T. 2017. Pharmacotherapy pearls for emergency neurological life support, *Neurocritical Care*, 27(suppl 1), pp. 51–73. Available at: https://doi.org/10.1007/s12028-017-0456-x
13. Epilepsy Action Australia. 2020. *What Is Epilepsy?* [online]. Available at: https://www.epilepsy.org.au/about-epilepsy/understanding-epilepsy/what-is-epilepsy/

SECTION 4 Disability

14. Trinka, E, Cock, H, Hesdorffer, D et al. A definition and classification of status epilepticus—Report of the ILAE Task Force on Classification of Status Epilepticus. *Epilepsia*. , 2015, 56(10), pp. 1515-1523.
15. Ambulance Victoria. 2020. *Clinical Practice Guidelines: Seizures*. Available at: https://cpg.ambulance.vic.gov.au/#/tabs/tab-0/info
16. Therapeutic Guidelines 2020. *Tricyclic Antidepressant (TCA) Poisoning*, eTG. Available at: https://tgldcdp.tg.org.au.acs.hcn.com.au/viewTopic?etgAccess=true&guidelinePage=Toxicology%20and%20Toxinology&topicfile=toxicology-TCA&guidelinename=Toxicology%20and%20Toxinology&sectionId=toc_d1e183#toc_d1e183/
17. Therapeutic Guidelines 2022. *Acute Management of Seizures and Status Epilepticus*, eTG. Available at: <https://tgldcdp.tg.org.au.acs.hcn.com.au/viewTopic?topicfile=acute-management-of-seizures-and-status-epilepticus&guidelineName=Neurology&topicNavigation=navigateTopic/>
18. Chamberlain, J, Kapur, J, Shinnar, S et al. 2020. Efficacy of levetiracetam, fosphenytoin, and valproate for established status epilepticus by age group (ESETT): a double-blind, responsive-adaptive, randomized controlled trial, *Lancet*, 395(10231), pp. 1217–1224. Available at: https://doi.org/10.1016/S0140-6736(20)30611-5
19. Dalziel, S, Borland, M, Furyk, J et al. 2019. Levetiracetam versus phenytoin for second-line treatment of convulsive status epilepticus in children (ConSEPT): an open-label, multicentre, randomised controlled trial, *Lancet*, 393(10186), pp. 2135–2145. Available at: https://doi.org/10.1016/S0140-6736(19)30722-6
20. Lyttle, M, Rainford, N, Gamble, C et al. 2019. Levetiracetam versus phenytoin for second-line treatment of paediatric convulsive status epilepticus (EcLiPSE): a multicentre, open-label, randomised trial, *Lancet*, 393(10186), pp. 2125–2134. Available at: https://doi.org/10.1016/S0140-6736(19)30724-X
21. Glauser, T, Shinnar, S, Gloss, D et al. 2016. Evidence-based guideline: treatment of convulsive status epilepticus in children and adults: report of the Guideline Committee of the American Epilepsy Society, *Epilepsy Currents*, 16(1), pp. 48–61. Available at: https://doi.org/10.5698/1535-7597-16.1.48
22. Joint British Diabetes Societies Inpatient Care Group. 2023. *The Hospital Management of Hypoglycaemia in Adults with Diabetes Mellitus* [online]. Available at: https://diabetes-resources-production.s3.eu-west-1.amazonaws.com/resources-s3/public/2023-03/JBDS%2001%20Hypo%20Guideline%20with%20qr%20code.pdf
23. Nickson, C. 2020. Hyponatraemia, *Life in the Fast Lane* [Online]. Available at: https://litfl.com/hyponatraemia/
24. Carney, N, Totten, A, O'Reilly, C et al. 2017. Guidelines for the management of severe traumatic brain injury, *Neurosurgery*, 80(1), pp. 6–15. Available at: https://10.1093/neuros/nyx148
25. Therapeutic Guidelines 2022. *Meningitis*, eTG. Available at: https://tgldcdp.tg.org.au.acs.hcn.com.au/viewTopic?etgAccess=true&guidelinePage=Antibiotic&topicfile=meningitis&guidelinename=Antibiotic&sectionId=toc_d1e134#toc_d1e134/.
26. Nickson, C. 2023. Status epilepticus, *Life in the Fast Lane* [Online]. Available at: https://litfl.com/status-epilepticus/
27. Wolfe, C, Wood, D, Dines, A et al. 2019. Seizures as a complication of recreational drug use: analysis of the Euro-DEN Plus data-set, *Neurotoxicology*, 73, pp. 183–187. Available at: https://10.1016/j.neuro.2019.02.008
28. Buckley, N, Dawson, A and Isbister, G. 2014. Serotonin syndrome, *British Medical Journal*, 348, pp. g1626. Available at: https://10.1016/j.neuro.2019.02.008
29. The Royal Women's Hospital. 2020. Magnesium sulphate – management of hypertensive disorders of pregnancy. Available at: https://thewomens.r.worldssl.net/images/uploads/downloadable-records/clinical-guidelines/magnesium-sulphate-management-of-hypertensive-disorders-of-pregnancy_280720.pdf

Severe Traumatic Brain Injury

16

*James Manktelow and Virginia Newcombe**

In this chapter you will learn:
- How to assess a traumatic brain injury (TBI)
- Early recognition and identification of key head injury red flags
- Neuroprotective measures to prevent secondary injury
- Preparation for appropriate further care and transfer of patients with severe TBI.

Case Details

Dispatch
70-year-old female, fallen down one flight of stairs, unconscious.

History
A 70-year-old female was found at the bottom of a flight of stairs by her husband after he heard a noise. Her husband called for an ambulance and advised the call-taker that the patient had blood on her head and face, as well as a bleeding nose. She had also recently been unwell with a urinary tract infection. She was groaning but by the time of the call was not answering any of her husband's questions. A double-crewed ambulance and a critical care paramedic are dispatched.

On Arrival of the First Crew
The scene is safe and the patient is lying on her side at the foot of a staircase. There is an obvious scalp wound with a large pool of blood on the floor. There is some slight bleeding from her nose. The patient's primary survey findings and initial vital signs are:

---

*Declarations: JM has no DOI to declare. VFJN reports holding a grant with Roche Pharmaceuticals on biomarkers which is unrelated to this chapter and is supported by a National Institute for Health and Care Research (NIHR) Advanced Fellowship. VFJN was a member of the Update Committee for the below NICE Guideline and represented the Royal College of Emergency Medicine to review the UK Concussion Guidelines for Grassroots Sport.

The head injury: assessment and early management guideline referred to in this chapter was produced by the National Institute for Health and Care Excellence (NICE). The views expressed in this article are those of the authors and not necessarily those of NICE.

National Institute for Health and Care Excellence (2023) Head injury: assessment and early management. Available from https://www.nice.org.uk/guidance/ng232

SECTION 4   Disability

Airway	Patent
Breathing	RR 13–16, irregular, SpO$_2$ 88% on air
Circulation	Peripheral pulses present, HR 54, BP 110/55, warm peripheries
Disability	GCS E3, V4, M5 (12), pupils 3 mm and sluggish, BGL 6.3 mmol/L
Environmental	Temp 37.1 °C

On Your Arrival as the Critical Care Paramedic

The initial paramedic crew are struggling to manage the patient, as she is agitated and combative. They have been unable to maintain spinal precautions.

AMPLE

This patient has a past medical history of atrial fibrillation. She is on bisoprolol and apixaban.

Allergies	NKDA
Medications	Bisoprolol 5 mg Apixaban 5 mg twice daily
Past history	Atrial fibrillation
Last ins and outs	Normal
Events	Fall down one flight of stairs

Decision Point 1

What are your clinical priorities in this situation?

With the decreased GCS she needs to be assessed for a potential TBI. She also needs to have the scalp wound bleeding stopped. Her agitation may make management difficult.

As you are trying to put pressure on her scalp wound, she becomes more obtunded, with a GCS of 8 (E1, V2, M5). You notice her right pupil is 4 mm larger than the left and is not reactive.

Decision Point 2

What is your provisional diagnosis and plan of action?

This patient likely has a space-occupying lesion causing raised intracranial pressure. She needs urgent management for raised intracranial pressure (ICP), rapid sequence induction for intubation and to be conveyed to a centre capable of neurosurgery as soon as possible.

PRACTICE TIPS

For patients with a severe TBI, even with a GCS of 3, always give appropriate RSI induction agents to present uncontrolled rises in ICP on laryngoscopy.

CHAPTER 16   Severe Traumatic Brain Injury

Question 1: How Should a Patient with Suspected Severe TBI be Assessed?

After initial assessment and correction of any issues involving airway, breathing and circulation, a neurological assessment should be performed. The aims of this assessment are to determine the level of consciousness and to note the presence or absence of focal or lateralising neurological signs. This usually comprises an assessment of consciousness via the Glasgow Coma Score (GCS), pupillary assessment and neurological examination for focal neurology. Key components are discussed below, and the GCS is described in **Table 16.1**.

Table 16.1   Components of the Glasgow Coma Score

Best response	Eye response	Verbal response	Motor response
1	No eye opening	No verbal response	No motor response
2	To pain	Incomprehensible words	Extension response to pain
3	To verbal command	Inappropriate words	Flexion response to pain
4	Spontaneously	Confused	Withdraws from pain
5	N/A	Orientated	Localises pain
6	N/A	N/A	Obeys command

The Glasgow Coma Score was first published in 1974 by Graham Teasdale and Bryan Jennett. It was developed specifically for patients after trauma with suspected traumatic brain injury and is the most commonly used scale to assess the level of consciousness/depth of coma for these patients.[1,2] The GCS ranges from 3 to 15 and may be used to categorise TBI severity; classically mild TBI is considered GCS 12 to 15, moderate 9 to 12 and severe 8 and below. However, GCS 13 patients are considered in some guidelines to be moderate, given their higher mortality compared to patients with a higher GCS.[3] It is important to note each component of the GCS individually, as in the context of TBI, the motor score contains the most prognostic information.[4] It has previously been common teaching that a GCS of 8 or below requires intubation and ventilation; however, increasingly it is recognised that some patients with a low GCS due to a known and reversible cause (such as a sedative drug overdose) may not benefit from intubation, whereas a combative, agitated, hypoxic patient with a severe TBI and GCS of 12 may benefit from intubation. It should also be considered in patients at risk of neuro-worsening (a drop on the GCS of 2 or more points) and who have other extracranial injuries that require intubation to aid management.

PRACTICE TIP

Older patients with TBI may have a discordantly high GCS at the scene of the accident in relation to the severity of the injury shown on subsequent neuro-imaging. Be mindful of this when deciding treatment and disposition.

SECTION 4 Disability

Pupillary reaction to light, size and symmetry should be assessed regularly. A difference of >1 mm in diameter is considered abnormal. Raised ICP may cause herniation of the uncus of the temporal lobe through the tentorial notch, which leads to compression of cranial nerve three (oculomotor nerve), causing dilation (mydriasis) and loss of pupil reactivity ('blown pupil'). Direct trauma to the eye may also cause mydriasis, although in the context of suspected TBI it should be assumed that it is secondary to raised ICP until proven otherwise.

> **PRACTICE TIP**
>
> If a patient has a fixed and dilated pupil that does not become reactive after a single dose of mannitol or hypertonic saline, a second dose can be considered.

Where possible, a brief neurological assessment should be performed looking for any evidence of focal abnormalities. Concurrent spinal fractures and/or cord injuries are relatively common, with 18% of patients who required critical care management for TBI having a spinal injury (unspecified) in a large European cohort study (CENTER-TBI).[5] Assume all patients with a head injury have fractures of the spine (especially c-spine) until this is ruled out. Noting the presence or absence of limb movement (and power if you are able to ascertain this) prior to intubation can be particularly useful in patients who may have spinal cord injury.

A head-to-toe assessment should be performed. Other signs of potential head injury/TBI may include:

- Signs of base of skull fractures – periorbital haematomas, mastoid bruising, CSF rhinorrhoea or otorrhoea.
- Open injuries of the cranial vault with CSF leakage or cerebral debris (particularly after gunshot wounds or stabbing).
- Maxillofacial injuries and injuries to the eyes.

Question 2: What Is the Epidemiology of TBI and how may this Affect Presentation and Assessment in the Prehospital Environment?

Traditionally TBI was considered to be predominantly a younger adult disease with a smaller peak of older patients. However, there is clear and consistent evidence worldwide, especially in higher income countries, that older people now comprise the largest group and the numbers are rising.[6] Younger patients tend to sustain a TBI secondary to high-velocity injuries (such as road traffic collisions) and assaults.[5] In contrast, older people will more commonly have low-velocity falls from standing or heights (for example, falling down stairs/ladders).

Consideration of mechanism is important for both the TBI and the likely pattern of extra-cranial injury. Fall-related TBIs more commonly result in mass lesions, such as contusions and/or subdural haemorrhage, with lower rates of intraparenchymal injuries.[7] Alcohol has been found to contribute to falls twice as often as road traffic incidents and may also confound

CHAPTER 16 Severe Traumatic Brain Injury

GCS measurement, making it artificially low for a given injury.[5,8] In the elderly, there is a lower incidence of raised ICP, which is thought to be secondary to age-related cerebral atrophy, although the incidence of post-traumatic seizures is higher.[6] Motor vehicle accident-related TBIs more commonly result in or have a component of traumatic (diffuse) axonal injury, and there is also an increased incidence of extradural haematoma.[9]

Higher morbidity and mortality rates among older versus younger individuals with TBI may contribute to an assumption of futility about aggressive management of the elderly patient with TBI. However, it is important to be mindful of this being a potential self-fulfilling prophecy, where older patients are denied aggressive treatment, including transfer to neurosurgical centres, operations or monitoring for example, purely on an age basis rather than being evidence based.[10] Elderly patients may also have an increased incidence of co-morbidities and, in particular, antiplatelet and anticoagulant use. Use of these is associated with higher rates of haemorrhagic progression and expansion of extra-axial lesions.[11] In addition, it is the extent of frailty rather than simply chronological age that may be a more important predictor of outcome.[12] As most interventional studies have inclusion criteria with age cut-offs of 60 or 65 years, there is little evidence to help guide the treatment for older patients.

Current prehospital triage systems, having been designed to identify those at significant risk after high-velocity injuries and in younger populations, are consequently poor at identifying the elderly at risk of injuries.[13] In addition, the GCS may be inappropriately high in older patients, where they may present with a higher GCS than younger patients for the same injury severity seen on computed tomography.[14] Under-triaging secondary to these factors may lead to treatment by less experienced staff and a delay in appropriate treatments and transfers to major trauma and neurosurgical centres.[14]

PRACTICE TIPS

Ketamine will (in general) reduce ICP. There was an old belief that it would increase ICP but there is much evidence in the TBI setting that this is not true, and it can be safely given.

Question 3: What Are the 'Red Flags' with TBI and how can they be Managed in the Prehospital Environment?

'Red flags' are symptoms and signs that indicate the need for a patient to be assessed in an emergency department. These are listed in **Table 16.2**. In some patient groups it can be particularly challenging to decide whether transport to hospital is required. For example, patients with cognitive impairment or dementia who live in nursing homes where it is unclear if they hit their heads, or patients on anticoagulants with no other signs of a head injury and a fall that was not witnessed. In these cases, a shared decision-making approach may be warranted, where the healthcare professional and patient or their 'next of care' work together to make an informed decision. If in doubt, a cautious approach with further assessment is advised.

SECTION 4 Disability

Table 16.2 Red flags indicating patients who should be referred to the emergency department (ED) for hospital assessment

Management	Clinical signs and symptoms since the injury
Refer/transport to an ED if there is:	• GCS less than 15 on initial assessment • Any loss of consciousness because of the injury (even if now alert) • Focal neurological deficit • Suspicion of skull fracture or penetrating head injury • Amnesia (pre- or post injury) • Persistent headache • Any vomiting episodes since the injury (clinical judgement should be used for those <12 years old) • Seizure • Any previous brain injury • High-energy head injury • History of bleeding or clotting disorder • Current anticoagulant and antiplatelet (except aspirin monotherapy) treatment • Current drug or alcohol intoxication • Safeguarding concerns • Ongoing concern of the professional about the diagnosis
In the absence of the above, consider referral if there is:	• Irritability or altered behaviour • Visible trauma to the head of concern to the assessing clinician • No one able to observe the patient at home • Ongoing concern from the patient or patient's family/carer concerning diagnosis

Source: National Institute for Health and Care Excellence. Head injury: Assessment and early management [NG232]. 2023. Available at: https://www.nice.org.uk/guidance/ng232

Question 4: What Are the Basic Physiological and Pathophysiological Principles After a Severe TBI that Underpin Early Management Strategies?

Primary injury refers to the injury that occurs at the time of impact from the biomechanical forces of the impact, including acceleration–deceleration forces, direct blow to the head, penetrating force or blast. Types of injury include skull fracture, contusion, extra-axial haematomas, vascular injuries, subarachnoid haemorrhage and diffuse axonal injury. Secondary brain injuries are the indirect damage that occurs after the initial insult from evolving pathophysiological consequences which worsen the brain injury. Causes include inadequate cerebral perfusion, hypoxia, hypoglycaemia, seizures, raised ICP and cerebral oedema. Therefore, many of the principles of early management are aimed at maintaining normal physiology and adequate cerebral perfusion in the acute phase after TBI to prevent secondary injury where possible. This is important, for

CHAPTER 16 Severe Traumatic Brain Injury

example, as there is consistent evidence that even a single episode of early hypoxia and/or hypotension is associated with an increased probability of worse long-term outcomes.[6]

Intracranial pressure may become elevated after a TBI. In the hyperacute phase this is often due to the presence of a space-occupying lesion, including an extradural haematoma or an acute subdural haematoma, although cerebral oedema in severe cases may also be rapid. If there is a high ICP, cerebral perfusion pressure (CPP) may become low, leading to cerebral ischemia. The relationship of CPP to blood pressure and ICP is as follows:

Cerebral perfusion pressure (CPP) = mean arterial pressure (MAP) − intracranial pressure (ICP)

Many treatments are therefore aimed at ensuring that intracranial pressure is maintained within safe limits and that blood pressure is high enough to maintain CPP.

Question 5: What Can be done to Aid Neuroprotection and Help Prevent Brain Injury Progression in the Prehospital Environment?

There are several measures that can be performed in the prehospital environment that may help to avoid extension of secondary injury in those with an acute brain injury of any aetiology. These include the following.

- Sit the patient up at 30–45 degrees to improve cerebral venous drainage. If this is not possible due to other injuries and/or transport requirements, when it is feasible, the entire bed can be tilted.
- Avoid jugular compression by facing the head forward.
- Ensure any ties for the endotracheal tube and the cervical spine collar are not too tight, as they may impede venous return.
- Aim for normocapnia with ventilation ($EtCO_2$ 30–33.8 mmHg).[15] The correlation between arterial and end-tidal CO_2 may be reduced in patients with significant physiological or anatomical derangement – for example, in those with significant chest trauma.[16]
- Ensure adequate sedation and analgesia.
- Consider maintaining paralysis.
- Avoid hypoxia.
- Avoid hypotension. If there is no concern for major haemorrhage (where a high blood pressure may drive further bleeding), aim for a MAP target >80–90 mmHg, where feasible. This may assist adequate cerebral perfusion in the context of (as yet) unknown raised intracranial pressure.
- Ensure blood glucose is within the normal range.
- Ensure adequate fluid resuscitation. Normal saline is the crystalloid of choice in patients with TBI, and there is randomised controlled trial evidence supporting use of normal saline in this context.[17,18]

SECTION 4 Disability

Question 6: What Are Signs of Raised Intracranial Pressure and What can be done in the Prehospital Environment to Reduce it?

Acute signs of raised ICP include:

- Headache
- Nausea and vomiting
- Restlessness/agitation
- Drowsiness (including worsening GCS)
- Abnormal posturing – decerebrate (abnormal flexion/flexor posturing) or decorticate (abnormal extension/extensor posturing)
- Sluggish, dilated pupil(s) that may become fixed ('blown pupil'); may be unilateral or bilateral (may progress from one to the other)
- Cushing's response – a triad of systolic hypertension, bradycardia and irregular breathing, which indicates impending coning (cerebral herniation through the foramen magnum causing brainstem compression). This may be masked somewhat in the context of a patient being on a beta-blocker. However, they tend to become more bradycardic than at their baseline.

Raised intracranial pressure is a time-critical emergency and a list of potential steps may be seen in **Figure 16.1**.

In the case of raised intracranial pressure, consider doing any/all of the following.

- Ensure basic neuroprotective measures are being followed (for example, raise head and ensure collar or ETT ties are not causing venous obstruction).
- Increase sedation.
- Administer a bolus of hypertonic saline or mannitol. These may be repeated if necessary and in case of a long transfer time.
- In the out-of-hospital setting hyperventilation to as low as 22 mmHg may be life saving while waiting for definitive management to reduce ICP. It should be carried out for as short a period as possible (30 minutes or less), as it may lead to brain ischaemia and is associated with poorer outcomes.
- Increase FiO_2 to 1.0 (which may help mitigate against ischaemia).
- Administer a 500 mL cold normal saline bolus if available.
- Paralyse if the patient is not already so.
- Consider a thiopentone bolus (1–2 mg/kg IV or 125 mg).
- Pre-alert the expecting ED at the earliest opportunity that emergent CT head and neurosurgical intervention may be required.

Figure 16.1 Emergent management of raised intracranial pressure.

Osmotherapy is typically given, with the most common form being mannitol (0.25–2.0 g/kg, usually given as a 20% solution) or hypertonic saline (HTS) to help reduce acute rises in ICP. HTS is available in different concentrations, from 3% up to 28.4%; usual doses are

CHAPTER 16   Severe Traumatic Brain Injury

approximately 2 mL/kg of 5% saline or 10 mL/kg of 28.4% HTS. In practice, it is common to give mannitol or the lower-concentration HTS solutions (7.5% and below) on presentation of a patient before central venous access has been established.

> **PRACTICE TIP**
>
> If mannitol is given and the transfer time to a hospital environment is long, the osmotic diuresis should be anticipated and early fluid resuscitation commenced.

The exact mechanism of action for osmotherapy is unclear. Traditionally such therapy is thought to raise plasma osmolality and so cause an osmotic withdrawal of cerebral water through an intact blood–brain barrier. However, it may also reduce erythrocyte and endothelial cell size, improve erythrocyte deformability and affect leucocyte adhesion. These effects are believed to contribute to improved microvascular flow.

The osmotic diuresis after mannitol administration may lead to hypernatraemia, intravascular depletion and hypotension. It is important to anticipate this and to consider starting adequate fluid resuscitation. These side-effects mean it is increasingly common for HTS to be used; however, it is unclear which (if either) is better to improve outcome after TBI. An RCT comparing management with either mannitol or HTS is currently under way in the UK (Sugar or Salt (SOS), Registration Number: ISRCTN16075091; https://warwick.ac.uk/fac/sci/med/research/ctu/trials/sos/).

Key Evidence

Systematic Review/Meta-Analyses

Alqurashi N, Alotaibi A, Bell S et al. The diagnostic accuracy of prehospital triage tools in identifying patients with traumatic brain injury: A systematic review. *Injury*. 2022;53(6):2060–2068. Available at: https://pubmed.ncbi.nlm.nih.gov/35190184/

Fuller G, Pandor A, Essat M et al. Diagnostic accuracy of prehospital triage tools for identifying major trauma in elderly injured patients: A systematic review. *Journal of Trauma and Acute Care Surgery*. 2021;90(2):403–412. Available at: https://pubmed.ncbi.nlm.nih.gov/33502151/

Lamperti M, Lobo FA, Tufegdzic B. Salted or sweet? Hypertonic saline or mannitol for treatment of intracranial hypertension. *Current Opinions on Anaesthesiology*. 2022;35(5):555–561. Available at: https://pubmed.ncbi.nlm.nih.gov/35787533/

Randomised Controlled Trials

CRASH-3 Collaborators. Effects of tranexamic acid on death, disability, vascular occlusive events and other morbidities in patients with acute traumatic brain injury (CRASH-3): A randomised, placebo-controlled trial. *Lancet*. 2019;394(10210):1713–1723. Available at: https://pubmed.ncbi.nlm.nih.gov/31623894/

Rowell SE, Meier EN, McKnight B et al. Effect of out-of-hospital tranexamic acid vs placebo on 6-month functional neurologic outcomes in patients with moderate or severe traumatic brain injury. *JAMA*. 2020;324(10):961–974. Available at: https://pubmed.ncbi.nlm.nih.gov/32897344/

Zampieri FG, Machado FR, Biondi RS et al. Effect of slower vs faster intravenous fluid bolus rates on mortality in critically ill patients: The BaSICS randomized clinical trial. *JAMA*. 2021;326(9):830–838. Available at: https://pubmed.ncbi.nlm.nih.gov/34547081/

SECTION 4   Disability

Guidelines for TBI Management

Hawryluk GWJ, Aguilera S, Buki A et al. A management algorithm for patients with intracranial pressure monitoring: The Seattle International Severe Traumatic Brain Injury Consensus Conference (SIBICC). *Intensive Care Medicine*. 2019;45:1783–1794.

National Institute for Health and Care Excellence. Head injury: Assessment and early management [NG232]. 2023. Available at: https://www.nice.org.uk/guidance/ng232

Self-Reflection Questions

1. How would you perform the initial assessment of a patient who may have a severe TBI?
2. What would you try to optimise in a patient with suspected TBI?
3. What things would you do if a patient developed unilateral or bilateral large non-reactive pupils?
4. What are potential differences between high- and low-velocity trauma?
5. These complex patients require a detailed handover when you arrive at the hospital. Using the table below, prepare a handover of the patient described using the IMIST AMBO format.

Introduction	
Mechanism	
Injuries	
Symptoms	
Treatment	
Allergies	
Medications	
Background history	
Other information	

References

1. Teasdale G, Jennett B. Assessment of coma and impaired consciousness. A practical scale. *Lancet*. 1974;2:81–84.
2. Mehta R, Chinthapalli K. Glasgow Coma Scale explained. *British Medical Journal*. 2019;365:1296.
3. Haydel MJ, Lauro AJ. Assessment of traumatic brain injury, acute. BMJ Best Practice [online]. 2021. Available at: https://bestpractice.bmj.com/topics/en-gb/515
4. Dijkland SA, Helmrich I, Nieboer D et al. Outcome prediction after moderate and severe traumatic brain injury: External validation of two established prognostic models in 1742 European patients. *Journal of Neurotrauma*. 2021;38(10):1377–1388.
5. Steyerberg EW, Wiegers E, Sewalt C et al. Case-mix, care pathways, and outcomes in patients with traumatic brain injury in CENTER-TBI: A European prospective, multicentre, longitudinal, cohort study. *Lancet Neurology*. 2019;18(10):923–934.
6. Maas AIR, Menon DK, Manley GT et al. Traumatic brain injury: Progress and challenges in prevention, clinical care, and research. *Lancet Neurology*. 2022;21(11):1004–1060.
7. Stocchetti N, Paterno R, Citerio G et al. Traumatic brain injury in an aging population. *Journal of Neurotrauma*. 2012;29(6):1119–1125.
8. DiGiorgio AM, Wittenberg BA, Crutcher CL et al. The impact of drug and alcohol intoxication on Glasgow Coma Scale assessment in patients with traumatic brain injury. *World Neurosurgery*. 2020;135:e664–e670.

9. Gardner RC, Dams-O'Connor K, Morrissey MR et al. Geriatric traumatic brain injury: Epidemiology, outcomes, knowledge gaps, and future directions. *Journal of Neurotrauma*. 2018;35(7):889–906.
10. Giordano KR, Rojas-Valencia LM, Bhargava V et al. Beyond binary: Influence of sex and gender on outcome after traumatic brain injury. *Journal of Neurotrauma*. 2020;37(23):2454–2459.
11. Mathieu F, Guting H, Gravesteijn B et al. Impact of antithrombotic agents on radiological lesion progression in acute traumatic brain injury: A CENTER-TBI propensity-matched cohort analysis. *Journal of Neurotrauma*. 2020;37(19):2069–2080.
12. Galimberti S, Graziano F, Maas AIR et al. Effect of frailty on 6-month outcome after traumatic brain injury: A multicentre cohort study with external validation. *Lancet Neurology*. 2022;21(2):153–162.
13. Fuller G, Pandor A, Essat M et al. Diagnostic accuracy of prehospital triage tools for identifying major trauma in elderly injured patients: A systematic review. *Journal of Trauma and Acute Care Surgery*. 2021;90(2):403–412.
14. Kehoe A, Smith JE, Bouamra O et al. Older patients with traumatic brain injury present with a higher GCS score than younger patients for a given severity of injury. *Emergency Medicine Journal*. 2016; 33(6):381–385.
15. Lockey DJ, Crewdson K, Davies G et al. AAGBI: Safer pre-hospital anaesthesia 2017: Association of Anaesthetists of Great Britain and Ireland. *Anaesthesia*. 2017;72(3):379–390.
16. Price J, Sandbach DD, Ercole A et al. End-tidal and arterial carbon dioxide gradient in serious traumatic brain injury after prehospital emergency anaesthesia: A retrospective observational study. *Emergency Medicine Journal*. 2020;37(11):674–679.
17. Zampieri FG, Machado FR, Biondi RS et al. Effect of intravenous fluid treatment with a balanced solution vs 0.9% saline solution on mortality in critically ill patients: The BaSICS randomized clinical trial. *JAMA*. 2021;326(9):1–12.
18. Hammond NE, Zampieri FG, Di Tanna GL et al. Balanced crystalloids versus saline in critically ill adults – A systematic review with meta-analysis. *NEJM Evidence*. 2022;1(2).

17 Assessment and Management of Acute Ischaemic Stroke

Skye Coote and Henry Zhao

> **In this chapter you will learn:**
> - Common clinical presentations associated with stroke
> - The difference in stroke diagnostic tools used to diagnose stroke
> - The role of brain imaging in stroke diagnosis
> - The role of mobile stroke units in improving patient outcomes
> - Current stroke treatments
> - The role of the paramedic in prehospital stroke care.

Case Details

Dispatch
76-year-old male, collapse to floor, right-sided weakness, possible stroke.

History
At 0810 hours, Hassan, a 76-year-old man, was found lying on the kitchen floor by his wife, Uma. Uma tried to get him up but could not manage due to weakness on Hassan's right side. Uma called her children, who insisted she call an ambulance. Uma told the call-taker that Hassan couldn't get up and was not talking. A double-crewed ambulance is dispatched on a Code 1 (lights and sirens).

On Arrival of the First Crew
The scene is assessed as safe, with Hassan lying on his right side near the kitchen bench. Uma tells the paramedics that both she and Hassan are up to date with their COVID-19 vaccinations and have no current or recent cold or flu symptoms. The patient's primary survey findings and initial vital signs are:

Airway	Patent
Breathing	RR 15, SpO$_2$ 95% on room air
Circulation	Peripheral pulses present, HR 126, irregular, BP 196/103, warm peripheries
Disability	GCS E4, V1, M5 (10), pupils 4 mm and equal, BGL 7.2 mmol/L
Environmental	Temp 36.6 °C

CHAPTER 17   Assessment and Management of Acute Ischaemic Stroke

Secondary survey

The patient has no obvious limb deformities or pain on movement or on palpation. His skin is intact, with no lacerations or cranial or facial haematomas. The patient has obvious dense right-sided arm and leg weakness, a right-sided facial droop and he is aphasic. Further findings are:

- Cardiac monitoring shows atrial fibrillation (AF)
- Temperature 36.3 °C
- BGL 5.6 mmol/L
- SpO_2 96% on room air.

Further history

Uma found Hassan when she came downstairs for breakfast at 0750 hours. She heard him get up at 0600 as usual, have his shower and take the dog for a walk. The dog still has his lead on.

The first paramedic crew call for a critical care paramedic, as the patient's GCS is low with a score of 10.

On Your Arrival as the Critical Care Paramedic

On your arrival you note that Hassan remains on the floor in the kitchen, he is mildly agitated and is struggling to get up. He is not obeying commands but is localising to painful stimuli with his left hand. The paramedics are next to him, talking to him and trying to keep him still. Uma is in the kitchen, along with her two sons and daughters-in-law, who have just arrived.

AMPLE

Hassan has a past medical history of hypertension, AF, hypercholesterolaemia and diabetes, all of which he is medicated for, although his apixaban has been withheld for the last 72 hours, as he is due for a dental procedure later that day. He has no known allergies.

Hassan is a retired school teacher and is physically active, walking his dog every day. He drives and still gardens.

Allergies	NKDA
Medications	Irbesartan 150 mg daily PO Perindopril 4 mg daily PO Apixaban 5 mg BD PO (withheld for 72 hours) Atorvastatin 40 mg daily PO Metformin 500 mg BD PO
Past history	Hypertension AF Hypercholesterolaemia Diabetes
Last ins and outs	Normal
Events prior	Unwitnessed collapse, no evidence of head strike or seizure

SECTION 4   Disability

Decision Point
What are your clinical priorities in this situation?

With a GCS of 10 and initial signs consistent with stroke, it is imperative to perform a full neurological and stroke assessment to determine if there is any risk of head injury or airway compromise. In any patient with suspected acute stroke, it is important to rule out common stroke mimics, particularly hypoglycaemia and seizure activity.

Question 1: What Types of Stroke Screening Tools are Used by Paramedics and What is the Role of the GCS in Assessing Stroke?

In this chapter we will be focusing on acute ischaemic stroke. Other types of stroke, such as haemorrhagic stroke and subarachnoid haemorrhage, will not be discussed.

Stroke is, first and foremost, a clinical diagnosis. Stroke symptom presentations are some of the most complex and varied in medicine. The clinical history is the most important part of the assessment and can provide key indicators that can immediately differentiate a stroke from a stroke mimic.[1] Commonly used stroke assessment tools can be insufficient when used in isolation, and should therefore be used as part of a broader clinical approach to diagnose stroke.[2]

Clinical stroke diagnostic tools used by paramedics generally fall into two categories:

1. General stroke screening tools – for example, FAST, ROSIER, CPSS, MASS[3]
2. Severity-based triaging tools for the detection of patients likely to be eligible for endovascular thrombectomy – for example, RACE, LAMS, ACT-FAST.[4]

General Stroke Screening Tools

These tools assist in differentiating a stroke from a non-stroke presentation; that is, asking the question is it likely that the patient is having a stroke? Most of these tools use similar assessment items, typically a combination of facial weakness, arm/hand weakness and speech/language disturbance (dysphasia and/or dysarthria). This constellation of symptoms is associated with strokes affecting the middle cerebral artery (MCA) territory in the brain (the most common type of ischaemic stroke).[3] It is not necessary for the patient to display all three symptoms to receive a diagnosis of stroke.

General assessment tools do not assess for symptoms originating from the posterior circulation (affecting the occipital lobes, brainstem and cerebellum), nor do they assess the extent or severity of the stroke.[5] As such, the diagnostic utility of these tools varies widely, with sensitivities of 60–90% and specificities of 70–95% for a hospital diagnosis of stroke, depending on the study population.[6] **Table 17.1** demonstrates the Cincinnati Prehospital Stroke Scale (CPSS), which is a general stroke screening tool.

Severity-Based Triage Tools

These tools were developed following the dawn of endovascular thrombectomy to treat large vessel arterial occlusions. Much like percutaneous coronary intervention for myocardial infarction, the need for specialist and costly angiogram suites and highly trained neuro-interventionalists means that thrombectomy is only available in specialised comprehensive stroke centres around the world.[4,7]

CHAPTER 17 Assessment and Management of Acute Ischaemic Stroke

Table 17.1 Cincinnati Prehospital Stroke Scale

Assessment item	Normal assessment	Abnormal assessment
Facial droop	Both sides of the face move equally	One side of the face does not move at all or moves less than the other side
Arm weakness	Both arms move equally	One arm does not move at all or has less strength than the other arm
Dysarthria	Speech is clear without signs of slurring	Speech is slurred

Source: Zohrevandi, B., Monsef Kasmaie, V., Asadl, P. et al. 2015. Diagnostic accuracy of Cincinnati Pre-Hospital Stroke Scale. *Emergency (Tehran)*, 3, 95–98.

Severity-based tools work on the premise that large-vessel occlusions cause a greater region of cerebral ischaemia, and therefore more severe deficits. A positive result thereby predicts a need for thrombectomy and can facilitate triage with direct transportation to an endovascular centre, negating the need for costly and lengthy secondary inter-hospital transfers. This can result in faster definitive treatment and improved patient outcomes.[4,7]

While the performance of these tools also varies, a positive result correctly predicts large-vessel occlusion in 40–60% of cases (depending on the tool used) and up to 80% if intracranial haemorrhages are included.[4] This is a substantial improvement compared to using a general stroke screening tool alone. As large haemorrhages (for example, intracerebral haematoma (ICH) or subdural haemorrhages (SDH)) can present with similarly severe symptoms, these severity-based tools can be useful for triaging patients to a comprehensive stroke centre with co-located neurosurgical services.

Glasgow Coma Scale (GCS)

This is a tool that is used to assess the level and extent of impaired consciousness through the assessment of three key items: eye opening, motor response and verbal response. In the prehospital setting, a low GCS can be an indicator for advanced airway management, including intubation. Developed originally for traumatic brain injury, its role in acute stroke assessment is limited.[8]

As it assesses the patient's 'best' response, a dense hemiplegia may not be scored if the patient can obey commands on their non-stroke affected side. Conversely, an aphasic patient will score one (losing four points), even if they are conscious and alert. This inaccuracy has prompted some protocols to warn against the use of GCS as an indicator of consciousness and airway management in acute stroke patients.[9]

In this case study, Hassan has a presumptive diagnosis of stroke, as he has a facial droop, arm weakness and speech disturbance. Given the severity of his symptoms, there is a strong suspicion of large-vessel occlusion (needing endovascular thrombectomy) or intracerebral haemorrhage (potentially needing neurosurgical management).

SECTION 4 Disability

Using the ACT-FAST severity-based tool as an example (**Figure 17.1**), Hassan's assessment is as follows.

- Step 1 positive – Hassan is unable to move the right arm, therefore automatically fulfilling the criteria for one arm dropping to stretcher <10 seconds.
- Step 2 positive – Hassan is mute (language is assessed due to the arm weakness being on the right side).
- Step 3 positive – This step assesses whether the patient would be a good candidate for prehospital bypass to a thrombectomy centre:
  - Symptom onset was acute today and symptoms are not pre-existing.
  - Onset is less than 24 hours, as Hassan was last known well at 0600 when he got up.
  - He is independent in all activities of daily living.
  - He has no history of brain cancer or seizures, he is euglycaemic and he is not comatose.

Despite the GCS of 10, which was the prompt for the critical care paramedic request, Hassan does not have impaired consciousness and does not need advanced airway management. His low GCS is a result of global aphasia rendering him mute and unable to understand or obey commands. The GCS does not detect his motor weakness given he can localise with his left hand and arm. In Hassan's case, the GCS does accurately reflect his clinical presentation.

ACT-FAST Stroke Algorithm

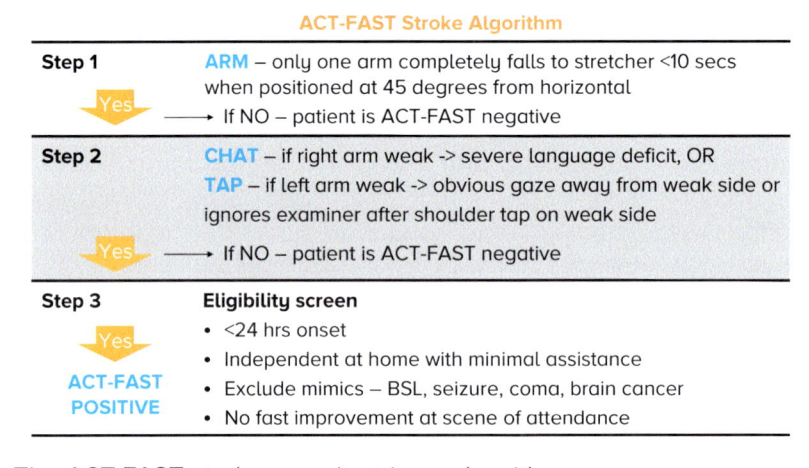

Step 1 — **ARM** – only one arm completely falls to stretcher <10 secs when positioned at 45 degrees from horizontal
Yes ↓ If NO – patient is ACT-FAST negative

Step 2 — **CHAT** – if right arm weak -> severe language deficit, OR
TAP – if left arm weak -> obvious gaze away from weak side or ignores examiner after shoulder tap on weak side
Yes ↓ If NO – patient is ACT-FAST negative

Step 3 — **Eligibility screen**
- <24 hrs onset
- Independent at home with minimal assistance
- Exclude mimics – BSL, seizure, coma, brain cancer
- No fast improvement at scene of attendance

Yes ↓ **ACT-FAST POSITIVE**

Figure 17.1 The ACT-FAST stroke severity triage algorithm.
Source: Henry Zhao.

Question 2: If Stroke is a Clinical Diagnosis, What is the Role of Brain Imaging?

Cerebrovascular anatomy is generally similar between individuals and stroke deficits often form recognisable patterns, making it possible to clinically diagnose stroke based on the patient's presenting symptoms and their clinical history. These patterns apply regardless of the type of the stroke – ischaemic or haemorrhagic.[1]

CHAPTER 17 Assessment and Management of Acute Ischaemic Stroke

For example:

- **Right hemispheric stroke** generally causes left-sided weakness/numbness, left-sided neglect, left hemianopia (loss of vision in the left visual field of *both* eyes) and gaze deviation to the right (from weakness of the left extraocular muscles) (**Figure 17.2**).
- **Left hemispheric stroke** generally causes right-sided weakness/numbness, right hemianopia and language deficits – receptive, expressive or global aphasia (even in most left-handed people).
- **Cerebellar stroke** will cause loss of balance, disequilibrium, gait ataxia and dizziness without motor weakness or numbness.
- **Brainstem stroke** typically causes eye movement and cranial nerve deficits, and may affect consciousness and haemodynamic status. Early symptoms seen by paramedics may also include nausea and dizziness. Due to a shared vascular supply, cerebellar and brainstem strokes often occur together, in which case you can see mixed brainstem and cerebellar symptoms.[10]

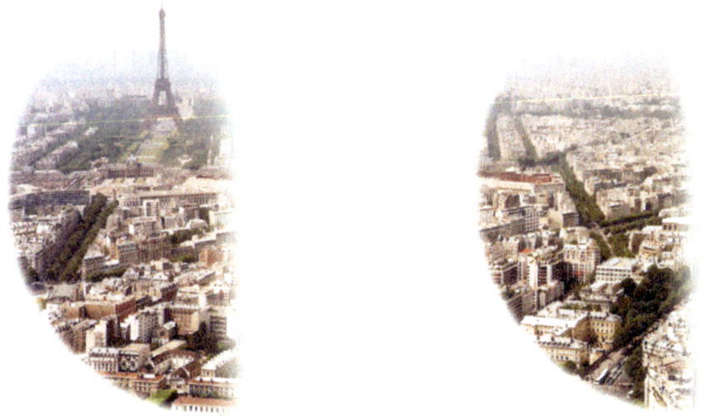

Figure 17.2 An example of a left-sided hemianopia with a loss of vision in the left visual field of both eyes (a binocular defect). A hemianopia is typically caused by a stroke in the contralateral hemisphere in the brain.
Source: https://en.wikipedia.org/wiki/Homonymous_hemianopsia

Due to these patterns, skilled clinicians can predict the arterial origin of the stroke based on the patient's clinical presentation. These patterns also help to distinguish stroke mimics from true stroke symptoms. For example, a patient exhibiting symptoms that localise to more than one vascular territory (for example, loss of language with *left* arm weakness and altered consciousness) is more likely to have a non-stroke cause of their symptoms, as stroke typically affects a single blood vessel.

These clinical patterns, however, will not differentiate between an ischaemic stroke and a haemorrhagic stroke. An intracerebral or subarachnoid haemorrhage can more commonly present with a severe headache, profuse vomiting, hypertension, Cushing's triad and a rapidly progressive loss of consciousness. However, these symptoms are not exclusive to a haemorrhagic stroke and can be seen with an ischaemic stroke, particularly severe strokes or brainstem strokes.[1]

SECTION 4 Disability

As there are no completely reliable clinical signs that will differentiate ischaemia from a haemorrhage, the only method to diagnose the type of stroke is brain imaging (CT or MRI).[1] It is for this reason that, until the recent advent of the Mobile Stroke Unit (MSU), acute stroke treatment has remained within the hospital setting.

MSUs are custom-built specialist ambulances that are equipped with a portable CT scanner and carry an expert multidisciplinary team. Generally, this team consists of paramedic(s), a neurologist (either physically on board the vehicle or working remotely via tele-medicine), an advanced practice nurse and a radiographer.[11,12] MSUs allow the team to rapidly assess and diagnose stroke at the roadside, removing delays to stroke treatments, including thrombolysis, and improving prehospital triage through immediate identification of large-vessel occlusions or haemorrhagic strokes requiring advanced treatment. MSUs have been proven to significantly improve patient outcomes through rapid diagnosis, treatment, triage and transfer, even within metropolitan areas.[13,14]

It is hoped that as technology advances, smaller portable helmet-like imaging devices may be rolled out across ambulance services (**Figure 17.3**). These devices, along with in-field tele-neurology consultations, may soon allow paramedics to administer intravenous thrombolytics for acute ischaemic stroke patients in the field.[15,16]

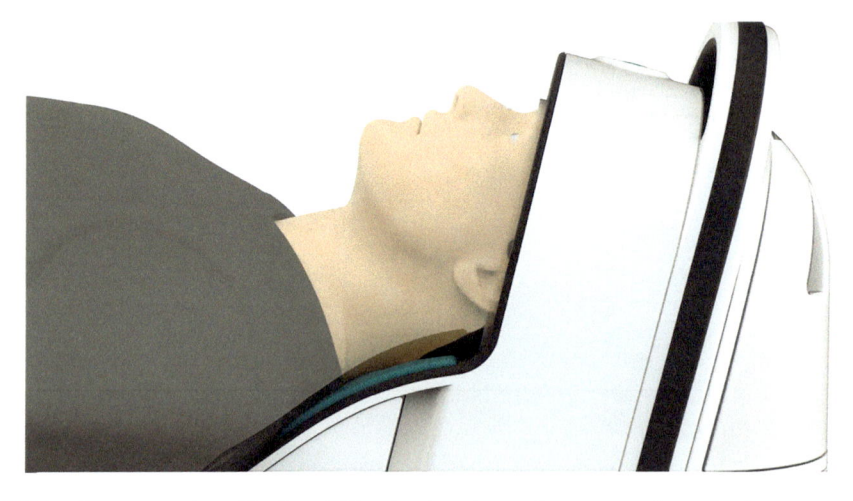

Figure 17.3 An example of helmet-like technology for assessing stroke.
Source: EM Vision: https://emvision.com.au/products/. Reproduced with permission.

In this case study, Hassan's symptoms are consistent with a proximal left middle cerebral artery (MCA) occlusion. However, without brain imaging, a conclusive diagnosis of an ischaemic stroke is not possible, and haemorrhage remains a possibility. This would be an ideal case for the MSU to attend if one was available in Hassan's area. The MSU could definitively diagnose Hassan and commence thrombolysis if indicated, all while transporting him to a thrombectomy centre if the scan demonstrated a large-vessel occlusion.

CHAPTER 17 Assessment and Management of Acute Ischaemic Stroke

Question 3: What Are the Current Treatment Options for Acute Ischaemic Stroke?

The principles of hyperacute stroke treatment are to reduce death and disability through the rapid provision of targeted stroke treatments. In the case of an ischaemic stroke the aim is vessel recanalisation using thrombolysis and/or thrombectomy, while for haemorrhagic stroke the priority is to prevent haematoma expansion through blood pressure control, anticoagulant reversal and/or neurosurgery.

Thrombolysis

This is a proven medical treatment for use in acute ischaemic stroke up to 4.5 hours from stroke onset or the time the person was last known to be free from stroke deficits. It is administered once a CT or MRI scan has eliminated a haemorrhagic cause of the symptoms and following a safety screen.[17] Recent research has shown that for patients with favourable brain imaging (those showing minimal stroke damage and ongoing viable tissue), thrombolysis is safe and effective, resulting in improved outcomes up to nine hours from onset/last known well time, including in patients who wake with symptoms ('wake-up strokes'). However, the earlier thrombolysis is administered, the better the chances of the patient having a good outcome. Therefore, all delays to treatment must be minimised.

Thrombolysis works by targeting the fibrin strands that bind a clot together. Tissue plasminogen activators (alteplase and tenecteplase) convert plasminogen to plasmin, a naturally occurring fibrinolytic agent. Alteplase has been the mainstay of stroke thrombolysis treatment since 1995,[18] but recent trials have been investigating the use of tenecteplase as an alternative agent. Tenecteplase has greater fibrin specificity than alteplase, making it more effective at clot dissolution. It also has a longer half-life, allowing it to be given as a bolus-only dose, rather than a bolus and infusion, which is required with alteplase, making it ideally suited to the prehospital setting. Recent research has found that across all ischaemic strokes, tenecteplase is non-inferior to alteplase, but it is superior in large-vessel occlusions. Therefore, international guidelines generally recommend tenecteplase as the drug of choice in large-vessel occlusions and an equivalent choice to alteplase for all other types of stroke.[19–21]

Endovascular Thrombectomy

This is a procedure that mechanically removes a clot from the patient's brain using a device, usually stent-retriever or aspiration. Arterial access is generally gained via the femoral artery, but other approaches can include the radial, brachial or carotid artery. Cerebral vasculature is more fragile with smaller diameters than cardiac vessels, so thrombectomy was initially performed in large vessels, specifically the carotid artery, proximal middle cerebral artery segments and the basilar artery (**Figure 17.4**).[22] Trials to show efficacy in smaller, medium-vessel occlusions are currently ongoing (**Figure 17.5**).

Thrombectomy is a powerful treatment, showing an improvement in disability in one patient out of every 2.6 patients treated.[23] Like intravenous thrombolysis, the benefit of thrombectomy is front-end loaded, meaning it is most effective when initiated as early as possible after stroke onset. Therefore, prehospital identification of patients with severe

SECTION 4 Disability

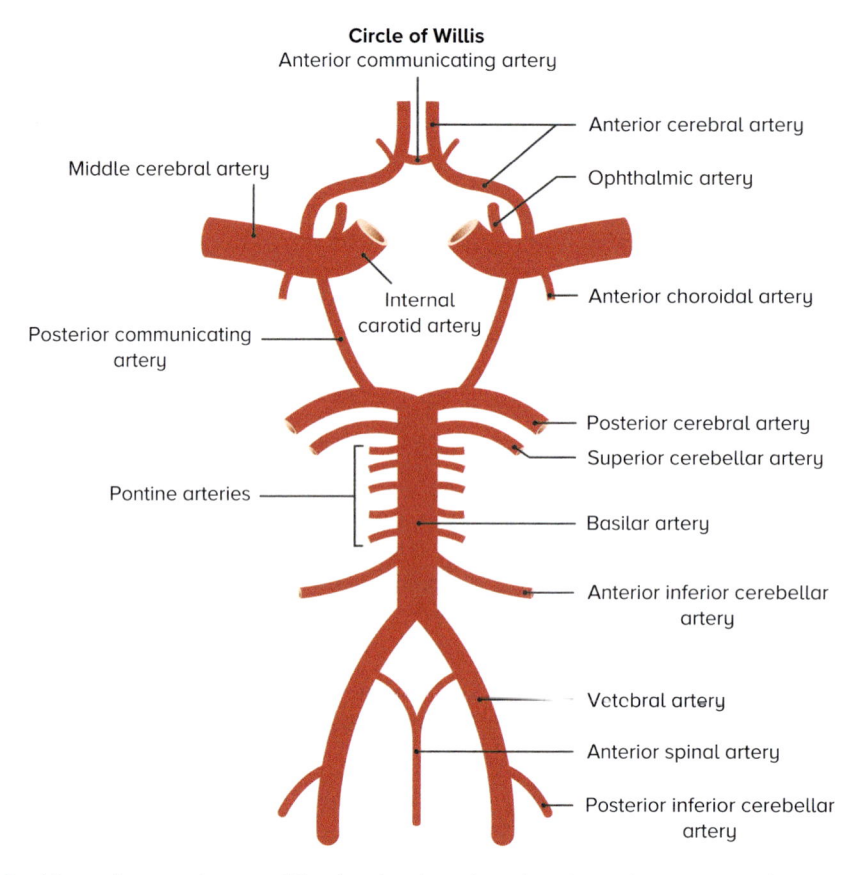

Figure 17.4 Vascular anatomy of the brain showing the three large vessels currently treated with thrombectomy.
Source: Jeniffer Fontan/Shutterstock.

deficits likely to need thrombectomy, and appropriate hospital bypass, is a crucial element in improving patient outcomes. Thrombectomy is proven to be effective up to 24 hours after onset but theoretically could be performed after this time in carefully selected patients with excellent collateral circulation and salvageable tissue.[23-26]

Unlike ischaemic stroke, there is no current standardised treatment for haemorrhagic stroke. Instead, recommendations are around supportive care and management.

Neurosurgery

Surgery can be important for a small percentage of haemorrhagic strokes, though limiting factors include patient age and premorbid health, the size and location of the haematoma, the presenting symptoms and level of consciousness. Historically, neurosurgery has reduced initial mortality rates but has not reduced the level of permanent disability caused by the bleed.[27,28] However, a new study trialling minimally invasive surgery using new technology

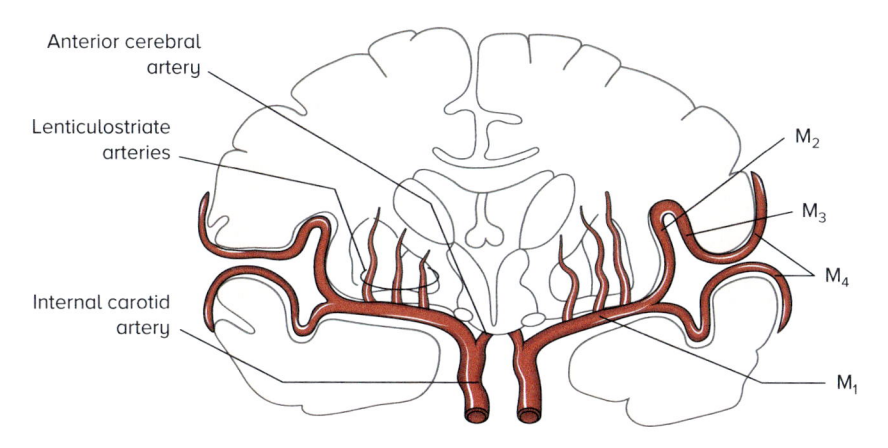

CHAPTER 17 Assessment and Management of Acute Ischaemic Stroke

Figure 17.5 The divisions of the middle cerebral artery. The lower the number, the more proximal the segment is to the circle of Willis.

has recorded improved patient outcomes six months after their stroke when the bleed is located more superficially in the brain.[29] Prehospital detection and triage of haemorrhagic stroke using portable imaging devices will therefore be an important step in resource allocation in the future.

Additional treatments

Hyperglycaemia and blood pressure management and potential anticoagulation reversal are additional treatments for all acute stroke patients. Hypoglycaemia is a known mimic for stroke. Patients presenting with low blood glucose levels should have their glucose corrected and be re-evaluated before any treatment begins.[19] Hyperglycaemia is common in the initial phases of a stroke and if left untreated, it is associated with poorer outcomes. International guidelines now recommend that all patients with stroke have their blood glucose levels normalised and maintained less than or equal to 10 mmol/L (180 mg/dL).[19,20,27,30] Prehospital monitoring and correction of hypoglycaemia are standard in most ambulance guidelines as a result.

Blood pressure management varies by stroke type and treatment; however, definitive values are lacking. In the setting of thrombolysis, uncontrolled hypertension is associated with haemorrhagic transformation – bleeding within the infarcted tissue – which contributes to morbidity and mortality. For this reason, the current recommendation for patients undergoing thrombolysis is a blood pressure less than or equal to 185/110 mmHg prior to and for 24 hours after treatment. Permissive hypertension, up to 220/120 mmHg, is accepted for non-thrombolysed ischaemic cases to maintain cerebral perfusion pressure and prevent worsening ischaemia through reduced flow. Conversely, it is recommended that patients with an intracerebral haemorrhage have their systolic blood pressure reduced to approximately 140 mmHg (but no lower) to reduce haematoma growth.[19,20,27] While not currently feasible, diagnosing the stroke type in the prehospital setting would allow critical care paramedics to

SECTION 4 Disability

manage blood pressure en route to hospital. This could further improve treatment times and outcome measures.

Anticoagulation reversal is recommended for patients who present with an intracerebral haemorrhage. In the case of a direct oral anticoagulant, this should be the specific reversal agent, for example, idarucizumab for dabigatran, andexanet alfa for rivaroxaban or apixaban, vitamin K and prothrombin complex concentrate for warfarin.[27] Current trials are examining the effectiveness of tranexamic acid for use in intracerebral haemorrhage.

Patients with demonstrated subtherapeutic levels of anticoagulants or who are known to have not had their medication for at least 48 hours (drug-dependent) may be safely thrombolysed if they present with an ischaemic stroke. Patients on dabigatran can safely have their anticoagulation reversed with idarucizumab and be immediately treated with thrombolysis;[31] however, warfarin is never reversed to allow thrombolysis administration.

For our case study, Hassan is hypertensive (BP 196/103), which would need to be treated before thrombolysis was commenced. While Hassan has previously been on apixaban, this has been withheld for 72 hours, meaning he will be subtherapeutic and would be safe to thrombolyse.[32] Even if thrombectomy was required, thrombolysis is generally still administered concurrently, as the combined approach shows some advantage in vessel reopening.[33,34]

Question 4: What Are Paramedic Responsibilities in Prehospital Management?

Paramedics have a vital role in the patient's stroke journey and significantly contribute to improving treatment times and patient outcomes. They are uniquely situated to assess the patient, determining the clinical history and onset time from on-scene eyewitnesses. Being in the patient's home allows them to make informed assessments of the patient's premorbid level of functioning, initial symptoms and any changes over time – key elements used in making a treatment decision. Critical care paramedics may also have a role in the interhospital transfer of patients from a smaller hospital to a tertiary hospital for an intervention.

Determining onset time or the time the patient was last known to be well is nuanced. When asked about onset time, patients often provide the time they first noticed their symptoms. This can be quite different from the actual onset time, especially if the patient woke with symptoms, or if their symptoms are mild or not immediately apparent, such as a dysarthria or mild aphasia.[35] To get an accurate onset time, repeated questioning may be needed, regarding the time the patient went to bed, if they got up in the middle of the night, if they spoke to someone during the day, if they were able to drive or get dressed, or do their normal chores before symptoms started. In some cases, an onset time may never be established, which greatly reduces treatment options for the patient.

Ascertaining an accurate past medical and medication history is a vital step that is required before treatment can commence. Potential risks to the patient must be identified, such as recent major surgery or trauma, known bleeding diathesis, recent stroke, use of anticoagulants, for example. Paramedics are best placed to establish a comprehensive history while in the patient's house with access to not only the patient, but also their family or friends, who can provide supplementary information.

CHAPTER 17 Assessment and Management of Acute Ischaemic Stroke

Prehospital notification by paramedics has been proven to improve treatment times for stroke patients.[35–37] Pre-notification allows the emergency department to allocate staff and resources, hold the CT table, organise pathways and pre-order tests and investigations where possible.[37] Ideally as part of the pre-notification, the patient's name and date of birth are provided, along with onset time, symptoms and significant vital signs. Providing patient identifiers allows hospital staff to look up electronic medical records, assess the patient's past medical history and medications and even pre-screen for treatment, all of which reduce door-to-needle and door-to-groin puncture times.

In this case, the key elements for paramedics to establish, pre-notify and handover include the following.

- Hassan is positive on both general stroke screening tools and severity-based triage tools.
- His last known well time was 0600 hours (unless paramedics can establish a more definitive onset time after talking to Uma).
- A brief description of his symptoms.
- He has a history of anticoagulated AF, but his anticoagulant has been withheld for three days.
- Hassan has known stroke risk factors including hypertension, hypercholesterolaemia and diabetes.
- He is normally independent in all aspects of self-care and requires no assistance with any activities of daily living.
- He is hypertensive, which will need to be addressed pre-treatment.
- All other vital signs are within normal limits.
- The type of dental procedure he was due to have.

Key Evidence

Campbell, B. C. V., Ma, H., Ringleb, P. A. et al. 2019. Extending thrombolysis to 4.5–9 h and wake-up stroke using perfusion imaging: a systematic review and meta-analysis of individual patient data. *Lancet*, 394(10193), 139–147. Available at: https://pubmed.ncbi.nlm.nih.gov/31128925/

Ebinger, M., Siegerink, B., Kunz, A. et al. 2021. Association between dispatch of mobile stroke units and functional outcomes among patients with acute ischemic stroke in Berlin. *JAMA*, 325(5), 454–466.

Goyal, M., Menon, B. K., van Zwam, W. H. et al. 2016. Endovascular thrombectomy after large-vessel ischaemic stroke: a meta-analysis of individual patient data from five randomised trials. *Lancet*, 387(10029), 1723–1731. Available at: https://pubmed.ncbi.nlm.nih.gov/26898852/

Grotta, J. C., Yamal, J.-M., Parker, S. A. et al. 2021. Prospective, multicenter, controlled trial of mobile stroke units. *New England Journal of Medicine*, 385(11), 971–981. Available at: https://pubmed.ncbi.nlm.nih.gov/34496173/

Hacke, W., Kaste, M., Bluhmki, E. et al. 2008. Thrombolysis with alteplase 3 to 4.5 hours after acute ischemic stroke. *New England Journal of Medicine*, 359(13), 1317–1329. Available at: http://www.nejm.org/doi/full/10.1056/NEJMoa0804656

Meretoja, A., Weir, L., Ugalde, M. et al. 2013. Helsinki model cut stroke thrombolysis delays to 25 minutes in Melbourne in only 4 months. *Neurology*, 81(12), 1071–1076. Available at: http://n.neurology.org/content/neurology/early/2013/08/14/WNL.0b013e3182a4a4d2.full.pdf

The National Institute of Neurological Disorders and Stroke rt-PA stroke study group. 1995. Tissue plasminogen activator for acute ischemic stroke. *New England Journal of Medicine*, 333(24), 1581–1587.

Zhao, H., Coote, S., Pesavento, L. et al. 2017. Large vessel occlusion scales increase delivery to endovascular centers without excessive harm from misclassifications. *Stroke*, 48(3), 568–573. Available at: https://pubmed.ncbi.nlm.nih.gov/28232591/

SECTION 4 Disability

Self-Reflection Questions

1. How have stroke patients you have cared for presented? Were their symptoms similar to Hassan's?
2. Have you used either general stroke assessment tools or stroke severity tools? How did you find them?
3. Can you think of a patient who was diagnosed with a stroke at hospital, but who did not score on prehospital assessment tools?
   a. If so, what were their symptoms? Did you appreciate those symptoms at the time of your assessment?
4. Have you assessed a patient with stroke who was diagnosed with a stroke mimic at hospital?
   a. On reflection, were there any red flags in their presentation that could have indicated a stroke mimic?
   b. Would this now change your management?

References

1. Musuka, T. D., Wilton, S. B., Traboulsi, M. et al. 2015. Diagnosis and management of acute ischemic stroke: speed is critical. *Canadian Medical Association Journal,* 187, 887–893.
2. Bray, J. E., Coughlan, K., Barger, B. et al. 2010. Paramedic diagnosis of stroke: examining long-term use of the Melbourne Ambulance Stroke Screen (MASS) in the field. *Stroke,* 41, 1363–1366.
3. Zohrevandi, B., Monsef Kasmaie, V., Asadi, P. et al. 2015. Diagnostic accuracy of Cincinnati Pre-Hospital Stroke Scale. *Emergency (Tehran),* 3, 95–98.
4. Zhao, H., Smith, K., Bernard, S. et al. 2021. Utility of severity-based prehospital triage for endovascular thrombectomy. *Stroke,* 52, 70–79.
5. Aroor, S., Singh, R. and Goldstein, L. B. 2017. BE-FAST (balance, eyes, face, arm, speech, time): reducing the proportion of strokes missed using the FAST mnemonic. *Stroke,* 48, 479–481.
6. Antipova, D., Eadie, L., Macaden, A. et al. 2019. Diagnostic accuracy of clinical tools for assessment of acute stroke: a systematic review. *BMC Emergency Medicine,* 19, 49.
7. Zhao, H., Coote, S., Pesavento, L. et al. 2017. Large vessel occlusion scales increase delivery to endovascular centers without excessive harm from misclassifications. *Stroke,* 48, 568–573.
8. Jain, S. and Iverson, L. M. 2023. *Glasgow Coma Scale* [Online]. StatPearls. Available at: https://www.ncbi.nlm.nih.gov/books/NBK513298/
9. Safer Care Victoria, 2018. *Endovascular Clot Retrieval for Acute Stroke. Statewide Service Protocol for Victoria.* 2nd edn. Victoria, Australia: Victorian Government.
10. Coote, S. and Alexandrov, A. W. 2017. Acute and critical stroke care. In: Goldsworthy, S., Kleinpell, R. and Williams, G. (eds.) *International Best Practices in Critical Care.* 2nd edn.
11. Kostopoulos, P., Walter, S., Haass, A. et al. 2012. Mobile stroke unit for diagnosis-based triage of persons with suspected stroke. *Neurology,* 78, 1849–1852.
12. Walter, S., Ragoschke-Schumm, A., Lesmeister, M. et al. 2018a. Mobile stroke unit use for prehospital stroke treatment – an update. *Der Radiologe,* 58, 24–28.
13. Ebinger, M., Siegerink, B., Kunz, A. et al. 2021. Association between dispatch of mobile stroke units and functional outcomes among patients with acute ischemic stroke in Berlin. *JAMA,* 325, 454–466.
14. Grotta, J. C., Yamal, J.-M., Parker, S. A. et al. 2021. Prospective, multicenter, controlled trial of mobile stroke units. *New England Journal of Medicine,* 385, 971–981.
15. Walter, S., Fassbender, K., Easton, D. et al. 2021. Stroke care equity in rural and remote areas – novel strategies. *Vessel Plus,* 5, 27.
16. Walter, S., Zhao, H., Easton, D. et al. 2018b. Air-mobile stroke unit for access to stroke treatment in rural regions. *International Journal of Stroke,* 13, 568–575.
17. Upton, D., Upton, P., Busby-Grant, J. et al. 2016. *Systematic Review of Intravenous Thrombolyis in Acute Ischaemic Stroke.* University of Canberra, Health Research Institute.
18. The National Institute of Neurological Disorders and Stroke rt-PA Stroke Study Group. 1995. Tissue plasminogen activator for acute ischemic stroke. *New England Journal of Medicine,* 333, 1581–1587.

CHAPTER 17 Assessment and Management of Acute Ischaemic Stroke

19. Powers, W. J., Rabinstein, A. A., Ackerson, T. et al. 2019. Guidelines for the early management of patients with acute ischemic stroke: 2019 update to the 2018 guidelines for the early management of acute ischemic stroke: a guideline for healthcare professionals from the American Heart Association/American Stroke Association. *Stroke,* 50, e344–e418.
20. Stroke Foundation. 2022. *Clincial guidelines for stroke management* [Online]. Available at: https://informme.org.au/guidelines/living-clinical-guidelines-for-stroke-management#
21. Heart and Stroke Foundation of Canada. 2023. *Stroke best practices.* [Online]. Available at: https://www.strokebestpractices.ca/
22. Papanagiotou, P. and Ntaios, G. 2018. Endovascular thrombectomy in acute ischemic stroke. *Circulation: Cardiovascular Interventions,* 11, e005362.
23. Goyal, M., Menon, B. K., van Zwam, W. H. et al. 2016. Endovascular thrombectomy after large-vessel ischaemic stroke: a meta-analysis of individual patient data from five randomised trials. *Lancet*, 387(10029), 1723–1731.
24. Sarraj, A., Hassan, A. E., Abraham, M. G. et al, 2023. Trial of endovascular thrombectomy for large ischemic strokes. *New England Journal of Medicine,* 388, 1259–1271.
25. Nogueira, R. G., Jadhav, A. P., Haussen, D. C. et al. 2018. Thrombectomy 6 to 24 hours after stroke with a mismatch between deficit and infarct. *New England Journal of Medicine,* 378, 11–21.
26. Albers, G. W., Marks, M. P., Kemp, S. et al. 2018. Thrombectomy for stroke at 6 to 16 hours with selection by perfusion imaging. *New England Journal of Medicine,* 378, 708–718.
27. Greenberg, S. M., Ziai, W. C., Cordonnier, C. et al. 2022. 2022 guideline for the management of patients with spontaneous intracerebral hemorrhage: a guideline from the American Heart Association/American Stroke Association. *Stroke,* 53, e282–e361.
28. Hanley, D. F., Thompson, R. E., Rosenblum, M. et al. 2019. Efficacy and safety of minimally invasive surgery with thrombolysis in intracerebral haemorrhage evacuation (MISTIE III): a randomised, controlled, open-label, blinded endpoint phase 3 trial. *Lancet,* 393, 1021–1032.
29. Pradilla, G., Ratcliff, J., Hall, A. et al. 2023, Very early minimally invasive removal of intracerebral haemorrhage: The ENRICH trial. European Stroke Organisation Conference, 25/5/23, Munich, Germany.
30. Middleton, S., McElduff, P., Ward, J. et al. 2011. Implementation of evidence-based treatment protocols to manage fever, hyperglycaemia, and swallowing dysfunction in acute stroke (QASC): a cluster randomised controlled trial. *Lancet,* 378, 1699–1706.
31. Zhao, H., Coote, S., Pesavento, L. et al. 2019. Prehospital idarucizumab prior to intravenous thrombolysis in a mobile stroke unit. *International Journal of Stroke*, 14, 265–269.
32. Sikorska, J. and Uprichard, J. 2017. Direct oral anticoagulants: a quick guide. *European Cardiology*, 12, 40–45.
33. Mitchell, P. J., Yan, B., Churilov, L. et al. 2022. Endovascular thrombectomy versus standard bridging thrombolytic with endovascular thrombectomy within 4·5 h of stroke onset: an open-label, blinded-endpoint, randomised non-inferiority trial. *Lancet*, 400, 116–125.
34. Fischer, U., Kaesmacher, J., Strbian, D. et al. 2022. Thrombectomy alone versus intravenous alteplase plus thrombectomy in patients with stroke: an open-label, blinded-outcome, randomised non-inferiority trial. *Lancet*, 400, 104–115.
35. Meretoja, A., Strbian, D., Mustanoja, S. et al. 2012. Reducing in-hospital delay to 20 minutes in stroke thrombolysis. *Neurology*, 79, 306–313.
36. Fassbender, K., Balucani, C., Walter, S. et al. 2013. Streamlining of prehospital stroke management: the golden hour. *Lancet Neurology*, 12, 585–596.
37. Zhang, S., Zhang, J., Zhang, M. et al. 2018. Prehospital notification procedure improves stroke outcome by shortening onset to needle time in Chinese urban area. *Aging and Disease*, 9, 426–434.

18 Severe/Uncontrolled Pain

Todd Blackburn

In this chapter you will learn:
- What multimodal analgesia is and how to apply this to a critically unwell patient
- What a dosing regimen is and whether there is a standard approach to a patient with severe pain
- The potential risks and complications of aggressive analgesia in the polytrauma patient
- What procedural sedation is and about the principles of care for maintaining safe boundaries while providing best care
- Ethical decision making and whether ICPs should consider drug-facilitated intubation for the patient with severe, uncontrolled traumatic pain.

Case Details

Dispatch
25-year-old male, single occupant of motor vehicle, high-speed collision into barrier, trapped.

History
A 25-year-old male was witnessed driving at high speed and erratically. The patient lost control of the vehicle and it hit a barrier head on. There is significant cabin intrusion and the patient is heavily trapped from the waist down. A double-crewed ambulance and a critical care paramedic crew are dispatched. HEMS are available if required.

On Arrival of the First Crew
The 25-year-old male is still trapped in the vehicle. The scene has been made safe by the police and fire services. Traffic has been stopped. The patient is sitting in the driver's seat. He is agitated and difficult to manage. His primary survey findings and initial vital signs are:

Airway	Patent
Breathing	RR 30, SpO$_2$ 93% on air
Circulation	Peripheral pulses present, HR 140, regular, BP 143/91, warm peripheries
Disability	GCS E3, V4, M6 (13), BGL 7.3 mmol/L
Environmental	Temp 37.1 °C

CHAPTER 18 Severe/Uncontrolled Pain

The first paramedic crew are able to obtain some simple monitoring, obtain an IV and administer some intranasal fentanyl with no effect. The patient is difficult to assess due to mechanical entrapment but the paramedics are considering the possibility of a pelvic fracture.

On Your Arrival as the Critical Care Paramedic

The patient remains trapped in the vehicle from the waist down. You are able to ascertain that he probably has a fractured pelvis and multiple long-bone fractures. His agitation may be due to his pain or a potential head injury.

AMPLE

The patient is difficult to manage but you are able to ascertain that his only past medical history is asthma. He is allergic to midazolam.

Allergies	Midazolam
Medications	Ventolin and Symbicort
Past history	Asthma, well controlled
Last ins and outs	Normal
Events	High-speed MVA

Decision Point

What are your clinical priorities in this situation?

The patient has been involved in a high-speed MVA and is mechanically trapped, with multiple long-bone fractures. He is at high risk of deterioration and needs expedient transport to a major trauma service.

Consider:

- How you are going to get the patient out safely
- How you are going to adequately provide aggressive, yet appropriate, analgesia to the patient
- Whether there are any risks with your management plan.

Question 1: What Is the Evidence to Support Multimodal Analgesia? Is there a Perfect Dosing Regimen?

Multimodal analgesia is a proven concept in many areas of medical care.[1] There is a paucity of good-quality research in the prehospital environment.[2–4] The principles of care that should be utilised in the prehospital environment should focus on the immediate care and also demonstrate an understanding of the complexities of pain management. Literature suggests that if a multimodal approach is used in the acute setting, it leads to a number of positive outcomes for patients.[1] These outcomes include an overall reduction in opioid use, lower requirements of ongoing opioids post incident, less time spent in hospital, reduction in the likelihood of opioid addiction and a reduction in the chances of developing post-traumatic stress disorder.[1,4] The evidence is strong and a multimodal approach is considered superior to using a single dosing regimen alone.[5] Multimodal analgesia leads to better outcomes for our patients, as they receive adequate analgesia, via different mechanisms of action. This leads to lower doses of medications, such as opioids, to achieve the same results. Ultimately, the clinician needs to consider the multiple pathways that are available when it comes to their service and their skillset.

> **PRACTICE TIP**
>
> The key to appropriate analgesia in these patients is to rapidly score them into a category – such as mild, moderate or severe. Once a clinician has decided what level of severity the patient's injuries/pain score is, this will allow for forward thinking and delegation to other paramedics to prepare the medication.

As prehospital clinicians, our goal should be to act in the best interests of the patient, be as humane as possible and provide the patient with the best clinical benefit – whether that be a reduction in pain, reduction of length in hospital, reducing ongoing analgesic requirements or helping avoid long-term opioid use. The overwhelming shift in the literature suggests that as a cohort, paramedics have the greatest ability to see a reduction in pain, and now we have more analgesic options available to us with many different mechanisms in order to guide our prehospital care and directly benefit our patients.

The use of a rating system is helpful to guide the clinician in initial decision making as to how aggressive they are with their analgesia.[6] It would be prudent, first and foremost, to remember the basics. Consider the administration of an inhalational analgesic if possible. Its ease of use, fast administration and rapid effects can be useful as the clinician moves towards securing vascular access. The clinician should weigh up the risks/benefits of using this approach initially, for example, poor patient compliance. Other options in this initial stage include IN fentanyl or IM morphine or fentanyl. The clinician should be cautious in considering ketamine as a first-line medication to treat these patients due to the increased risk of emergence reactions.[7] Moving forward, once vascular access has been gained, the options become more widely available.

Standard dosing regimens are shown in **Table 18.1**. Consider first-line intravenous opioids such as morphine or fentanyl. The clinician can consider the patient's underlying haemodynamic status to guide decision making and the choice of which medication might be more appropriate for their clinical setting. Fentanyl has fewer haemodynamic effects and also has a lower likelihood of inducing nausea and vomiting.[8] The limitation of using fentanyl is its lower duration of action, which might be undesirable in these types of patients. This is not suggesting that you should not use it, rather that a clinician needs to be mindful that these patients will require more frequent dosing in order to ensure adequate analgesia.

Supposing our patient has been given an initial regime that includes an inhalational anaesthetic and some intravenous morphine or fentanyl, the evidence supports using another analgesic option to improve pain relief and reduce the overall likelihood of undesirable side-effects.[1] If the clinician is presented with a patient in severe pain who is refractory to first- and second-line analgesic options, most prehospital services support the transition to a different medication, such as ketamine. Ketamine is proven to be an effective prehospital option in patients with refractory pain, provided it is used appropriately.[9] Consider the patient's

CHAPTER 18 Severe/Uncontrolled Pain

underlying condition and their environment. Smaller doses are able to achieve adequate analgesia and the clinician can also consider setting up an infusion to maintain analgesia. It is prudent to consider the dosing and reaching the therapeutic index in a timely manner. Ketamine is a great option given its side-effect profile including haemodynamic stability and preservation of respiratory function and airway tone.[9] The risks will be covered under Question 2.

There is not a perfect dosing regimen for multimodal analgesia, and it will ultimately depend on the patient's presentation. Interestingly, for patients with mild to moderate pain, the combination therapy of paracetamol and ibuprofen has been shown to have excellent benefits when compared to opioid therapy alone.[10] This has always been discounted as an option for the patients that could take oral analgesia. For the unconscious patients, or patients unable to administer oral medications, consider the use of IV paracetamol. Older literature originally suggested a greater benefit of IV paracetamol in these patients; however,

Table 18.1 Multimodal analgesia dosing regimens

Drug	Dose (Adult) >60 kg	Timing	Side-effects of significance
Paracetamol	0.5–1 g	Single dose only	Nil
NSAID (ibuprofen)	400 mg	Single dose only	Nausea, GI ulceration or bleeding
Morphine	Up to 5 mg	5/60	Nausea and vomiting, drowsiness, dizziness, dose-related respiratory depression, bradycardia
Fentanyl	Up to 50 mcg	5/60	Nausea and vomiting, drowsiness, dizziness, dose-related respiratory depression
Ketamine	10–20 mg analgesic dose Infusion – 0.1–0.3 mg/kg/hour	10/60	Respiratory depression may occur with overdosage or too rapid a rate of administration
			Concern with emergence reactions – dreams, restlessness, confusion, hallucinations, irrational behaviour. Treatment with small doses of benzodiazepines for severe reactions
Parecoxib or variant (if unable to take oral NSAID)	40 mg	Single dose only	Nausea, GI ulceration or bleeding

Source: Adapted from Buckley N, Australasian Society of Clinical and Experimental Pharmacologists and Toxicologists, The Royal Australian College of General Practitioners, Pharmaceutical Society of Australia. *Australian Medicines Handbook*. Adelaide: AMH Pty Ltd, 2016.

more contemporary literature suggests that there is no benefit in the different methods of administration.[11] One of the limitations of IV paracetamol is that it costs considerably more than oral paracetamol; however, this should not affect the clinician's decision making.

In severe pain and traumatic settings, the clinician should consider the use of IV paracetamol with the addition of IV opioids, IV ketamine and an IV coxib (or alternative) in acute trauma. There is a lack of evidence to support the use of each of these; however, as clinicians we understand that all of these medications will have a synergistic effect on patients with intractable pain, due to each of their main mechanisms of action. This ultimately results in less of each medication being administered and a reduced likelihood of side-effects (**Table 18.1**).

Question 2: What Is the Role for, and Evidence Behind, Methoxyflurane?

Administered at low concentrations, methoxyflurane is an inhalational anaesthetic.[12] It is widely used within the Australian prehospital environment and has been proven to be safe and effective in pain management.[13] It is considered a desirable analgesic because of its ease of use, fast action, patient empowerment and control. Inhalational analgesics are an excellent first-line analgesic option for the patient that presents in severe pain. Literature suggests that the onset of duration is 4–5 minutes,[14] and it can most certainly give the clinician time to establish vascular access and progress to opioid therapy as required. Methoxyflurane is not without risk, although an experienced clinician will use a risk–benefit approach to utilising this in the trauma environment. The evidence suggests that the side-effects are extremely rare, as this is typically associated with high doses.[15] The most common side-effects seen are headache, nausea and dizziness.[14] Consider an inhalational anaesthetic such as methoxyflurane as a bridge to more permanent analgesia. Inhalational agents may also have benefits, and the synergistic effects when combined with an opioid make them a perfect addition to a pain management regime.

Question 3: What Are the Risks Associated with Rapid Administration of Analgesics?

In this case study, it will be imperative and advisable that a timely and aggressive dosing schedule should be considered in order to gain control over the patient. A suggested dosing regimen for this patient presenting with severe trauma is shown in **Table 18.2**.

Overall, the patient who presents with polytrauma or a significant pain-producing injury has the physiological capacity to deal with large doses of analgesia. With good practice, a clinician should always consider the risks and benefits of each of their interventions.

Initially, the clinician should consider a pain score for the patient, as this will help to guide their decision making as to what analgesic route they will take, and this should help with the forward momentum of the case. The patient who presents with moderate to severe pain should be aggressively managed in the prehospital setting.[6]

Paracetamol and an NSAID, such as ibuprofen, are unlikely to have any side-effects that will be seen in the prehospital setting, related to their main mechanisms of action and are not associated with rapid administration. The prehospital clinician should be aware of the medications that do produce dose-dependent side-effects. Higher doses of opioids have the

CHAPTER 18 Severe/Uncontrolled Pain

Table 18.2 Analgesia dosing regimen for a patient presenting with severe trauma

Drug		Dose
First line	IN fentanyl	200 mcg with repeat 50 mcg 5/60.
	Methoxyflurane (if tolerated)	3 ml.
Second line	IV fentanyl	50 mcg as required. Rough guide should be 5/60 but might need to be more aggressive to gain control.
Third line	IV ketamine	20 mg every 10/60. Balance this with fentanyl administration.
Fourth line	IV paracetamol	1 g every 4–6 hours (unlikely for repeat doses).
Fifth line	IV parecoxib	40 mg single dose only. Rationale for being fourth line is longer onset time. Be aggressive with alternative options to gain control. This will allow for reduced doses during transport.

Source: Adapted from Buckley N, Australasian Society of Clinical and Experimental Pharmacologists and Toxicologists, The Royal Australian College of General Practitioners, Pharmaceutical Society of Australia. *Australian Medicines Handbook.* Adelaide: AMH Pty Ltd, 2016.

ability to produce dose-dependent side-effects, such as central nervous system depression, hypotension, bradycardia or respiratory depression. Ketamine also has dose-dependent side-effects, and higher doses and administration more frequently lead patients towards disassociation and anaesthesia. Ketamine also has a side-effect profile and, when rapidly administered, can cause respiratory depression and apnoea.[12] This should be at the forefront of the clinician's decision making and the clinician should consider diluting these smaller doses so that they can be administered over a longer period of time, which will assist in improving the safety profile.

Preparation is key in the management of these patients. Be aware of the risks associated with high doses of opioids and ketamine. Prepare the patient with oxygen therapy and always prepare another paramedic with a bag-valve-mask and airway adjuncts for the unlikely event that the patient needs assisted ventilation following administration.

PRACTICE TIP

Always be prepared. As discussed, opioids and ketamine *can* have dose-dependent side-effects if given too rapidly. Note that this is not necessarily a problem; it is just something that a good clinician should be aware of and delegate another paramedic to be watching for predictable side-effects.

Hypotension and bradycardia are unlikely to be seen in the prehospital setting from the administration of opioids; however, it is something a clinician should be aware of. In the patient who presents with polytrauma, their derangement in vital signs is more likely to be associated with their injuries than with the analgesia. If the clinician is concerned regarding haemodynamic stability, the preferred choice in this setting should be fentanyl and ketamine

SECTION 4 Disability

as analgesic options. Fentanyl should produce fewer haemodynamic effects and ketamine produces a slight catecholamine release, which will improve its safety profile.

Question 4: What Is the Rationale Behind Procedural Sedation/Analgesia?

Procedural sedation refers to a technique of administering sedatives or dissociative agents with or without analgesics to induce a state that allows the patient to tolerate unpleasant procedures while maintaining cardiorespiratory function. Procedural analgesia or sedation has five main principles that clinicians should abide by and which should guide their decision making. These are:

1. Patient safety
2. Minimising pain and anxiety associated with the procedure
3. Minimising patient motion during the procedure
4. Maximising the chances of success with a procedure
5. Returning the patient to presentation state as quickly as possible.[16]

As clinicians, if we abide by these principles, we should feel comfortable to perform procedural sedation in the prehospital environment. Indications could include fracture reduction, thoracostomy and extrication of the polytrauma patient. The literature supports several approaches to the procedure; however, it should be noted that in the prehospital environment, we might be limited to propofol, midazolam or ketamine as our methods of choice.

Each medication comes with some level of risk. The literature supports that propofol and midazolam both risk dose-dependent respiratory depression and a very negative effect on overall haemodynamics, so the clinician should consider using an alternative agent, such as ketamine, for the patient who is poorly perfused in the setting of trauma.[17] A suggested dosing regimen for adults (>60 kg) can be found in **Table 18.3**.

Table 18.3 A suggested procedural sedation dosing regimen for adults (>60 kg)

Medication	Dose	Risks	Benefits
Propofol IV	0.5–1.0 mg/kg over 1–5 minutes, then 1.5–3.0 mg/kg per hour	Pain at injection site, bradycardia, hypotension, apnoea	Rapid onset and offset
Midazolam IV	2.0–2.5 mg then wait 3/60. If required 1 mg bolus titrated to patient effect	Hypotension, respiratory depression, apnoea	Anxiolytic effect, anterograde amnesia from procedure
Ketamine IV	1.0–1.5 mg/kg titrated to effect over 2–5 minutes, then half dose every 10 minutes if required	Salivation, nausea and vomiting, apnoea (rapid administration)	Preserve cardiovascular and respiratory function; provides analgesia concurrently

Source: Adapted from Buckley N, Australasian Society of Clinical and Experimental Pharmacologists and Toxicologists, The Royal Australian College of General Practitioners, Pharmaceutical Society of Australia. *Australian Medicines Handbook*. Adelaide: AMH Pty Ltd, 2016.

CHAPTER 18 Severe/Uncontrolled Pain

Question 5: Once the Patient is Extricated, What is the Ongoing Plan for Analgesia?

Let us refer to our case study and consider that the clinician has given intranasal fentanyl, intravenous fentanyl and intravenous ketamine for analgesia. Depending on the patient's response to this, the critical care paramedic (CCP) might have needed to give a dose of procedural sedation to allow extrication from the vehicle. The clinician, being diligent with their decision making, has administered a bolus dose of ketamine to facilitate the rapid extrication of this patient. Once extricated, the CCP needs to consider the ongoing analgesic requirements of the patient. With the long bones and pelvis appropriately splinted and stabilised, and the patient in the vehicle en route to a major trauma centre, the CCP should consider using a ketamine infusion and administration of fourth- and fifth-line analgesic options. As previously discussed, the establishment of a ketamine infusion will depend on the patient's weight, but a reasonable starting point could be 0.2 mg/kg/hour. The bolus doses of ketamine would have placed the patient into a therapeutic range, and this will allow the sustained effects with a very safe safety profile. The fourth-line suggestion is an IV NSAID and this is the time for this administration, if not earlier in the patient management, depending on your crew resource management. The rationale for leaving this as an additional therapy is that these types of NSAID have a longer onset when compared to other pharmacological options that prehospital clinicians carry. We have explored the idea that using combination therapy for these patients is beneficial and could potentially decrease the ongoing analgesic requirement, as well as reduce hospital stay and the need for ongoing analgesia once discharged.

> **PRACTICE TIP**
>
> In paramedic practice we rarely have the ability to see the immediate positive results of our treatment, especially in the multi-trauma patient. Be aggressive and humane in your approach and do not forget the basics, especially when you have the ability, knowledge and medication to have a profound impact on the patient's overall trajectory.

Question 6: What Does the Evidence Suggest is Practical for Humane Purposes of Analgesia Management? Does the Evidence Support Prehospital Intubation?

There is a dearth of high-quality literature surrounding the evidence for prehospital intubation for analgesia management in the trauma patient. The practice, or consideration, of intubation has been removed from the paramedic thought process for most trauma patients following the expansion of prehospital analgesic options including ketamine. Current CCPs have multiple lines of analgesic options and have the flexibility and freedom to administer high doses and aggressive analgesia to gain patient control in this cohort.

If a clinician was to consider the humane purpose in this setting, they could consider this for a patient that has experienced extensive burns. Realistically this decision is multifactorial and comprises a number of different angles. These patients, depending on the types of burns, will potentially have an element of respiratory involvement. Intubating this patient will ensure that airway patency will be maintained during prehospital care. As CCPs we can also anticipate the ongoing care and the probable clinical course of these patients. Early intubation can facilitate expedient movement through the emergency department to surgery if required. The benefits of intubation in this cohort are that it will allow high doses of opioids without respiratory concern and clinicians can adequately maintain haemodynamic stability with fluid and vasopressors if required. This particular situation is rare, though, and the practice of intubation to facilitate high-dose analgesia should be a very carefully considered decision, weighing up all risks and benefits.

Key Evidence

Bansal A, Miller M, Ferguson I et al. Ketamine as a prehospital analgesic: a systematic review. *Prehospital Disaster Medicine*. 2020;35(3):314–321.

Galinski M, Hoffman L, Bregeaud D et al. Procedural sedation and analgesia in trauma patients in an out-of-hospital emergency setting: a prospective multicenter observational study. *Prehospital Emergency Care*. 2018;22(4):497–505.

Hanson S, Hanson A, Aldington D. Pain priorities in pre-hospital care. *Anaesthesia and Intensive Care Medicine*. 2020;21(8):387–389.

Self-Reflection Questions

1. What methods for analgesia do you have in your service?
2. Consider the future – do you think that there will be the ability to give local anaesthesia nerve block for certain injuries?
3. What are some signs of 'undersedation' or 'underanalgesia' in this cohort?
4. Where do you place splinting as part of your analgesic regime?
5. How might you prepare your medications and delegate your crew resources to ensure appropriate timing and momentum in your practice?

References

1. Singer KE, Philpott CD, Bercz AP et al. Impact of a multimodal analgesia protocol on inpatient and outpatient opioid use in acute trauma. *Journal of Surgical Research*. 2021;268:9–16.
2. Dalton MK, Semco RS, Ordoobadi AJ et al. Opioid administration in the prehospital setting for patients sustaining traumatic injuries: an evaluation of national emergency medical services data. *Injury*. 2022;53(9):2923–2929.
3. Hollis GJ, Keene TM, Ardlie RM et al. Prehospital ketamine use by paramedics in the Australian Capital Territory: a 12-month retrospective analysis. *Emergency Medicine Australasia*. 2017;29(1):89–95.
4. Eimer C, Reifferscheid F, Jung P et al. Pre-hospital analgesia in pediatric trauma and critically ill patients: an analysis of a German air rescue service. *Scandinavian Journal of Trauma, Resuscitation and Emergency Medicine*. 2023;31(1):5.
5. Hamrick KL, Beyer CA, Lee JA et al. Multimodal analgesia and opioid use in critically ill trauma patients. *Journal of the American College of Surgeons*. 2019;228(5):769–775 e1.
6. Hanson S, Hanson A, Aldington D. Pain priorities in pre-hospital care. *Anaesthesia and Intensive Care Medicine*. 2020;21(8):387–389.
7. Jennings PA, Cameron P, Bernard S et al. Morphine and ketamine is superior to morphine alone for out-of-hospital trauma analgesia: a randomized controlled trial. *Annals of Emergency Medicine*. 2012;59(6):497–503.

8. Friesgaard KD, Kirkegaard H, Rasmussen CH et al. Prehospital intravenous fentanyl administered by ambulance personnel: a cluster-randomised comparison of two treatment protocols. *Scandinavian Journal of Trauma, Resuscitation and Emergency Medicine*. 2019;27(1):11.
9. Bansal A, Miller M, Ferguson I et al. Ketamine as a prehospital analgesic: a systematic review. *Prehospital Disaster Medicine*. 2020;35(3):314–321.
10. Graudins A, Meek R, Parkinson J et al. A randomised controlled trial of paracetamol and ibuprofen with or without codeine or oxycodone as initial analgesia for adults with moderate pain from limb injury. *Emergency Medicine Australasia*. 2016;28(6):666–672.
11. Mallama M, Valencia A, Rijs K et al. A systematic review and trial sequential analysis of intravenous vs. oral peri-operative paracetamol. *Anaesthesia*. 2021;76(2):270–276.
12. Buckley N, Australasian Society of Clinical and Experimental Pharmacologists and Toxicologists, The Royal Australian College of General Practitioners, Pharmaceutical Society of Australia. *Australian Medicines Handbook*. Adelaide: AMH Pty Ltd, 2016.
13. Jacobs I. Health effects of patients given methoxyflurane in the pre-hospital setting: a data linkage study. *Open Emergency Medicine Journal*. 2010;3:7–13.
14. Coffey F, Wright J, Hartshorn S et al. STOP!: a randomised, double-blind, placebo-controlled study of the efficacy and safety of methoxyflurane for the treatment of acute pain. *Emergency Medicine Journal*. 2014;31(8):613–618.
15. Porter KM, Dayan AD, Dickerson S et al. The role of inhaled methoxyflurane in acute pain management. *Open Access Emergency Medicine*. 2018;10:149–164.
16. Sheta SA. Procedural sedation analgesia. *Saudi Journal of Anaesthesia*. 2010;4(1):11–16.
17. Galinski M, Hoffman L, Bregeaud D et al. Procedural sedation and analgesia in trauma patients in an out-of-hospital emergency setting: a prospective multicenter observational study. *Prehospital Emergency Care*. 2018;22(4):497–505.

SECTION 5

Exposure

Hypothermia and Hyperthermia

19

Eystein Grusd and Justin Hensley

> **In this chapter you will learn:**
> - About the evidence base for hypothermia and hyperthermia in out-of-hospital care
> - The consequences of hypothermia and hyperthermia
> - How to identify hypothermia and hyperthermia
> - How to treat hypothermia and hyperthermia.

Case Details

Dispatch
53-year-old male, injured right ankle, minor abrasions.

History
A 53-year-old hiker has fallen from the track and is injured in a ravine, a 30-minute hike from the trail head. The weather is 5 °C and the conditions prohibit an air response.

On Arrival of the First Crew
The scene is safe, and the patient is easily accessible. The patient's vital signs are:

Airway	Patent
Breathing	RR 22, SpO_2 99% on air
Circulation	HR 105, regular, BP 143/89
Disability	GCS E4, V5, M6 (15)
Environmental	Outdoors, 5 °C

The patient's right ankle has an obvious deformity. The patient is dressed in light hiking clothes and tells the paramedic he is cold. Secondary survey reveals no other injuries.

On Your Arrival as the Critical Care Paramedic
The patient has been carried up to the trail by the first attending crew and bystanders. He is now sitting against a tree. There is a moulded splint on the injured ankle, and one cannula has been placed in situ. The patient is shivering.

SECTION 5 Exposure

AMPLE

The patient has high blood pressure. His only medication is ramipril 5 mg daily.

Allergies	NKDA
Medications	Ramipril 5 mg PO daily
Past history	Hypertension
Last ins and outs	Normal
Events	Fall from a hiking trail

Decision Point

What are your clinical priorities in this situation?

When the patient tells the paramedic that he is 'freezing', temperature conservation should be the first priority, especially when the timeframe for evacuation is at least 30 minutes. Pain management, combined with repositioning the ankle, should be the second priority.

Question 1: What Are the Stages of Hypothermia?

Hypothermia, a condition marked by dangerously low body temperatures, presents with varying symptoms at different stages of severity. Mild hypothermia, characterised by body temperatures ranging from 32 to 35 degrees Celsius, typically manifests with peripheral vasoconstriction and centralised circulation, resulting in white skin, a cold-to-touch sensation and slow capillary refill. Patients may also experience shivering and may exhibit behavioural changes. Moving into the moderate hypothermia range (32–28 °C), patients often display a weak and thready pulse and respiratory rates slower than the standard. Additionally, their moods can become irritable. As hypothermia progresses, confusion sets in, leading to increasingly bizarre behaviour. Severe or profound hypothermia, with temperatures below 28 °C, presents more dramatically, with an absent pulse and respirations, giving the appearance of clinical death. Patients in this state will lose consciousness, and their bodies may become more rigid. Recognising these distinct stages of hypothermia is crucial for timely intervention and appropriate medical care.[1,2]

PRACTICE TIP

Be aware of hypothermia, even in warm months.

Question 2: In What Ways Does Heat Loss Occur?

Various mechanisms govern the transfer of heat energy, and understanding these processes is essential for comprehending how our bodies regulate temperature. Radiation is the transfer of energy through electromagnetic waves. Although prevalent in various natural phenomena, its significance in affecting human body temperature is relatively minimal. Conversely, evaporative

CHAPTER 19   Hypothermia and Hyperthermia

heat transfer plays a crucial role in our thermoregulation. This process involves the conversion of fluids, such as sweat, into vapour, leading to a cooling effect on the body. Another mechanism is convection, where heat is transferred by the movement of fluids, such as warm air rising and being replaced by cooler air. Finally, conduction involves the direct transfer of heat energy through physical contact, for instance, feeling cold when lying on a chilly surface.

Question 3: What Is the Treatment for Hypothermia?

Managing hypothermia requires a tailored approach based on its severity, as different degrees of hypothermia demand distinct interventions. For patients experiencing mild hypothermia, active rewarming may not be necessary. However, it is crucial to protect them from further heat loss by removing wet clothing, elevating them off the cold ground and providing a thermal barrier around their body. As they may be shivering, high-energy foods and drinks can help replace any glucose being used during shivering. Trauma patients, alternatively, should receive active warming measures if they are hypothermic, whether mild or moderate.

In the case of moderate hypothermia, preventing further heat loss is essential, and patients may or may not be shivering. Due to their altered mental status, oral intake might not be feasible, necessitating other warming methods. Active rewarming should be initiated through the use of heat packs or bottles applied to the skin of the torso or forced air methods. Warmed intravenous or intraosseous fluids containing glucose (at 40–42 °C) can also aid in raising their body temperature.

Severe hypothermia poses more critical challenges, as patients may appear to have lost their pulse and respiration. The cold myocardium can be highly irritable, making any movement potentially induce dysrhythmias. It is crucial to determine if actual asystole or other non-perfusing rhythms are present before initiating CPR. If warranted, CPR should be started and continued until the patient's core temperature reaches 32–34°C, if possible. In cases where extrication is difficult, intermittent or delayed CPR may be considered. However, defibrillation or antiarrhythmic drugs should not be used multiple times until the core temperature has significantly increased. In certain circumstances, local protocols may involve considering eCPR (extracorporeal cardiopulmonary resuscitation).[3,4]

It is essential to note that there are contraindications to resuscitating certain hypothermia patients. If traumatic injuries are inconsistent with life, or if snow/ice is obstructing their airway, the patient may be pronounced life extinct without resuscitation attempts. Proper evaluation and understanding of the severity of hypothermia will guide the appropriate interventions and decisions to optimise patient outcomes.[1,2,4]

> **PRACTICE TIP**
>
> Remove anything wet, as conductive heat loss has the most rapid effect.

Question 4: What Are the Stages of Hyperthermia?

Heat-related illnesses encompass a spectrum of conditions, each with distinct characteristics and severity. Heat cramps may occur as involuntary contractions of large muscles, often associated with exertion in hot conditions. These cramps are linked to electrolyte imbalances

SECTION 5 Exposure

and dehydration. Heat syncope involves a transient loss of consciousness resulting from dehydration and peripheral vasodilation. Heat exhaustion manifests as weakness and fatigue, followed by symptoms such as headaches, nausea, dizziness and muscle aches. Heat stroke, the most critical condition, can include any of the previously mentioned symptoms combined with altered mental status due to hyperthermia. This life-threatening condition typically occurs when body temperatures rise above 40 °C and can present as encephalopathy, seizures, coma or even death. Proper awareness and preventive measures, such as recognising early stages of hyperthermia, appropriate cooling, rest and first aid, are crucial in managing these heat-related illnesses.[5,6]

> **PRACTICE TIP**
>
> Don't rely on standard methods of measuring exact temperature; they may be inaccurate in both the hyperthermic and hypothermic patient.

Question 5: How Is Hyperthermia Treated?

Heat-related conditions require varying degrees of intervention and cooling measures. Heat cramps, typically mild, can often be managed effectively with oral rehydration to restore electrolyte balance. Heat syncope, considered moderate, necessitates removal from the heat source and passive cooling, such as seeking shade to reduce heat exposure.

For heat exhaustion, more active cooling methods are essential. Removing the individual from the heat source remains crucial, but now cooling should be actively pursued. This can be achieved through evaporative cooling, such as using a wet sheet and fanning it to promote heat loss, conductive cooling by placing the person on a cool surface or insulating them from hot surfaces, or convective cooling through methods like fanning, air conditioning and removing tight-fitting clothing. Hospitalisation may not be necessary at this stage.

Heat stroke, however, demands urgent and immediate attention, as it is a life-threatening emergency. Airway, breathing and circulation support are critical. The primary method of cooling in this situation is cold water immersion. Starting cooling therapy within 60 minutes of onset is crucial, as delayed cooling can significantly increase mortality. If ice packs are used, it is essential to cover the entire body to optimise cooling rather than limiting it to just the groin and armpits. Swift and appropriate measures can make a substantial difference in the outcome of heat stroke cases. Altered mental status, seizures or coma should be managed aggressively.[5,6]

> **PRACTICE TIP**
>
> Hyperthermia needs to be treated more aggressively than hypothermia.

CHAPTER 19 Hypothermia and Hyperthermia

Key Evidence

Perkins GD, Graesner JT, Semeraro F et al. European Resuscitation Council Guidelines 2021: Executive summary. *Resuscitation*. 2021 Apr;161:1–60. Available at: https://pubmed.ncbi.nlm.nih.gov/33773824/. Erratum in: *Resuscitation*. 2021 May 4;163:97–98.

Haverkamp FJC, Giesbrecht GG, Tan ECTH. The prehospital management of hypothermia – An up-to-date overview. *Injury*. 2018 Feb;49(2):149–164. Available at: https://pubmed.ncbi.nlm.nih.gov/29162267/

Knapik JJ, Epstein Y. Exertional heat stroke: Pathophysiology, epidemiology, diagnosis, treatment, and prevention. *Journal of Special Operations Medicine*. 2019 Summer;19(2):108–116. Available at: https://pubmed.ncbi.nlm.nih.gov/31201762/

Self-Reflection Questions

1. How will you evaluate for hypothermia in patients?
2. What changes would hypothermia make in your management of patients?
3. How can you identify hyperthermia?

References

1. Musi ME, Sheets A, Zafren K et al. Clinical staging of accidental hypothermia: The revised Swiss system: Recommendation of the International Commission for Mountain Emergency Medicine (ICAR MedCom). *Resuscitation*. 2021 May;162:182–187. Available at: https://pubmed.ncbi.nlm.nih.gov/33675869/
2. Dow J, Giesbrecht GG, Danzl DF et al. Wilderness Medical Society clinical practice guidelines for the out-of-hospital evaluation and treatment of accidental hypothermia: 2019 update. *Wilderness Environment Medicine*. 2019 Dec;30(4S):S47–S69. Available at: https://pubmed.ncbi.nlm.nih.gov/31740369/
3. Haverkamp FJC, Giesbrecht GG, Tan ECTH. The prehospital management of hypothermia – An up-to-date overview. *Injury*. 2018 Feb;49(2):149–164. Available at: https://pubmed.ncbi.nlm.nih.gov/29162267/
4. Perkins GD, Graesner JT, Semeraro F et al. European Resuscitation Council Guidelines 2021: Executive summary. *Resuscitation*. 2021 Apr;161:1–60. Available at: https://pubmed.ncbi.nlm.nih.gov/33773824/. Erratum in: *Resuscitation*. 2021 May 4;163:97–98.
5. Knapik JJ, Epstein Y. Exertional heat stroke: Pathophysiology, epidemiology, diagnosis, treatment, and prevention. *Journal of Special Operations Medicine*. 2019 Summer;19(2):108–116. Available at: https://pubmed.ncbi.nlm.nih.gov/31201762/
6. Lipman GS, Gaudio FG, Eifling KP et al. Wilderness Medical Society clinical practice guidelines for the prevention and treatment of heat illness: 2019 update. *Wilderness Environment Medicine*. 2019 Dec;30(4S):S33–S46. Available at: https://pubmed.ncbi.nlm.nih.gov/31221601/

20

Prehospital Sepsis Management

Daniel Cudini and Judit Orosz

> **In this chapter you will learn:**
> - Contemporary sepsis assessment and management in accordance with current guidelines, recommendations and evidence
> - Common aetiologies and prevalence of prehospital sepsis presentations
> - Challenges relating to paramedic sepsis care and recognition
> - The latest sepsis definitions and the relevance of 'sepsis care pathways' for the prehospital environment.

Case Details

Dispatch

58-year-old female, altered conscious state, short of breath.

History

A 58-year-old female has not been seen by friends for the past week. She had previously received community nursing care for a wound on her right foot. A friend visited today and found her drowsy, diaphoretic and breathless. A double-crewed ambulance and a critical care paramedic are dispatched.

On Arrival of the First Crew

The scene is safe, and the patient is lying, semi-recumbent, on the couch. Her primary survey findings and initial vital signs are:

Airway	Patent
Breathing	RR 24, SpO_2 96% on room air
Circulation	Peripheral pulses weak, HR 128, BP 70/40, warm peripheries
Disability	GCS E3, V4, M5 (12), pupils 4 mm and equally reactive, BGL 11 mmol/L
Environmental	Temp 37.8 °C

The first paramedic crew arrive, leave the patient in the semi-recumbent position, and apply high-flow oxygen via a non-rebreather mask. The secondary survey reveals a right foot wound with an erythematous border and obvious exudate. The right lower leg is hot to touch.

CHAPTER 20   Prehospital Sepsis Management

On Your Arrival as the Critical Care Paramedic

One of the paramedics is inserting an 18 gauge IV in the left forearm and upon observing the patient, you see that she appears diaphoretic, dyspnoeic at rest and in an altered conscious state. Further assessment of the patient's cardiovascular state reveals weak peripheral pulses and a central capillary refill >2 seconds. The patient's SpO_2 has increased to 98% and no other abnormalities are evident upon performing a 12-lead ECG.

AMPLE

The patient has a past medical history of type 2 diabetes mellitus, anxiety and depression. Her only medication is metformin and sertraline. She has no known allergies, lives alone and is currently unemployed.

Allergies	NKDA
Medications	Metformin 500 mg PO twice a day Sertraline 25 mg PO once a day
Past history	T2DM, anxiety and depression
Last ins and outs	Normal
Events	Not seen for a week and now presents in an altered conscious state

Decision Point

What are your clinical priorities in this situation?

It would appear the patient presents in a shocked state, with organ dysfunction likely due to sepsis. Early recognition of sepsis and commencement of rapid care are crucial in this setting to prevent further morbidity and mortality. The focus of prehospital care should be oxygenation and fluid resuscitation with consideration of inotropes or vasopressors. Importantly, although not without its limitations or controversy, early IV antibiotic administration should also be considered.

Question 1: What Are the Aetiologies, Incidence and Impact of Sepsis?

Sepsis is a global health problem, and it is hard to estimate the impact it has on healthcare. Data from the Sepsis Global Burden of Diseases Study estimated that in 2017 around 11 million deaths (19.7% of all global deaths) were related to sepsis.[1] Importantly, sepsis burden is disproportionately higher among people living in regions with a lower socio-demographic index.

Sepsis can occur on a background of both communicable and non-communicable diseases and, worldwide, the most common underlying cause of sepsis was diarrhoeal disease. The most common non-communicable diseases complicated by sepsis were maternal disorders. Overall, the incidence of sepsis-related deaths exhibited two peaks, one during early childhood and another among older adults. Globally, for both sexes and all age groups, the most common underlying cause of death in relation to sepsis was lower respiratory infection.

SECTION 5 Exposure

The global impact of sepsis cannot be overestimated, as it is a major cause of morbidity and mortality, and it significantly contributes to hospital costs. People who survive sepsis often suffer from physical, psychological and cognitive long-term effects of the disease.[2]

Regardless of location, patients with sepsis often present for urgent medical care with undifferentiated symptoms and providers need to be able to recognise sepsis in a timely fashion to be able to initiate treatment.

> **PRACTICE TIP**
>
> In the absence of an alternative diagnosis, always ask the question:
>
> COULD THIS BE SEPSIS?

> **PRACTICE TIP**
>
> Always treat sepsis as a time-critical emergency.

Question 2: What Is the Current Definition of Sepsis?

Sepsis is a clinical syndrome in patients with suspected infection. What differentiates sepsis from a simple infection is the abnormal host response to the infection, resulting in organ dysfunction.

The Third International Consensus Definitions for Sepsis and Septic Shock (Sepsis-3) defined sepsis as a life-threatening organ dysfunction due to a dysregulated host response to infection.[3] The Sepsis-3 definition recommends the use of the SOFA (sequential or sepsis-related organ failure assessment) score to estimate the degree of organ failure. SOFA utilises laboratory and clinical data, where higher scores represent increased likelihood of mortality. Calculating the SOFA score is not currently possible in the prehospital setting, and its usefulness is also limited in the initial phase of hospital assessment prior to laboratory test results. A presumptive diagnosis has to be made early, based on a combination of vital signs and clinical features, to start resuscitation and administer antibiotics promptly.

Sepsis presents on a spectrum of severity. Septic shock is a subset of sepsis where there are underlying circulatory and cellular (metabolic) abnormalities. Septic shock is defined as a lactate of >2 mmol/L despite adequate fluid resuscitation and a requirement for vasopressor therapy to elevate MAP over 65 mmHg.[3]

Sepsis should be considered in an unwell patient with a suspicion of infection and any degree of organ dysfunction. When sepsis is a possibility, uncertainty about the diagnosis should not delay the initiation of treatment, as there is a potential for rapid deterioration.

In the prehospital setting sepsis screening tools usually rely on vital signs and clinical features and their specificity and sensitivity are variable.[4] Overall, when patients have moderate- or high-risk criteria for sepsis outside the acute hospital setting, they should be assessed and referred to urgent medical care if they cannot be treated safely outside hospital.[5] In addition, early hospital pre-notification systems should be considered when patients are at high risk of sepsis or septic shock to ensure timely treatment and investigations.

CHAPTER 20   Prehospital Sepsis Management

Question 3: What Is the Current Management of Sepsis?

Sepsis and septic shock are life-threatening and time-critical medical emergencies. Early recognition, targeted management and supportive therapy are key to preventing bad outcomes.

The definitive therapy of sepsis is treating the underlying infection. Perform a thorough clinical examination to identify a source (or sources) of infection. Treatment and resuscitation should commence immediately when sepsis is diagnosed or suspected.[6] It is recommended to administer antibiotics effective against the likely source within one hour.[6] To choose effective antibiotics, identification of the likely source is vital. The need for antibiotic administration has to be balanced against the potential harm caused by unnecessary antibiotic administration (for example, allergic reactions, increased antibiotic resistance, Clostridium difficile infection). Ideally, blood cultures should be obtained before antibiotic administration; however, this should not delay emergent management.

When patients need fluid resuscitation, use crystalloid fluid boluses that contain sodium 130–154 mmol/L.[5] Over- and under-resuscitation should be avoided as both have deleterious consequences. Frequent reassessment and repeated boluses may be necessary to restore adequate volume status.

In prehospital care it may not be possible to identify the potential source of infection. Once initial management and resuscitation are provided, the patient should be transferred to a centre where further tests can be carried out and treatment or source control can be provided. If the source is identified, definitive source control should be undertaken (for example, drainage of abscess or removal of infected devices).

An initial target of MAP >65 mmHg should be achieved. In Cases of septic shock, a vasopressor is needed to achieve this target. Depending on availability in the prehospital setting, noradrenaline, metaraminol or adrenaline can be used for this purpose.

Clinical standards are used worldwide to ensure timely care and diagnosis in the hospital setting.[5,7] Healthcare organisations continue to develop sepsis care bundles and locally approved clinical pathways, which include criteria to support clinical decision making to enable recognition of sepsis and elements of initial management (such as use of fluids, lactate measurement, obtaining blood cultures, antimicrobial therapy and guidance on source control, monitoring and other aspects of care).[8,9]

Question 4: What Are the Benefits and Challenges Associated with Prehospital Antibiotic Administration?

Critical care paramedics may play a key role in the management of sepsis by reducing time to antibiotic treatment. Evidence from observational studies and contemporary evidence-based guidelines have found the time between the onset of hypotension to administration of antibiotics has a significant impact on mortality in patients with sepsis.[3,6,7,8,10,11] As stated, it is recommended that rapid administration of appropriate antibiotic therapy be provided within one hour from onset of diagnosed sepsis or septic shock.[3,6,7,10]

In an eminent study undertaken by Kumar et al., initiation of effective antimicrobial therapy within the first hour following onset of septic shock-related hypotension was associated with 79.9% survival to hospital discharge. As a result, mortality increased by 7.6% for every hour

SECTION 5   Exposure

of delay in starting antibiotic therapy after the onset of hypotension.[10] A paramedicine study found the median time to first antibiotic administration in the ED from loading the patient into the ambulance was 107 (74–160) minutes. This was associated with a median transport time of 29 (20–42) minutes, suggesting a significant delay weighted towards the in-hospital setting.[12]

The 2021 Surviving Sepsis Campaign guidelines recommend that for adults with sepsis or septic shock, antimicrobials should be administered immediately, ideally within one hour of recognition. They also acknowledge that a balance must exist to mitigate the potential harms associated with administering unnecessary antimicrobials to patients without infection.[6] This is also reflected in the Sepsis Clinical Care Standard released by the Australian Commission on Safety and Quality in Health Care. It highlights that, when signs of infection-related organ dysfunction are present, appropriate antimicrobials should be administered within 60 minutes, importantly noting that a patient with suspected sepsis must have blood cultures collected immediately and that this collection must not delay the administration of appropriate antimicrobial therapy.[7]

Several challenges exist relating to prehospital antimicrobial administration:

- Variation in sensitive and specific prehospital sepsis identification criteria
- Access and feasibility of prehospital blood culture collection prior to broad-spectrum antibiotic administration
- Access to the appropriate antibiotics for treating specific sources of infection
- Prehospital antimicrobial stewardship:
    - Access to various antibiotics to treat different infective sources versus administration of broad-spectrum antibiotics for all suspected prehospital infections
- Antimicrobial resistance:
    - Potential consequences of administering unnecessary antimicrobials to patients without infection
- Lack of RCTs highlighting a mortality benefit from prehospital antibiotic administration.

In 2018, the PHANTASi trial was published in *The Lancet*.[13] It was the first large prehospital RCT determining the impact of blood culture collection and subsequent antibiotic administration on survival. The intervention group received antibiotics 26 minutes (median) before arriving at the ED, versus the usual care group, who received antibiotics at 70 minutes (median). The PHANTASi investigators concluded that administering antibiotics in the prehospital setting did not lead to improved survival (28-day mortality 8% versus 8% for intervention and usual care groups, respectively). The methodology of this study should be considered, as only SIRS criteria were used to enrol patients, regardless of illness severity, and there existed an imbalance of patients enrolled in the intervention group. Sterling et al. undertook a systematic review and meta-analysis looking at the impact and timing of antibiotic administration on outcomes in sepsis and septic shock. Based on the studies reviewed, they also found no significant mortality benefit from administering antibiotics within three hours of ED triage or within one hour of shock recognition.[14]

> **PRACTICE TIP**
>
> The presence of SIRS alone does not imply sepsis. Sepsis is likely when two or more of the following organ dysfunction criteria are present +/- SIRS criteria: hypotension, altered conscious state, metabolic disturbance (blood lactate >2 mmol/L).

CHAPTER 20 Prehospital Sepsis Management

> **PRACTICE TIP**
>
> Many emergency medical services have broad-spectrum antibiotics available and often with no provision or guidelines to allow blood culture collection prior to administration. If a patient presents with suspected prehospital sepsis, in the absence of a specific clinical practice guideline, paramedics should consult the receiving hospital or doctor and discuss antibiotic administration. This decision is based on the risks and benefits of early treatment versus the difficulty of identifying the pathogen and its sensitivities in the absence of blood culture collection.

Conversely, recent studies have reported positive mortality benefits when prehospital broad-spectrum antibiotics were administered. Varney et al. published a systematic review and meta-analysis reviewing prehospital administration of broad-spectrum antibiotics for sepsis. They included 19 studies for systematic review and four for meta-analysis (three cohort and one clinical trial). Their findings revealed that prehospital antibiotic administration to patients with sepsis can significantly lower mortality compared to patients who do not receive prehospital antibiotics.[15] In a retrospective study, Martel and colleagues compared outcomes of patients meeting sepsis criteria assessed by paramedics who were treated with IV fluids and antibiotics, versus those who were administered prehospital fluids and antibiotics in the ED. They found a statistically significant lower mortality in the study cohort when compared to the control group (approximate 66% decrease in in-hospital mortality between the groups). The authors concluded that prehospital IV administration of antibiotics significantly improves outcome in EMS patients who meet sepsis criteria based on a modified qSOFA score.[16]

From an evidence base point of view, the mortality and morbidity benefit from prehospital antibiotic administration remains inconclusive. This certainly warrants further prehospital randomised trials with more contemporary and sensitive or specific enrolment criteria to validate or disprove the above findings.

Question 5: Why Is Blood Lactate Used in Sepsis Recognition, and Does it Have a Role in Prehospital Identification?

Prehospital point-of-care blood lactate assessment (POCBLA) when used in accordance with a sepsis guideline has been shown to enhance recognition and ultimately improve sepsis identification. Shiuh et al. reported that clinicians correctly identified 76.7% of sepsis presentations when using a prehospital sepsis protocol that included POCBLA.[17] In addition, Boland et al. reported that patients with elevated prehospital lactate were more likely to be admitted to the ICU (23% versus 15%) and to have been diagnosed with sepsis (38% versus 22%) than those with normal lactate levels; however, these differences were not statistically significant.[18] Van Beest et al. also found that by measuring serum lactate of prehospital sepsis patients, and then managing those patients who presented with signs of septic shock (based on the lactate level), less time was spent in ICU and the patients had improved long-term outcomes.[19]

In clinical practice, the value of POCBLA in prehospital sepsis identification and management has been much debated. Interestingly, lactate-enhanced qSOFA may also provide greater sensitivity than qSOFA alone and is easily used in the prehospital setting.[7,20] It is important to note that despite the association between rising lactate, hypotension and mortality, elevated

SECTION 5　Exposure

lactate can also be present in other conditions not specific to sepsis and should be considered in conjunction with clinical judgement and the patient's other presenting findings.[21,22]

Key Evidence

Australian Commission on Safety and Quality in Health Care, 2022. *Sepsis Clinical Care Standard 2022*. Sydney: ACSQHC. Available at: https://www.safetyandquality.gov.au/publications-and-resources/resource-library/sepsis-clinical-care-standard-2022

Evans, L., Rhodes, A., Alhazzani, W. et al., 2021. Surviving sepsis campaign: international guidelines for management of sepsis and septic shock 2021. *Intensive Care Medicine*, 47(11), pp. 1181–1247.

National Institute for Health and Care Excellence, 2016. Sepsis: recognition, diagnosis and early management [NG51]. NICE. Available at: https://www.nice.org.uk/guidance/ng51

Singer, M., Deutschman, C.S., Seymour, C.W. et al., 2016. The third international consensus definitions for sepsis and septic shock (Sepsis-3). *JAMA*, 315(8), pp. 801–810.

Smyth, M.A., Gallacher, D., Kimani, P.K. et al., 2019. Derivation and internal validation of the screening to enhance prehospital identification of sepsis (SEPSIS) score in adults on arrival at the emergency department. *Scandinavian Journal of Trauma, Resuscitation and Emergency Medicine*, 27, pp. 1–13.

Sterling, S.A., Miller, W.R., Pryor, J. et al., 2015. The impact of timing of antibiotics on outcomes in severe sepsis and septic shock: a systematic review and meta-analysis. *Critical Care Medicine*, 43(9), p. 1907.

Varney, J., Motawea, K.R., Kandil, O.A. et al., 2022. Prehospital administration of broad-spectrum antibiotics for sepsis patients: a systematic review and meta-analysis. *Health Science Reports*, 5(3), p. e582.

Self-Reflection Questions

1. What are some of the key things to identify when assessing a prehospital sepsis patient?
2. Adrenaline or noradrenaline infusion therapy is often used by critical care paramedics when managing sepsis. What are the risks and benefits of using adrenaline or noradrenaline as an inotrope and/or vasopressor in this group?
3. Some evidence suggests that large-volume fluid resuscitation in sepsis may worsen patient outcomes. What are the considerations and mechanisms for this and are there any implications for the prehospital environment?
4. What are the benefits and considerations relating to early antibiotic administration in sepsis patients? Is ceftriaxone an appropriate prehospital antibiotic for sepsis?
5. What are the benefits of point-of-care blood lactate in the prehospital sepsis recognition?

References

1. Rudd, K.E., Johnson, S.C., Agesa, K.M. et al., 2020. Global, regional, and national sepsis incidence and mortality, 1990–2017: analysis for the Global Burden of Disease Study. *Lancet*, 395(10219), pp. 200–211.
2. Winters, B.D., Eberlein, M., Leung, J. et al., 2010. Long-term mortality and quality of life in sepsis: a systematic review. *Critical Care Medicine*, 38(5), pp. 1276–1283.
3. Singer, M., Deutschman, C.S., Seymour, C.W. et al., 2016. The third international consensus definitions for sepsis and septic shock (Sepsis-3). *JAMA*, 315(8), pp. 801–810.
4. Smyth, M.A., Gallacher, D., Kimani, P.K. et al., 2019. Derivation and internal validation of the screening to enhance prehospital identification of sepsis (SEPSIS) score in adults on arrival at the emergency department. *Scandinavian Journal of Trauma, Resuscitation and Emergency Medicine*, 27, pp. 1–13.
5. National Institute for Health and Care Excellence (2016). Sepsis: recognition, diagnosis and early management [NG51]. NICE. Available at: https://www.nice.org.uk/guidance/ng51
6. Evans, L., Rhodes, A., Alhazzani, W. et al., 2021. Surviving sepsis campaign: international guidelines for management of sepsis and septic shock 2021. *Intensive Care Medicine*, 47(11), pp. 1181–1247.

CHAPTER 20 Prehospital Sepsis Management

7. Australian Commission on Safety and Quality in Health Care, 2022. *Sepsis Clinical Care Standard 2022*. Sydney: ACSQHC. Available at: https://www.safetyandquality.gov.au/publications-and-resources/resource-library/sepsis-clinical-care-standard-2022
8. Burrell, A.R., McLaws, M.L., Fullick, M. et al., 2016. SEPSIS KILLS: early intervention saves lives. *Medical Journal of Australia*, 204(2), pp. 73–73.
9. Daniels, R., Nutbeam, T., McNamara, G. et al., 2011. The sepsis six and the severe sepsis resuscitation bundle: a prospective observational cohort study. *Emergency Medicine Journal*, 28(6), pp. 507–512.
10. Kumar, A., Roberts, D., Wood, K.E. et al., 2006. Duration of hypotension before initiation of effective antimicrobial therapy is the critical determinant of survival in human septic shock. *Critical Care Medicine*, 34(6), pp. 1589–1596.
11. Ferrer, R., Martin-Loeches, I., Phillips, G. et al., 2014. Empiric antibiotic treatment reduces mortality in severe sepsis and septic shock from the first hour: results from a guideline-based performance improvement program. *Critical Care Medicine*, 42(8), pp. 1749–1755.
12. Cudini, D., Smith, K., Bernard, S. et al., 2019. Can pre-hospital administration reduce time to initial antibiotic therapy in septic patients? *Emergency Medicine Australasia*, 31(4), pp. 669–672.
13. Alam, N., Oskam, E., Stassen, P.M. et al., 2018. Prehospital antibiotics in the ambulance for sepsis: a multicentre, open label, randomised trial. *Lancet Respiratory Medicine*, 6(1), pp. 40–50.
14. Sterling, S.A., Miller, W.R., Pryor, J. et al., 2015. The impact of timing of antibiotics on outcomes in severe sepsis and septic shock: a systematic review and meta-analysis. *Critical Care Medicine*, 43(9), p. 1907.
15. Varney, J., Motawea, K.R., Kandil, O.A. et al., 2022. Prehospital administration of broad-spectrum antibiotics for sepsis patients: A systematic review and meta-analysis. *Health Science Reports*, 5(3), p. e582.
16. Martel, T., Melmer, M.N., Leaman, S.M. et al., 2020. Prehospital antibiotics improve morbidity and mortality of emergency medical service patients with sepsis. *HCA Healthcare Journal of Medicine*, 1(3), p. 10.
17. Shiuh, T., Sweeney, T., Rupp, R. et al., 2012. 120 An emergency medical services sepsis protocol with point-of-care lactate accurately identifies out-of-hospital patients with severe infection and sepsis. *Annals of Emergency Medicine*, 60(4), p. S44.
18. Boland, L.L., Hokanson, J.S., Fernstrom, K.M. et al., 2016. Prehospital lactate measurement by emergency medical services in patients meeting sepsis criteria. *Western Journal of Emergency Medicine*, 17(5), p. 648.
19. Van Beest, P.A., Mulder, P.J., Oetomo, S.B. et al., 2009. Measurement of lactate in a prehospital setting is related to outcome. *European Journal of Emergency Medicine*, 16(6), pp. 318–322.
20. Safe Care Victoria, 2019. Emergency Clinical Network Projects. Available at: https://www.bettersafercare.vic.gov.au/emergency-care-network/sepsis
21. Shapiro, N.I., Howell, M.D., Talmor, D. et al., 2005. Serum lactate as a predictor of mortality in emergency department patients with infection. *Annals of Emergency Medicine*, 45(5), pp. 524–528.
22. Trzeciak, S., Dellinger, R.P., Chansky, M.E. et al., 2007. Serum lactate as a predictor of mortality in patients with infection. *Intensive Care Medicine*, 33, pp. 970–977.

SECTION 6

Cardiac Arrest

High-Performance CPR

21

Belinda Delardes, Jack Howard and Ziad Nehme

> **In this chapter you will learn:**
> - The importance of high-performance CPR in resuscitation
> - The description of the elements that optimise CPR performance and patient outcomes
> - The role of choreography, education and training in resuscitation
> - The clinical utility of performance monitoring, feedback and debriefing in resuscitation
> - The importance of communication and team leadership.

Case Details

Dispatch
54-year-old female, collapsed and unresponsive, abnormal breathing (highest level response).

History
A 54-year-old female has collapsed unconscious at home. She was witnessed to complain of chest pain and nausea before collapsing in the presence of her husband. The patient has slow, gasping respirations and is unconscious. Her husband immediately made an emergency call for an ambulance and was advised by the call-taker to administer cardiopulmonary resuscitation (CPR). A three-tiered emergency response was activated by the emergency dispatcher, including basic life support trained fire-fighters, advanced life support paramedics and critical care paramedics.

On Arrival of the First Crew
The scene is safe, and the patient is lying in a supine position. Basic and advanced life support crews arrive at the scene simultaneously. A primary survey is undertaken by paramedics:

Airway	Patent
Breathing	Absent
Circulation	Central pulses absent, no major haemorrhage
Disability	GCS E1, V1, M1 (3)
Environmental	No environmental concerns

SECTION 6 Cardiac Arrest

Chest compressions are commenced by fire-fighters while paramedics apply defibrillation pads and prepare for the insertion of a supraglottic airway. A rhythm check is performed, which identifies the patient to be in ventricular fibrillation (VF). The patient is defibrillated at 200 joules and CPR is then resumed.

On Your Arrival as the Critical Care Paramedic

Paramedics have successfully inserted a supraglottic airway. An attempt to insert an intravenous cannula is unsuccessful. The patient has received two consecutive defibrillations and remains in VF. Resuscitation is being performed in a confined space, there is significant task saturation, and the quality of CPR is suboptimal.

AMPLE

The patient has no known medical history and is described as fit and well by family. She has a family history of ischaemic heart disease.

Allergies	NKDA
Medications	Rosuvastatin
Past history	Hyperlipidaemia
Last ins and outs	Normal
Events prior	Complained of chest pain and nausea prior to collapsing to the floor

Decision Point

What are your clinical priorities in this situation?

Successful resuscitations are dependent on clear communication, team leadership and choreography, with well-defined team roles. In this case, the team is spread thinly across multiple tasks and the quality of CPR is suboptimal. Immediate decisions need to be made.

1. Introduce yourself as the team leader and immediately define roles and responsibilities for basic and advanced life support crews.
2. Establish 360-degree access to the patient with appropriate placement of equipment.
3. Confirm supraglottic airway patency and ensure ventilation performance (rate, volume).
4. Allocate basic life support crews to champion CPR performance and provide active feedback around resuscitation metrics (rate, depth, recoil, pauses).
5. Designate an advanced life support paramedic to perform intravenous access.
6. Maintain two-minutely rhythm checks with minimal hands-off-chest time and changes in compressors.

Question 1: What Is High-Performance CPR?

High-performance CPR is an approach to resuscitation that optimises the delivery of high-quality CPR, underpinned by team leadership, choreography, real-time feedback on performance and clear communication. Often referred to as a 'pit crew' approach to

CHAPTER 21 High-Performance CPR

resuscitation, the purpose of high-performance CPR is to champion the delivery of CPR at the target rate and depth, with adequate recoil of the chest and minimal pauses in chest compressions. As the name suggests, pit crew CPR requires a commitment to regular team-based training, a designated team leader and ongoing monitoring and feedback on performance (both in real time and post event). High-performance CPR is both a clinical intervention and a cultural one – a system-wide culture of excellence drives patient outcomes.[1]

> **PRACTICE TIP**
>
> The bottom-tier response (usually basic life support responders) in your emergency medical service should always champion CPR performance. Create a culture that empowers staff to take accountability for key interventions at a resuscitation.

Question 2: What Are the Elements of High-Performance CPR and How Are They Prioritised?

Resuscitation utilising high-performance CPR has a clear focus on minimising hands-off-chest time and ensuring that compressions are delivered effectively. This requires the prioritisation and optimisation of basic life support as shown in **Figure 21.1**.

In the setting of two or more initial responders, defibrillation pads should be immediately placed by one of the responders, while another responder begins chest compressions. The defibrillator should be pre-emptively charged during compressions prior to the rhythm analysis to minimise hands-off-chest time and pre-shock pauses.[2]

Following the first rhythm analysis, the compressor should immediately swap to reduce the potential for fatigue, and an airway adjunct, such as a supraglottic airway, may be considered if the operator is trained in its use. A supraglottic airway can be inserted quickly and will allow for uninterrupted chest compressions at a ratio of 15:1. The alternative is to commence chest compression with bag-valve-mask ventilation at a ratio of 30:2, pausing briefly to administer ventilations. Both approaches require clear communication between operators to ensure that ventilations are being delivered adequately, while avoiding hyperventilation.

Advanced interventions, such as vascular access, medication administration or endotracheal intubation, should be deferred until the arrival of adequate responders on scene. This maintains the focus on maximising the effectiveness of basic life support interventions. Advanced skills should be considered according to local guidelines but should not result in hands-off-chest time.

> **PRACTICE TIP**
>
> Basic life support interventions are far more effective than advanced life support interventions at improving patient outcomes. Never perform advanced life support interventions unless there are sufficient responders on scene, and both CPR and defibrillation performance have been optimised.

SECTION 6 Cardiac Arrest

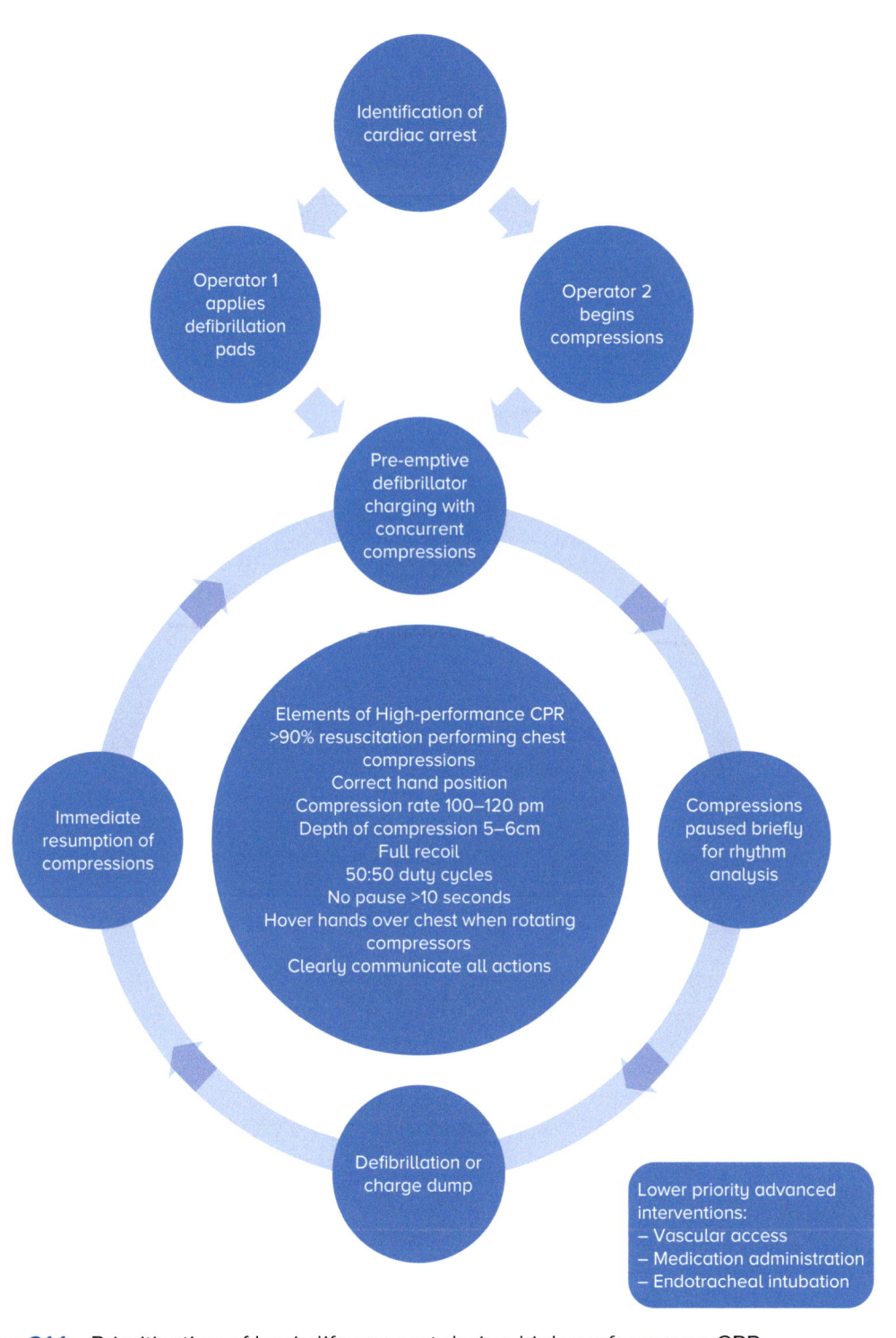

Figure 21.1 Prioritisation of basic life support during high-performance CPR.
Source: Image by Belinda Delardes and Ziad Nehme.

CHAPTER 21   High-Performance CPR

Question 3: What Is the Role of Choreography, Education and Training in High-Performance CPR?

Training and exposure to resuscitation are receiving increasing interest in the medical literature. The Global Resuscitation Alliance believes that high-performance CPR is strengthened by the collective performance of the team, achieved only with regular exposure to team-based training and well-defined choreography (for example, like 'pit crews', each team member knows exactly what to do with little wastage of time and effort).[3] A number of systems that have adopted these approaches to resuscitation training have shown significant improvements in clinical outcomes.

Exposure to resuscitation training is becoming of increasing importance, as real-life exposure to resuscitation declines for many paramedics.[4] There is evidence from randomised controlled trials and observational studies that training directed at the mastery of resuscitation skills can help improve CPR quality and reduce errors.[5] Similarly, data from observational studies indicate that participation in an accredited advanced life support course may improve the likelihood of return of spontaneous circulation and survival after cardiac arrest.[6] International consensus guidelines recommend that emergency medical service agencies monitor paramedic exposure to resuscitation and implement strategies to address low exposure.[7]

Question 4: What Is the Role of Feedback and Performance Monitoring in High-Performance CPR?

Real-time CPR feedback is intended to improve the chances of return of spontaneous circulation and survival by aligning chest compression rate, depth and recoil and hands-off-chest time with existing evidence-based guidelines. CPR feedback devices often consist of metronomes and audio and visual prompts (feedback) to guide rescuers during a resuscitation attempt (for example, 'push harder', 'good compressions'). Although high-level evidence for the benefit of these devices is lacking, international recommendations indicate that their use as part of a comprehensive quality improvement bundle, rather than an isolated intervention, may help to improve patient outcomes from cardiac arrest.[8] The Global Resuscitation Alliance also recommends the use of real-time CPR feedback devices to guide the delivery of optimal CPR during resuscitation.[3]

Most CPR feedback devices also provide a second-by-second and summary recording of CPR performance, which can also be used to enhance feedback and debriefing post cardiac arrest. Debriefing is a discussion that involves members of the resuscitation team after the event, which provides objective review of resuscitation performance with the aim of improving future performance.[7] International consensus is that post-event debriefing, which consists of data-driven objective feedback on resuscitation performance, can significantly improve survival to hospital discharge and return of spontaneous circulation when compared to no debriefing.[7] Furthermore, there is evidence from observational studies that debriefing also improves some components of CPR quality.[7]

Question 5: What Is the Impact of Team Leadership and Communication in High-Performance CPR?

Effective communication and team leadership are the cornerstone features of high-performance CPR that facilitate the pit crew approach. A clearly identified team leader is an essential component of a well-organised and high-performing resuscitation team and ensures that tasks are undertaken in a methodological and efficient manner, minimising delays and omissions of care. It is the responsibility of the team leader to control the dynamic flow of a resuscitation, be responsive to changes in the patient's condition and be prepared to manage those changes.

Leadership is an acquired skill that requires regular training and rehearsal to master.[9] Tasks or interventions carried out during a resuscitation should only be allocated to team members by the team leader. While members of the resuscitation team are often responsible for carrying out clinical interventions, it is the responsibility of the team leader to maintain overall supervision of the resuscitation and be free from task distraction. It is therefore recommended that the team leader take a prominent position at the foot-end of the patient, with complete visibility of the patient, the resuscitation team and the defibrillator.

One of the most important aspects of effective leadership is communication. Tasks or actions should be stated loudly and clearly and should be directed at the individual expected to carry out the task. Doing so avoids confusion, minimises errors of omission and duplication of interventions. It is also important to recognise that resuscitations are stressful events, and commonly result in clinical errors. Decision support tools, such as checklists, have been shown to be useful in mitigating decision-making stress and may also help to improve team leader communication during resuscitation attempts.[10]

PRACTICE TIP

High-performance CPR is both a clinical intervention and a cultural one. A system-wide culture of excellence around team-based training, feedback and debriefing, and communication will deliver the best patient outcomes.

Key Evidence

Considine J, Gazmuri RJ, Perkins GD et al. Chest compression components (rate, depth, chest wall recoil and leaning): a scoping review. *Resuscitation*. 2020;146:188–202.

Eisenburg M, Lippert F, Castren M et al. Acting on the call: improving survival from out-of-hospital cardiac arrest – 2018 update from the global resuscitation alliance [online]. Global Resuscitation Alliance. 2018. Available at: https://www.globalresuscitationalliance.org/wp-content/pdf/acting_on_the_call.pdf

Meaney PA, Bobrow BJ, Mancini ME et al. Cardiopulmonary resuscitation quality: improving cardiac resuscitation outcomes both inside and outside the hospital. *Circulation*. 2013;128:417–435.

Ng QX, Han MX, Lim YL et al. A systematic review and meta-analysis of the implementation of high-performance cardiopulmonary resuscitation on out-of-hospital cardiac arrest outcomes. *Journal of Clinical Medicine*. 2021;10:2098.

Olasveengen TM, Mancini ME, Perkins GD et al. Adult basic life support: 2020 international consensus on cardiopulmonary resuscitation and emergency cardiovascular care science with treatment recommendations. *Circulation*. 2020;142:S41–S91.

Self-Reflection Questions

1. What factors underpin the delivery of high-performance CPR?
2. How are the elements of high-performance CPR prioritised in a resuscitation attempt?
3. What sort of preparation is required to ensure familiarity with high-performance CPR?

References

1. Dyson K, Brown SP, May S et al. Community lessons to understand resuscitation excellence (culture): association between emergency medical services (EMS) culture and outcome after out-of-hospital cardiac arrest. *Resuscitation*. 2020;156:202–209.
2. Iversen BN, Meilandt C, Væggemose U et al. Pre-charging the defibrillator before rhythm analysis reduces hands-off time in patients with out-of-hospital cardiac arrest with shockable rhythm. *Resuscitation*. 2021;169:23–30.
3. Eisenburg M, Lippert F, Castren M et al. Acting on the call: improving survival from out-of-hospital cardiac arrest – 2018 update from the global resuscitation alliance [online]. Global Resuscitation Alliance. 2018. Available at: https://www.globalresuscitationalliance.org/wp-content/pdf/acting_on_the_call.pdf
4. Bray J, Nehme Z, Nguyen A et al. A systematic review of the impact of emergency medical service practitioner experience and exposure to out of hospital cardiac arrest on patient outcomes. *Resuscitation*. 2020;155:134–142.
5. Donoghue A, Navarro K, Diederich E et al. Deliberate practice and mastery learning in resuscitation education: a scoping review. *Resuscitation Plus*. 2021;6:100137.
6. Lockey A, Lin Y, Cheng A. Impact of adult advanced cardiac life support course participation on patient outcomes – a systematic review and meta-analysis. *Resuscitation*. 2018;129:48–54.
7. Greif R, Bhanji F, Bigham BL et al. Education, implementation, and teams: 2020 international consensus on cardiopulmonary resuscitation and emergency cardiovascular care science with treatment recommendations. *Resuscitation*. 2020;156:A188–a239.
8. Soar J, Berg KM, Andersen LW et al. Adult advanced life support: 2020 international consensus on cardiopulmonary resuscitation and emergency cardiovascular care science with treatment recommendations. *Resuscitation*. 2020;156:A80–a119.
9. Abildgren L, Lebahn-Hadidi M, Mogensen CB et al. The effectiveness of improving healthcare teams' human factor skills using simulation-based training: a systematic review. *Advances in Simulation*. 2022;7(1):12.
10. Groombridge CJ, Kim Y, Maini A et al. Stress and decision-making in resuscitation: a systematic review. *Resuscitation*. 2019;144:115–122.

22

Refractory Cardiac Arrest and Salvage Extracorporeal Cardiopulmonary Resuscitation (ECPR)

Matthew Thornton, Julia Coull and Sacha Richardson

> **In this chapter you will learn:**
> - The definition and incidence of refractory cardiac arrest
> - The operational challenges of refractory cardiac arrest
> - Underlying physiological principles of ECPR
> - Indications and contraindications for ECPR
> - What evidence and ECPR options are available.

Case Details

Dispatch

52-year-old male, collapsed, unconscious and apnoeic.

History

A 52-year-old man has suffered a witnessed collapse on a building site after appearing pale and diaphoretic; he was subsequently found to be in cardiac arrest. No significant traumatic injury was evident. A colleague rendered immediate assistance and commenced external chest compressions, with an initial attempt at defibrillation administered by an on-site AED. An ambulance staffed by two paramedics, two critical care paramedic solo responders and a team of fire brigade first responders have been dispatched.

On Arrival of the First Crew

The scene is safe, and the patient is lying supine with 360-degree access. The patient is in cardiac arrest, with ventricular fibrillation as the initial cardiac rhythm.

Airway	Patent
Breathing	Absent
Circulation	Central pulses absent, no major haemorrhage
Disability	GCS E1, V1, M1 (3)
Environmental	No environmental concerns

CHAPTER 22 Refractory Cardiac Arrest

The patient receives ongoing CPR and a further three attempts at defibrillation with no return of spontaneous circulation (ROSC) achieved. The paramedic crew position the airway ear-to-sternal notch and insert an appropriately sized supraglottic airway device (SAD). They also place a peripheral intravenous cannula in the right antecubital fossa, with 1 mg adrenaline administered prior to your arrival.

On Your Arrival as the Critical Care Paramedic

The paramedics are struggling to ventilate the patient, owing to vomitus in the airway and subsequent difficulty seating the SAD. CPR is effective, with high-quality chest compressions, minimal hands-off-chest time, and timely rhythm checks and defibrillation evident.

You suction the airway and intubate the trachea. You are subsequently able to ventilate the patient effectively. End-tidal capnography confirms tracheal ETT placement, with a sustained quantitative reading of 30 mmHg.

You are aware that the patient has now been in cardiac arrest for 14 minutes and has been unresponsive to initial advanced cardiac life support therapy (CPR, 5x DCCV defibrillation, 2 mg adrenaline, 300 mg amiodarone). Given the age of the patient, the witnessed arrest, good immediate bystander CPR and failure to achieve ROSC with conventional measures, you believe he is a candidate for extracorporeal CPR (ECPR). No prehospital ECPR capability is available to you, but the nearest ECPR-capable hospital is located nearby, with an estimated transport time of ten minutes.

Two further unsuccessful defibrillation attempts are made. Your fellow critical care paramedic also administers further doses of adrenaline and amiodarone. The cardiac rhythm remains ventricular fibrillation. It is now 20 minutes since the onset of arrest.

AMPLE

Allergies	NKDA
Medications	Irbesartan, atorvastatin
Past history	Hypertension and hypercholesterolaemia, recently diagnosed; otherwise well and physically active
Last eaten	Breakfast, four hours previously
Events	VF cardiac arrest

Decision Point
What are your clinical and logistical priorities in this situation?

Despite optimised ACLS resuscitation up to this point, you are concerned that the patient remains in refractory cardiac arrest. You continue to treat him as per guidelines, concurrently institute mechanical CPR (mCPR) therapy, and prepare for rapid extrication and transport to hospital for consideration of ECPR. Early pre-alert is essential to allow the destination hospital time to activate an ECPR team.

SECTION 6 Cardiac Arrest

Question 1: What Defines Refractory Cardiac Arrest, and What Logistical Implications Does It Have on Priorities at the Scene?

The definition of refractory cardiac arrest varies in the scientific literature. Failing to achieve ROSC despite conventional cardiopulmonary resuscitation (CCPR) with repeated defibrillation attempts is typical.[1] Shock refractory ventricular arrhythmia is usually defined as the need for more than three shocks.[2–4] CCPR durations beyond a range of 10–30 minutes may also be considered refractory.

In the case of out-of-hospital cardiac arrest (OHCA), many guidelines recommend CCPR at the scene until either ROSC is achieved or ongoing resuscitation attempts are considered futile and subsequently ceased, typically after 30–60 minutes. ECPR is a novel therapy for refractory cardiac arrests that may improve outcomes and extend viable resuscitation timeframes when compared to CCPR alone.[5]

Patient management at the scene may now include assessment for ECPR eligibility, early application of an mCPR device, and decisions regarding the timing of transport to a hospital with an ECPR capability.

Question 2: How Is Extracorporeal Membrane Oxygenation (ECMO) Beneficial in Refractory Cardiac Arrest?

ECMO is a temporary extracorporeal life support (ECLS) therapy, and ECPR refers to the commencement of veno-arterial (V-A) ECMO support while a patient is in cardiac arrest.

CPR and ECPR are not definitive therapies; they aim to provide organ perfusion until a perfusing rhythm with native cardiac output (ROSC) is achieved. ECPR is able to provide complete circulatory support, allowing maintenance of haemodynamics and gas exchange in the absence of any native cardiac function. This provides an extended timeframe to perform diagnostic and therapeutic interventions in order to achieve native ROSC and ultimately separation from ECMO (**Figure 22.1**).

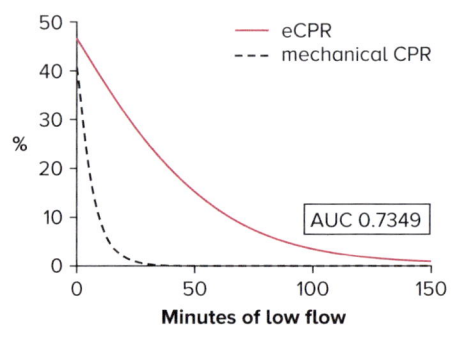

Figure 22.1 eCPR versus mechanical CPR survival with AUC curve.

Source: Wengenmayer T, Rombach S, Ramshorn F et al. Influence of low-flow time on survival after extracorporeal cardiopulmonary resuscitation (eCPR). *Critical Care*. 2017;21(1):157. Available at: https://ccforum.biomedcentral.com/articles/10.1186/s13054-017-1744-8

CHAPTER 22 Refractory Cardiac Arrest

V-A ECMO provides both cardiac and respiratory support. The large arterial and venous catheters that facilitate this therapy are typically inserted in the femoral vessels for ECPR. Deoxygenated blood is drained from the venous system, from the right atrium and inferior vena cava, via a centrifugal pump. It is then passed through a gas exchange membrane that facilitates diffusion of oxygen into the blood and removal of carbon dioxide. The oxygenated blood is returned under positive pressure to the arterial system, typically at the level of the distal aorta or proximal iliac artery. The returned blood flows retrograde (up the descending aorta) with continuous flow (i.e. without a pulse) and provides whole-body perfusion (**Figure 22.2**).[6]

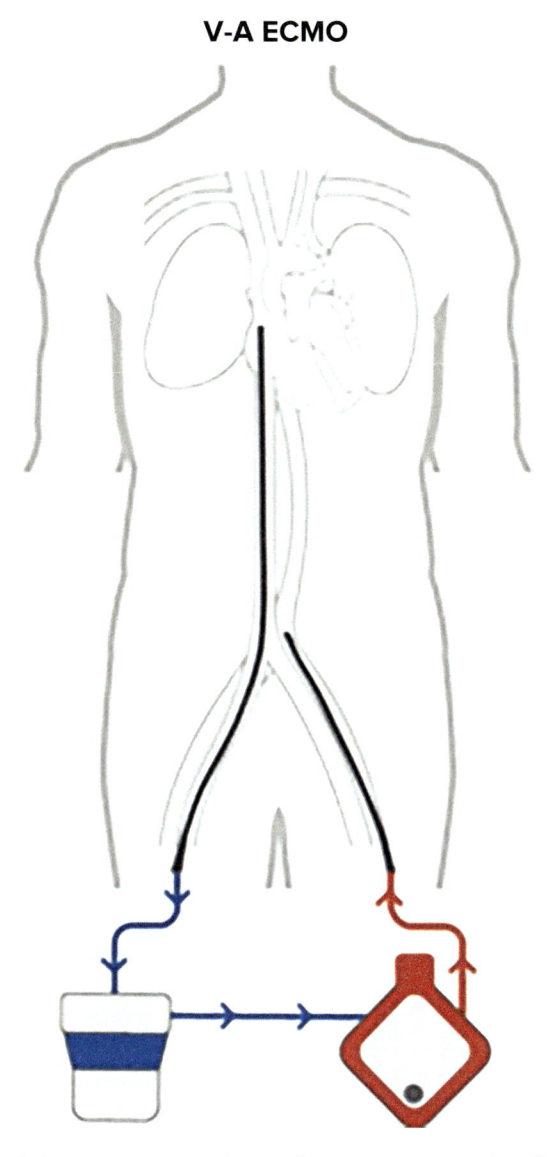

V-A ECMO

Figure 22.2 Veno-arterial extracorporeal membrane oxygenation (VA-ECMO) support (VA-ECMO) Support.

Source: Julia Coull.

221

SECTION 6 Cardiac Arrest

Question 3: Which Cases Should Be Considered for ECPR?

Optimum inclusion criteria have yet to be defined for refractory OHCA salvaged with ECPR. Survival rates reported in the literature range from 8% to 43%.[7,8] However, younger age (<70 years), witnessed arrests with good immediate bystander CPR and refractory VF/VT seem to have the best chances of survival and should be considered appropriate cases.[9,10] Some special circumstances, such as hypothermia and toxidrome-mediated cardiac arrests, may also be considered candidates.[11,12]

Timing of initiation of ECPR has also been variably reported. A useful model to identify potential candidates for ECPR focuses on the time course from onset of cardiac arrest. No-flow duration (NFD) is from cardiac arrest till the initiation of CPR, where no blood is circulating at all. Low-flow duration (LFD) is from commencement of CPR till ROSC or ECMO flow. It is noteworthy that high-quality CPR produces cerebral blood flow that is only 30–40% of native circulation (**Figure 22.3**).[13] Neurologically intact survival rates fall significantly where NFD exceeds five minutes[14] and LFD exceeds 60 minutes,[15] although some survivors have been reported beyond this.

> **PRACTICE TIP**
>
> Think about ECPR before arriving at all OHCA cases.

Such urgency poses major logistical hurdles for OHCA patients, who must be transported to an ECPR-capable facility with ongoing, high-quality resuscitation and arrive at a time point that allows for commencement of cannulation by an ECMO team. Experienced ECPR cannulators take approximately 15 minutes to achieve ECMO blood flow, so patients with refractory OHCA ideally need to be delivered to an ECPR-capable facility no later than 45 minutes from onset of arrest.

Survival from CCPR rapidly declines after the onset of cardiac arrest. Even the optimal cohort of patients, those with bystander witnessed VF/VT cardiac arrest who receive immediate CPR, have poor rates of survival-to-discharge once cardiac arrest is refractory to initial treatment. These rates fall from 37% for those still receiving CCPR at 20 minutes to 17% at 30 minutes (**Figure 22.4**).[16] Though the optimal time to deploy ECPR remains controversial, we would advocate for ECPR for appropriately selected patients who have had 20 minutes of ACLS therapies without sustained ROSC, those experiencing intermittent ROSC with multiple re-arrests, or those with refractory cardiac arrest and signs of life under CPR.[17]

Time course from OHCA to ECPR

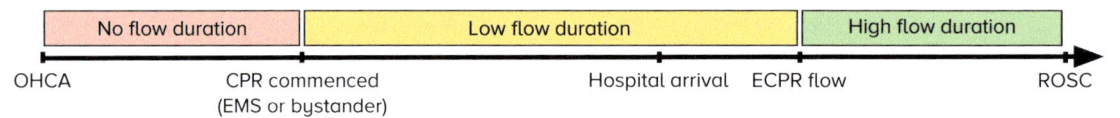

No flow duration	Low flow duration	High flow duration
OHCA — CPR commenced (EMS or bystander)	Hospital arrival — ECPR flow	ROSC

Figure 22.3 Time course from OHCA to ECPR.
Source: Image by Matthew Thornton.

CHAPTER 22 Refractory Cardiac Arrest

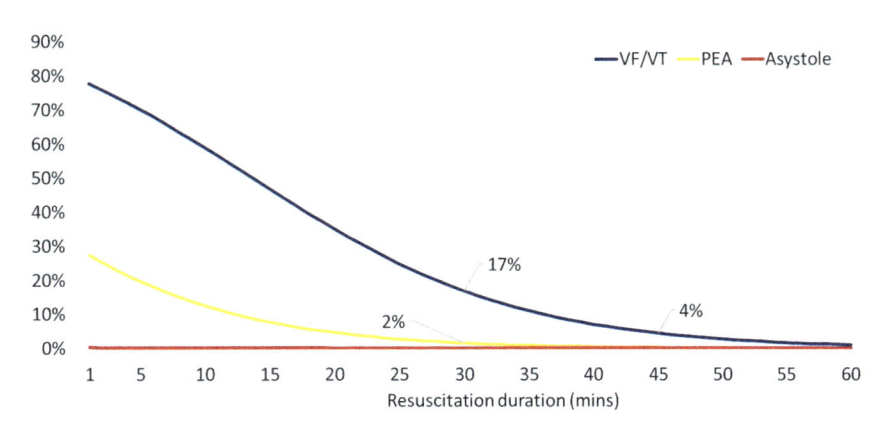

Figure 22.4 CPR survival curves.

Source: Victorian Ambulance Cardiac Arrest Registry, used with permission. Data from the Victorian Ambulance Cardiac Arrest Registry predicting probability of survival of the "average" patient (based on averaging of age, gender, aetiology, witness status, arrest location, response time, bystander CPR, region, initial arrest rhythm and arrest duration).

The following are examples of inclusion criteria for ECPR:[18]

- Age <70 years
- Witnessed arrest **with:**
    o No-flow duration <5 minutes
    o Initial cardiac rhythm of VF/pulseless VT/PEA
    o Low-flow duration <60 minutes
    o $EtCO_2$ >10 mmHg during CCPR
    o Intermittent ROSC or recurrent VF
    o Signs of life during CCPR
    o Absence of known life-limiting co-morbidities (for example, end-stage heart failure, chronic obstructive pulmonary disease, end-stage renal failure, liver failure, terminal illness)
    o Absence of aortic valve incompetence (> mild should be excluded).

Question 4: What Are the Different Delivery Models to Facilitate ECMO-CPR (Hospital versus Prehospital)?

ECPR may be initiated for both in- and out-of-hospital cardiac arrests. Suitable OHCA patients may be transported to an ECPR-capable facility while receiving mCPR on route. Some centres (Paris, Melbourne, Albuquerque, Minnesota, London) have a limited prehospital ECPR capability, whereby the ECMO team attends the scene of the arrest, assesses and cannulates the patient on site, then transfers the patient to hospital with V-A ECMO support. The goal of prehospital ECPR is to improve outcomes by minimising LFD.[19] It should be noted that at this time most prehospital ECPR programmes are undertaken in the context of research.

SECTION 6   Cardiac Arrest

> **PRACTICE TIP**
>
> Improved understanding of ECPR deployment, physiology and workflow will invariably lead to improved use and outcomes.

Question 5: How Can the Patient and the CCPR Team Be Optimised to Facilitate Integration with the ECPR Team?

Whether ECPR is undertaken at hospital or in the field, it is logistically challenging and requires 360-degree access to the patient. Clear lines of communication must be established between the CCPR and ECPR teams, with effective logistical planning, situational awareness and team leadership.

There are three phases to establishing ECPR for the patient in cardiac arrest: the first stage consists of CCPR only, the second allows for transitional care and the final stage consists of deployment of V-A ECMO.

Initially, the focus should be on high-quality CCPR to maximise the chances of early ROSC. If the ECPR team is present during this phase, they should assist in a supportive role.

During transitional care, changes are made to the resuscitation to prepare for the implantation of V-A ECMO. CCPR remains ongoing, but personnel in this team are relocated away from the patient's torso (ideally above the head and shoulders). The patient should be intubated. This is to protect the airway, minimise ongoing gastric insufflation and allow for optimised ventilation strategies once established on V-A ECMO. Manual compressions may be replaced with mCPR to improve access to the patient. The patient should be exposed from the navel to the ankles, and the ECPR team will sterilise both inguinal areas. A sterile field is then created and the equipment is set up (**Figure 22.5**).

In the final phase, the vessels are accessed, either by surgical or percutaneous Seldinger technique. The cannulas are inserted and connected to an ECMO circuit that is pre-primed with crystalloid fluid and then attached to the pump. V-A ECMO blood flow is subsequently established, and the circuit tubing is secured to the patient's thighs.[20,21]

Ongoing care is specialised and requires in-depth understanding of how ECMO interacts with the patient's native physiology. It is notable that after establishment of ECMO blood flow, an improvement in diastolic perfusion pressure to the coronary arteries and improving acid–base status may increase chances of achieving ROSC in the subsequent minutes. However, the primary role of V-A ECMO is to provide adequate organ perfusion until definitive care can be delivered. Thus, it is imperative that preparations to relocate the patient to a site capable of definitive care (for example, cardiac catheterisation laboratory) are made concurrently with the processes outlined above, in order to minimise delays and improve chances of neurologically intact survival.

Question 6: What Are the Early Complications and Challenges of ECPR?

Early complications of ECPR can be due to issues with the physical implantation of the cannulas, or from patient interaction with V-A ECMO physiology. Failure to cannulate, bleeding due to vascular injury and cannula dislodgement are usually fatal if not rapidly

CHAPTER 22 Refractory Cardiac Arrest

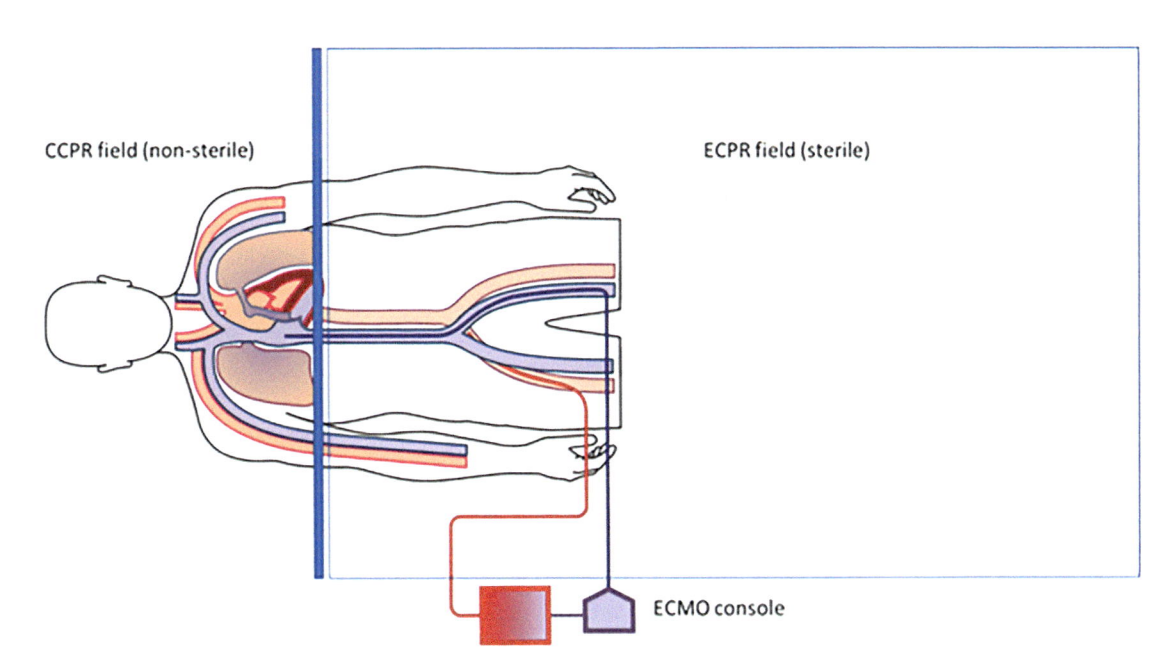

Figure 22.5 ECPR set-up.
Source: The Alfred Hospital: ecmo.icu. Reproduced with permission.

rectified. Some pathologies soon prove unsupportable on V-A ECMO; increased afterload with severe LV impairment can lead to LV overdistension, LV clot formation and pulmonary oedema. Ongoing complications of V-A ECMO include bleeding with coagulopathies, thrombus formation and infection.

Despite these complications, logistical challenges pose the greatest obstacle to increased uptake and success with ECPR programmes. Optimal outcomes from ECPR are attained with early deployment (<60 minutes from arrest onset), which is logistically challenging. Complicating this, refractory cardiac arrests have heterogeneous aetiologies, only some of which are amenable to salvage ECPR.

In highly selected cases, ECPR provides hope for increased neurologically intact survival from refractory cardiac arrest when compared with CCPR alone. With greater uptake, refinement and technological advancement, ECPR may become a cornerstone of management for refractory cardiac arrest in the future.

> **PRACTICE TIP**
> Simulation is key to optimising early resuscitation and to enable rapid transport for consideration of ECPR.

Key Evidence

ARREST trial: Yannopoulos D, Bartos J, Raveendran G et al. Advanced reperfusion strategies for patients with out-of-hospital cardiac arrest and refractory ventricular fibrillation (ARREST): a phase 2, single centre, open-label, randomised controlled trial. *Lancet*. 2020;396(10265):1807–1816. Available at: https://pubmed.ncbi.nlm.nih.gov/33197396/

SECTION 6   Cardiac Arrest

CHEER trial: Stub D, Bernard S, Pellegrino D et al. Refractory cardiac arrest treated with mechanical CPR, hypothermia, ECMO and early reperfusion. *Resuscitation*. 2015;86:88–94. Available at: https://pubmed.ncbi.nlm.nih.gov/25281189/

ELSO ECPR guidelines: Richardson ASC, Tonna JE, Nanjayya V, et al. Extracorporeal cardiopulmonary resuscitation in adults. Interim guideline consensus statement from the Extracorporeal Life Support Organization. *Journal of the American Society for Artificial Internal Organs*. 2021;67(3):221–228. Available at: https://pubmed.ncbi.nlm.nih.gov/33627592/

Inception trial: Suverein MM, Delnoij TSR, Lorusso R et al. Early extracorporeal CPR for refractory out-of-hospital cardiac arrest. *New England Journal of Medicine*. 2023;388:299–309. Available at: https://pubmed.ncbi.nlm.nih.gov/36720132/

Prague trial: Belohlavek J, Smalcova J, Rob D et al. Effect of intra-arrest transport, extracorporeal cardiopulmonary resuscitation, and immediate invasive assessment and treatment on functional neurologic outcome in refractory out-of-hospital cardiac arrest. *JAMA*. 2022;327(8):737–747.

Self-Reflection Questions

1. When should you think about the possibility of ECPR during an OHCA case?
2. What is the location of your nearest ECPR-capable hospital?
3. Are there established guidelines to access this service? If not, why not?
4. Do you know or can you access the local inclusion/exclusion criteria?
5. Have you simulated mCPR deployment and the logistics of rapid extrication in the past three months?

References

1. Sonneville R, Schmidt M. Extracorporeal cardiopulmonary resuscitation for adults with refractory out-of-hospital cardiac arrest: towards better neurological outcomes. *Circulation*. 2020;141(11):887–890. Available at: https://pubmed.ncbi.nlm.nih.gov/32176540/
2. Shanmugasundaram M, Lotun K. Refractory out of hospital cardiac arrest. *Current Cardiology Reviews*. 2018;14(2):109–114. Available at: https://pubmed.ncbi.nlm.nih.gov/29737259/
3. Siao FY, Chiu CC, Chiu CW et al. Managing cardiac arrest with refractory ventricular fibrillation in the emergency department: conventional cardiopulmonary resuscitation versus extracorporeal cardiopulmonary resuscitation. *Resuscitation*. 2015;92:70–76. Available at: https://pubmed.ncbi.nlm.nih.gov/25936930/
4. Hanneken K, Gaieski D, Hall R. Extracorporeal membrane oxygenation (ECMO) for refractory cardiac arrest. *Journal of Education and Teaching in Emergency Medicine*. 2020;5(4):S28–S58. Available at: https://www.researchgate.net/publication/372454523_Extracorporeal_Membrane_Oxygenation_ECMO_for_Refractory_Cardiac_Arrest
5. Patricio D, Peluso L, Brasseur A et al. Comparison of extracorporeal and conventional cardiopulmonary resuscitation: a retrospective propensity score matched study. *Critical Care*. 2019;23(1):27. Available at: https://pubmed.ncbi.nlm.nih.gov/30691512/
6. Riley B, Coull J. Extracorporeal support of the respiratory system. *Anaesthesia and Intensive Care Medicine*. 2022;23(10):642–646. Available at: https://www.sciencedirect.com/science/article/abs/pii/S1472029922001606
7. Bougouin W, Dumas F, Lamhaut L et al. Extracorporeal cardiopulmonary resuscitation in out-of-hospital cardiac arrest: a registry study. *European Heart Journal*. 2020;41(21):1961–1971. Available at: https://pubmed.ncbi.nlm.nih.gov/31670793/
8. Yannopoulos D, Bartos J, Raveendran G et al. Advanced reperfusion strategies for patients with out-of-hospital cardiac arrest and refractory ventricular fibrillation (ARREST): a phase 2, single centre, open-label, randomised controlled trial. *Lancet*. 2020;396(10265):1807–1816. Available at: https://pubmed.ncbi.nlm.nih.gov/33197396/

9. Wang J, Ma Q, Zhang H et al. Predictors of survival and neurologic outcome for adults with extracorporeal cardiopulmonary resuscitation: a systemic review and meta-analysis. *Medicine*. 2018;97(48):e13257. Available at: https://pubmed.ncbi.nlm.nih.gov/30508912/
10. Mochizuki K, Imamura H, Iwashita T et al. Neurological outcomes after extracorporeal cardiopulmonary resuscitation in patients with out-of-hospital cardiac arrest: a retrospective observational study in a rural tertiary care center. *Journal of Intensive Care*. 2014;2(1):33. Available at: https://pubmed.ncbi.nlm.nih.gov/25908986/
11. Kraai E, Wray TC, Ball E et al. E-CPR in cardiac arrest due to accidental hypothermia using intensivist cannulators: a case series of nine consecutive patients. *Journal of Intensive Care Medicine*. 2023;38(2):215–219. Available at: https://pubmed.ncbi.nlm.nih.gov/35876344/
12. Ng M, Wong ZY, Ponampalam R. Extracorporeal cardio-pulmonary resuscitation in poisoning: a scoping review article. *Resuscitation Plus*. 2023;13:100367. Available at: https://pubmed.ncbi.nlm.nih.gov/36860990/
13. Meaney PA, Bobrow BJ, Mancini ME et al. Cardiopulmonary resuscitation quality: improving cardiac resuscitation outcomes both inside and outside the hospital: a consensus statement from the American Heart Association. *Circulation*. 2013;128(4):417–435. Available at: https://pubmed.ncbi.nlm.nih.gov/23801105/
14. Murakami N, Kokubu N, Nagano N et al. Prognostic impact of no-flow time on 30-day neurological outcomes in patients with out-of-hospital cardiac arrest who received extracorporeal cardiopulmonary resuscitation. *Circulation Journal*. 2020;84(7):1097–1104. Available at: https://pubmed.ncbi.nlm.nih.gov/32522902/
15. Fagnoul D, Combes A, De Backer D. Extracorporeal cardiopulmonary resuscitation. *Current Opinions in Critical Care*. 2014;20(3):259–265. Available at: https://pubmed.ncbi.nlm.nih.gov/24785674/
16. Data from the Victorian Ambulance Cardiac Arrest Registry predicting probability of survival of the "average" patient (based on averaging of age, gender, aetiology, witness status, arrest location, response time, bystander CPR, region, initial arrest rhythm and arrest duration.
17. Lamhaut L, Hutin A, Puymirat E et al. A pre-hospital extracorporeal cardio pulmonary resuscitation (ECPR) strategy for treatment of refractory out hospital cardiac arrest: an observational study and propensity analysis. *Resuscitation*. 2017;117:109–117. Available at: https://pubmed.ncbi.nlm.nih.gov/28414164/
18. Richardson ASC, Tonna JE, Nanjayya V et al. Extracorporeal cardiopulmonary resuscitation in adults. Interim guideline consensus statement from the Extracorporeal Life Support Organization. *Journal of the American Society for Artificial Internal Organs*. 2021;67(3):221–228. Available at: https://pubmed.ncbi.nlm.nih.gov/33627592/
19. Singer B, Reynolds JC, Lockey DJ et al. Pre-hospital extra-corporeal cardiopulmonary resuscitation. *Scandinavian Journal of Trauma, Resuscitation and Emergency Medicine*. 2018;26(1):21. Available at: https://pubmed.ncbi.nlm.nih.gov/29587810/
20. Kumar KM. ECPR-extracorporeal cardiopulmonary resuscitation. *Indian Journal of Thoracic Cardiovascular Surgery*. 2021;37(Suppl 2):294–302. Available at: https://pubmed.ncbi.nlm.nih.gov/33432257/
21. Makdisi G, Wang IW. Extra corporeal membrane oxygenation (ECMO) review of a lifesaving technology. *Journal of Thoracic Disease*. 2015;7(7):E166–176. Available at: https://pubmed.ncbi.nlm.nih.gov/26380745/

23

Traumatic Cardiac Arrest

Zainab Alqudah and Brian Burns

> **In this chapter you will learn:**
> - Whether treating a patient with traumatic cardiac arrest (TCA) is futile
> - What evidence is related to prioritising addressing underlying causes of traumatic cardiac arrest prior to commencing external chest compressions and administration of adrenaline
> - What the optimal treatment for TCA is.

Case Details

Dispatch

43-year-old male, vehicle-related trauma (vehicle versus pedestrian), unconscious.

History

A 43-year-old male is reported to have been skateboarding along the mountain road with no helmet when he was struck by a car travelling at approximately 50 mph (80 kph). The driver of the vehicle stopped and immediately called emergency services. He said he saw the patient at the last minute and swerved to miss; however, he clipped him with the left front corner of his car. The patient struck the left windscreen and was thrown onto the road. A driver of a truck witnessed the incident, pulled over and commenced cardiopulmonary resuscitation (CPR), as the patient was in cardiac arrest. A double-crewed ambulance and a critical care paramedic are dispatched.

On Arrival of the First Crew

There is traffic at the scene and the street lighting is poor. The patient is lying supine in a concrete gutter on the side of the road. His primary survey findings and initial vital signs are:

Airway	Patent
Breathing	Absent, SpO_2 unreadable
Circulation	Peripheral pulses absent, BP unrecordable
Disability	GCS E1, V1, M1 (3)
Environmental	Outdoors, no specific concerns

CHAPTER 23   Traumatic Cardiac Arrest

The first paramedic crew to arrive positioned the patient on his back and confirmed that he was in pulseless electrical activity (PEA) arrest. After the secondary survey, the paramedic suspected head and cervical injuries due to blood coming from the mouth and a continuous need to suction the airway. The secondary survey also revealed crepitus to the lower jaw, damage to the patient's teeth and tongue, a deep laceration in the chin (approximately 3 cm long), bruising in upper chest and grazes and bruising to the back. The crew has performed the following intervention:

1. Bilateral chest decompression using pneumothorax set (result: positive on left side)
2. Applied SAM sling to pelvis
3. Gained intravenous access (IV) and commenced delivery of normal saline
4. CPR (30 comps: 2 vents) was begun while attempting to secure the airway by supraglottic airway (result: unsuccessful).

There were no other obvious injuries.

On Your Arrival as the Critical Care Paramedic

Airway management is handed over to you as the critical care paramedic (CCP) on your arrival for further management due to significant jaw and facial fractures and copious blood in the airway. Repeated suctioning is required throughout the case and performed as needed. Another attempt to open the airway with a supraglottic airway is undertaken (result: unsuccessful). The CCP is then switched to bag-valve-mask (BVM) ventilation, which turns out to be adequate. You are still unable to get an SpO_2 reading. The crew continue to provide normal saline via IV. One of the paramedics repositions the SAM splint. After 20 minutes of resuscitation, a sudden increase in $EtCO_2$ (25 mmHg) is recorded, although the patient remains in PEA. One dose of adrenaline is administered (1 mg), and spontaneous circulation is returned shortly after. Paramedics get a reading of 86% on 100% O_2, a pulse rate of 72, regular, and BP of 62/37 mmHg. A successful attempt to open the airway with a supraglottic airway is undertaken, and adequate ventilation is provided.

Further management by CCP includes continuing the normal saline IV, spinal motion restriction by a cervical collar, log rolling the patient onto a spine board to a stretcher and moving him into the back of the vehicle, then warming patient with heater blankets. You consult with a hospital clinician on adrenaline infusion, as the patient remains hypotensive despite giving the normal saline IV. The clinician advises giving an adrenaline infusion of 5–10 mcg/min IV to improve the patient's blood pressure.

AMPLE

The patient's past medical history is difficult to obtain due to his arrested status and the unavailability of family members.

Allergies	Unknown
Medications	Unknown
Past history	Unknown
Last ins and outs	Unknown
Events	Vehicle-related trauma (vehicle versus pedestrian)

SECTION 6 Cardiac Arrest

Decision Point
What are your clinical priorities in this situation?

Treatment priorities include addressing reversible causes of the patient's arrest; treating pneumothorax and managing the airway to correct the oxygen saturations and support circulation are of the utmost importance, followed by commencing CPR and giving adrenaline to restart the heart and maintain circulation.

Question 1: Is Treating a Patient with Traumatic Out-of-Hospital Cardiac Arrest (OHCA) Futile and Resource-Consuming?

The issue of futility in the resuscitation of a TCA is one that is often brought up when discussing the merits of resuscitation. A published systematic review of 34 studies (overall population of 5,391 patients) reported a low survival rate of 4.4%, with many survivors experiencing severe neurological disability at follow-up.[1] In 2013, a joint position article for withholding or termination of resuscitation of patients in cardiopulmonary arrest caused by trauma found that to achieve survival in OHCA, certain characteristics should be present, including witnessed arrest, early bystander CPR, an initial shockable rhythm, and ROSC within 20 minutes of collapse.[2] Unfortunately, the majority of traumatic OHCA do not present in an initial shockable rhythm and the victim is usually not witnessed to arrest.[3,4] In addition to poor prognosis, there is the high cost of resuscitation per individual patient and the issue of diverting resources from other time-critical patients.[2,5]

Irrespective of the high expenditure and the poor prognosis, it has been suggested that resuscitation after traumatic OHCA is just as essential as in medical patients, unless there are injuries that are incompatible with life.[6–8] Several recent studies from North America,[6] Germany,[9] England and Wales[7] have reported better survival rates, suggesting that prehospital resuscitation may not be entirely futile. The authors have attributed the improvement in survival to advancements in prehospital care, reduced EMS response time, and rapid access to designated trauma centres.[10–12] Therefore, withholding resuscitation should be based on the determination that there are no obvious signs of life, the injuries are incompatible with life, there is evidence of prolonged arrest and there is a lack of organised electrocardiographic activity (**Figure 23.1**).

PRACTICE TIP
Resuscitation is definitely not futile, and your ideal survival is a patient who was witnessed to arrest by EMS and has an initial shockable arrest rhythm.

Question 2: What Is the Evidence Related to Prioritising by Addressing Underlying Causes of Traumatic Cardiac Arrest prior to Commencing External Chest Compressions and Administration of Adrenaline?

The management of traumatic OHCA patients is different from that of medical cardiac arrest with other causes and underlying pathophysiology.[13] In medical cardiac arrest, the majority

> - It is appropriate to withhold resuscitative efforts for certain trauma patients for whom death is the predictable outcome.
> - Resuscitative efforts should be withheld for trauma patients with injuries that are obviously incompatible with life, such as decapitation or hemicorporectomy.
> - Resuscitative efforts should be withheld for patients of either blunt or penetrating trauma when there is evidence of prolonged cardiac arrest, including rigor mortis or dependent lividity.
> - Resuscitative efforts may be withheld for a blunt trauma patient who, on the arrival of EMS personnel, is found to be apnoeic, pulseless and without organised electrocardiographic activity.
> - Resuscitative efforts may be withheld for a penetrating trauma patient who, on arrival of EMS personnel, is found to be pulseless and apnoeic, with no other signs of life, including spontaneous movement, electrocardiographic activity and papillary response.
> - When the mechanism of injury does not correlate with the clinical condition, suggesting a non-traumatic cause of cardiac arrest, standard resuscitative measures should be followed.

Figure 23.1 The 2012 joint NAEMSP-ACSCOT position statements on withholding resuscitation in traumatic cardiopulmonary arrest.

Source: Millin MG, Galvagno SM, Khandker SR et al. Withholding and termination of resuscitation of adult cardiopulmonary arrest secondary to trauma: resource document to the joint NAEMSP-ACSCOT position statements. *Journal of Trauma and Acute Care Surgery*. 2013;75(3):459–467.

of adult patients have primary cardiac aetiology. In contrast, in traumatic cardiac arrest, the leading causes are major haemorrhage, head or chest injuries, or airway obstruction.[8,14,15] Until recently, protocols for the management of cardiac arrest have not differentiated between traumatic and medical aetiologies. Recent guidelines published for managing traumatic cardiac arrest have emphasised the need for rapid identification and correction of potentially reversible causes of arrest.[15,16] An example of these guidelines is presented in **Figure 23.2**.

Traumatic cardiac arrest is a time-critical condition, and survival depends on a well-established chain of care, including advanced prehospital and designated trauma centre care. The updated resuscitation guidelines are consensus based and focus on the simultaneous treatment of reversible causes, which takes priority over chest compressions.[8,16] It is vital that a medical cardiac arrest is not misdiagnosed as a traumatic cardiac arrest; the former must be treated with the universal advanced life support algorithm.

The development of algorithms for the management of TCA has focused on providing interventions specifically aimed at treating the underlying pathology, reflecting the more common causes of TCA, including:

- Hypovolaemia
- Hypoxia
- Tension pneumothorax
- Tamponade.

Hypovolaemia

Cardiac arrest occurring secondary to major haemorrhage has a very poor prognosis.[17] Therefore, all interventions other than definitive (surgical) haemorrhage control should occur in prehospital setting, including direct compression, tourniquets, topical haemostatic

SECTION 6 Cardiac Arrest

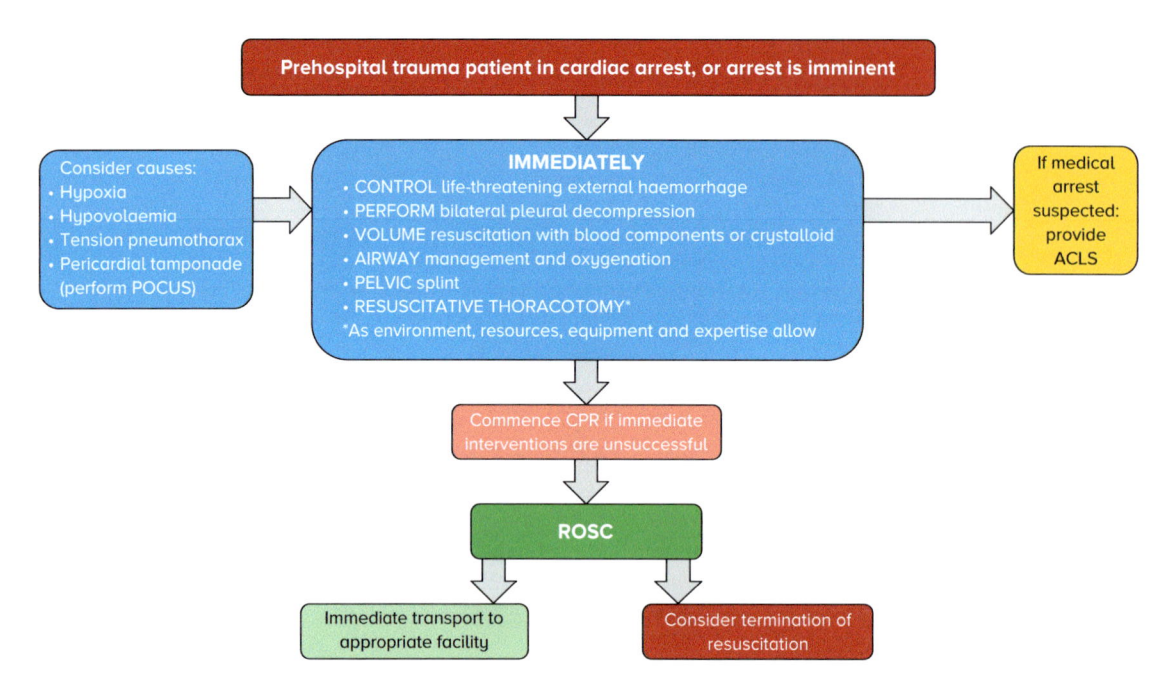

Figure 23.2 Traumatic cardiac arrest algorithm.
Source: Image by Ben Meadley, 2024.

agents, splinting of long bone and pelvic fractures and fluid replacement. While the control of obvious haemorrhage using tourniquets or topical haemostatic agents is shown to be beneficial in a military setting,[18] data on the survival benefit in civilian populations is lacking since, in contrast to military mechanisms of injury, blunt trauma rarely results in traumatic amputation. Therefore, control of internal haemorrhage using splinting and pelvic binders, where appropriate, could be significant.

Immediate aortic occlusion is recommended as a last resort in patients with exsanguination. This can be achieved through resuscitative endovascular balloon occlusion of the aorta or resuscitative thoracotomy.[19] In extremely rare circumstances, placing a resuscitative balloon for occlusion of the aorta by those trained in this technique may be lifesaving. Use of this device is recommended in hospital for severe trauma patients with intra-abdominal or retroperitoneal sources of haemorrhage until defensive therapy is possible.[20,21] However, it is not recommended in the prehospital setting due to a lack of supporting evidence.[20]

Patients in traumatic cardiac arrest as a result of hypovolaemia are unlikely to achieve ROSC unless haemorrhage control is performed in combination with intravascular volume replacement.[22] The use of blood products has become more common in the prehospital setting, and their inclusion in the bundle of care to control haemorrhage on the scene has been recommended and is likely to be more beneficial than crystalloid and colloid infusion in this patient group.[23,24] However, while the use of prehospital blood products has been associated with an improvement in short-term outcomes following traumatic cardiac arrest (allowing for ROSC, for example), a survival benefit has not been demonstrated[25] and further studies are warranted.

Hypoxia

Adequate oxygenation and ventilation must be immediately provided using basic or advanced airway interventions, depending on the provider's skill set, while not delaying blood volume expansion and decompression of tension pneumothorax.[15] The benefits of using prehospital advanced airway procedures in traumatic cardiac arrest remain controversial.[26,27] Several studies from North America reported wide regional variation in the use of prehospital advanced airways and survival outcomes.[6,28–30] For instance, a recent study by Evans et al. shows lower odds of surviving to hospital discharge after traumatic OHCA when inserting advanced airways compared with bag-mask ventilation.[6] Another study found that such interventions were associated with decreased mortality in EMS-witnessed arrest patients.[30]

Tension Pneumothorax and Resuscitative Thoracotomy

Tension pneumothorax has been reported in 13% of patients who are in traumatic cardiac arrest;[9] therefore, it must always be rapidly identified and treated. Because of positive pressure ventilation, performing bilateral finger thoracostomies, if required, is likely more effective than needle thoracostomies and faster than inserting a chest tube.[31] Resuscitation guidelines also recommend the use of a resuscitative emergency thoracotomy by adequately trained personnel, with ultrasound to assist with the assessment, as definitive care for suspected cardiac tamponade. While the majority of cardiac tamponade cases are secondary to penetrating injuries, cardiac injuries have been described in up to 20% of patients involved in traffic accidents,[32] and it should be considered in patients with significant blunt chest trauma. Resuscitative emergency thoracotomy is a time-critical procedure; the faster the intervention is performed for a patient with traumatic cardiac arrest due to penetrating trauma, the higher the chance of survival.[33,34]

> **PRACTICE TIP**
>
> For traumatic cardiac arrest patients, always remember not to delay interventions and to compress after HOTT (haemorrhage, oxygenation, tension pneumothorax/tamponade).

Question 3: Is Addressing Reversible Causes of Arrest prior to Chest Compression Considered an Optimal Treatment for Traumatic OHCA Patients?

The optimal treatment approaches for the traumatic OHCA population remain unclear. Many EMS systems have recently revised prehospital guidelines for managing this population.[15,16] The evidence to support the updated recommendations comes from both animal and human observational studies, which show that conventional resuscitation is unlikely to be helpful in achieving ROSC in patients with traumatic OHCA.[35–38] Despite the supporting evidence, limited studies have evaluated the impact of the new guideline recommendations on patient outcomes from traumatic OHCA. National registry studies from France[39] and Australia[40,41] found no improvement in survival following the updated guidelines, which raises some doubt over the effectiveness of the recent treatment recommendations. However, several factors

SECTION 6 Cardiac Arrest

may contribute to the lack of improvement in patient outcomes under the new treatment protocol, including and not limited to those described in **Table 23.1**.

It is still uncertain whether addressing potentially reversible causes ahead of traditional CPR is the optimal treatment approach. However, managing reversible causes is highly prioritised in TCA patients, and other approaches that simultaneously address reversible causes while performing CPR might lead to better outcomes in a specific traumatic cardiac arrest population with identified reversible causes.

Table 23.1 Factors contributing to unfavourable patient outcomes in traumatic cardiac arrest

Factor	Potential reasons for limiting the effect of new treatment protocol
The population's low survival rate	With a low survival rate, finding meaningful improvements in survival is difficult, even with effective treatments.
The population's high-risk mortality profile: • High traffic accident • Initial arrest rhythm of asystole	The high-risk mortality profile of traumatic OHCA populations has been associated with extremely low rates of survival to hospital discharge and rare neurologically intact survival, even if the patients are successfully resuscitated in the field.[7,42,43]
The prolonged downtime after traumatic OHCA	Prolonged downtime (duration between collapse and arrival of EMS is presumed to be greater than 15 minutes)[44] has been associated with poor survival outcomes even with aggressive resuscitation.[2]
Long EMS response time and delay in providing critical trauma-based interventions by paramedic	It is possible that the long response times and delays in providing crucial interventions in traumatic OHCA populations diminish the impact of the trauma-based interventions on survival, even if the reversal of the underlying causes of arrest leads to ROSC.
Limited exposure to traumatic OHCA and low competency	Traumatic resuscitation interventions require experience and/or periodic training to maintain competency. Low paramedic exposure rates to physiologically distressed trauma patients and traumatic OHCA, and limited training, may increase the possibility of delay in patient injury recognition and paramedics' performance errors.[45–47]

CHAPTER 23 Traumatic Cardiac Arrest

Key Evidence

This is the current evidence pool of high-quality studies to guide paramedic/prehospital resuscitation management in the setting of traumatic cardiac arrest. Search last updated May 2023.

Systematic Review/Meta-Analyses/Joint Position Statement

Millin MG, Galvagno SM, Khandker SR et al. Withholding and termination of resuscitation of adult cardiopulmonary arrest secondary to trauma: resource document to the joint NAEMSP-ACSCOT position statements. *Journal of Trauma and Acute Care Surgery*. 2013;75(3):459–467.

Tran A, Fernando SM, Rochwerg B et al. Pre-arrest and intra-arrest prognostic factors associated with survival following traumatic out-of-hospital cardiac arrest – a systematic review and meta-analysis. *Resuscitation*. 2020;153:119–135.

Zwingmann J, Mehlhorn AT, Hammer T et al. Survival and neurologic outcome after traumatic out-of-hospital cardiopulmonary arrest in a pediatric and adult population: a systematic review. *Critical Care*. 2012;16(4):R117.

Observational Studies

Alqudah Z, Nehme Z, Williams B et al. Impact of a trauma-focused resuscitation protocol on survival outcomes after traumatic out-of-hospital cardiac arrest: an interrupted time series analysis. *Resuscitation*. 2021 May 1;162:104–111.

Barnard E, Yates D, Edwards A et al. Epidemiology and aetiology of traumatic cardiac arrest in England and Wales – a retrospective database analysis. *Resuscitation*. 2017;110:90–94.

Benhamed A, Mercier E, Freyssenge J et al. Impact of the 2015 European guidelines for resuscitation on traumatic cardiac arrest outcomes and prehospital management: a French nationwide interrupted time-series analysis. *Resuscitation*. 2023;Mar 15:109763.

Evans C, Petersen A, Meier EN et al. Prehospital traumatic cardiac arrest: management and outcomes from the resuscitation outcomes consortium epistry-trauma and PROPHET registries. *Journal of Trauma and Acute Care Surgery*. 2016;81(2):285.

Randomised Controlled Trials

Guyette FX, Sperry JL, Peitzman AB et al. Prehospital blood product and crystalloid resuscitation in the severely injured patient: a secondary analysis of the prehospital air medical plasma trial. *Annals of Surgery*. 2021;273(2):358–364.

Tisherman SA, Alam HB, Rhee PM et al. Development of the emergency preservation and resuscitation for cardiac arrest from trauma clinical trial. *Journal of Trauma and Acute Care Surgery*. 2017;83(5):803–809.

Self-Reflection Questions

1. What do you think should determine the decision to resuscitate a traumatic OHCA patient?
2. What do you think about the recent trauma-based resuscitation guidelines?
3. Does the evidence support the benefits of the recent trauma-based resuscitation guidelines in improving survival?
4. What do you think is the optimal treatment protocol for this population?

References

1. Zwingmann J, Mehlhorn AT, Hammer T et al. Survival and neurologic outcome after traumatic out-of-hospital cardiopulmonary arrest in a pediatric and adult population: a systematic review. *Critical Care*. 2012;16(4):R117.

SECTION 6 Cardiac Arrest

2. Millin MG, Galvagno SM, Khandker SR et al. Withholding and termination of resuscitation of adult cardiopulmonary arrest secondary to trauma: resource document to the joint NAEMSP-ACSCOT position statements. *Journal of Trauma and Acute Care Surgery*. 2013;75(3):459–467.
3. Deasy C, Bray J, Smith K et al. Paediatric traumatic out-of-hospital cardiac arrests in Melbourne, Australia. *Resuscitation*. 2012;83(4):471–475.
4. Nehme Z, Namachivayam S, Forrest A et al. Trends in the incidence and outcome of paediatric out-of-hospital cardiac arrest: a 17-year observational study. *Resuscitation*. 2018;128:43–50.
5. Rosemurgy AS, Norris PA, Olson SM et al. Prehospital traumatic cardiac arrest: the cost of futility. *Journal of Trauma*. 1993;35(3):468–473; discussion 73–74.
6. Evans C, Petersen A, Meier EN et al. Prehospital traumatic cardiac arrest: management and outcomes from the resuscitation outcomes consortium epistry-trauma and PROPHET registries. *Journal of Trauma and Acute Care Surgery*. 2016;81(2):285.
7. Barnard E, Yates D, Edwards A et al. Epidemiology and aetiology of traumatic cardiac arrest in England and Wales – a retrospective database analysis. *Resuscitation*. 2017;110:90–94.
8. Truhlar A, Deakin CD, Soar J et al. European Resuscitation Council Guidelines for Resuscitation 2015: Section 4. Cardiac arrest in special circumstances. *Resuscitation*. 2015;95:148–201.
9. Kleber C, Giesecke MT, Lindner T et al. Requirement for a structured algorithm in cardiac arrest following major trauma: epidemiology, management errors, and preventability of traumatic deaths in Berlin. *Resuscitation*. 2014;85(3):405–410.
10. Beck B, Smith K, Mercier E et al. Clinical review of prehospital trauma deaths – the missing piece of the puzzle. *Injury*. 2017;48(5):971–972.
11. Pickens JJ, Copass MK, Bulger EM. Trauma patients receiving CPR: predictors of survival. *Journal of Trauma*. 2005;58(5):951–958.
12. Kleber C, Giesecke MT, Tsokos M et al. Trauma-related preventable deaths in Berlin 2010: need to change prehospital management strategies and trauma management education. *World Journal of Surgery*. 2013;37(5):1154–1161.
13. Deasy C, Bray J, Smith K et al. Traumatic out-of-hospital cardiac arrests in Melbourne, Australia. *Resuscitation*. 2012;83(4):465–470.
14. Vassallo J, Nutbeam T, Rickard AC et al. Paediatric traumatic cardiac arrest: the development of an algorithm to guide recognition, management and decisions to terminate resuscitation. *Emergency Medicine Journal*. 2018;35(11):669–674.
15. Australian Resuscitation Council. ANZCOR guideline 11.10. 1-management of cardiac arrest due to trauma [online]. 2016. Available at: https://www.anzcor.org/home/adult-advanced-life-support/guideline-11-10-1-management-of-cardiac-arrest-due-to-trauma/
16. Lavonas EJ, Drennan IR, Gabrielli A et al. Part 10: Special circumstances of resuscitation: 2015 American Heart Association guidelines update for cardiopulmonary resuscitation and emergency cardiovascular care. *Circulation*. 2015;132(18 Suppl 2):S501–18.
17. Lockey D, Crewdson K, Davies G. Traumatic cardiac arrest: who are the survivors? *Annals of Emergency Medicine*. 2006;48(3):240–244.
18. Kragh Jr JF, Walters TJ, Baer DG et al. Survival with emergency tourniquet use to stop bleeding in major limb trauma. *Annals of Surgery*. 2009;249(1):1–7.
19. Lott C, Truhlar A, Alfonzo A et al. European Resuscitation Council Guidelines 2021: Cardiac arrest in special circumstances. *Resuscitation*. 2021;161:152–219.
20. Bulger EM, Perina DG, Qasim Z et al. Clinical use of resuscitative endovascular balloon occlusion of the aorta (REBOA) in civilian trauma systems in the USA, 2019: a joint statement from the American College of Surgeons Committee on Trauma, the American College of Emergency Physicians, the National Association of Emergency Medical Services Physicians and the National Association of Emergency Medical Technicians. *Trauma Surgery and Acute Care Open*. 2019;4(1):e000376.
21. Osborn LA, Brenner ML, Prater SJ et al. Resuscitative endovascular balloon occlusion of the aorta: current evidence. *Open Access Emergency Medicine*. 2019;11:29–38.

22. Lockey DJ, Lyon RM, Davies GE. Development of a simple algorithm to guide the effective management of traumatic cardiac arrest. *Resuscitation*. 2013;84(6):738–42.
23. Lockey DJ, Weaver AE, Davies GE. Practical translation of hemorrhage control techniques to the civilian trauma scene. *Transfusion*. 2013;53 Suppl 1:17S–22S.
24. Ball CG, Salomone JP, Shaz B et al. Uncrossmatched blood transfusions for trauma patients in the emergency department: incidence, outcomes and recommendations. *Canadian Journal of Surgery*. 2011;54(2):111–115.
25. Brown JB, Sperry JL, Fombona A et al. Pre-trauma center red blood cell transfusion is associated with improved early outcomes in air medical trauma patients. *Journal of the American College of Surgeons*. 2015;220(5):797–808.
26. Cera SM, Mostafa G, Sing RF et al. Physiologic predictors of survival in post-traumatic arrest. *American Surgery*. 2003;69(2):140–144.
27. Seamon MJ, Fisher CA, Gaughan J et al. Prehospital procedures before emergency department thoracotomy: 'scoop and run' saves lives. *Journal of Trauma and Acute Care Surgery*. 2007;63(1):113–120.
28. Minei JP, Schmicker RH, Kerby JD et al. Severe traumatic injury: regional variation in incidence and outcome. *Annals of Surgery*. 2010;252(1):149–157.
29. Newgard CD, Koprowicz K, Wang H et al. Variation in the type, rate, and selection of patients for out-of-hospital airway procedures among injured children and adults. *Academic Emergency Medicine*. 2009;16(12):1269–1276.
30. Meizoso JP, Valle EJ, Allen CJ et al. Decreased mortality after prehospital interventions in severely injured trauma patients. *Journal of Trauma and Acute Care Surgery*. 2015;79(2):227–231.
31. Sherren PB, Reid C, Habig K et al. Algorithm for the resuscitation of traumatic cardiac arrest patients in a physician-staffed helicopter emergency medical service. *Critical Care*. 2013;17(2):308.
32. Fitzgerald M, Spencer J, Johnson F et al. Definitive management of acute cardiac tamponade secondary to blunt trauma. *Emergency Medicine Australasia*. 2005;17(5–6):494–499.
33. Moore EE, Knudson MM, Burlew CC et al. Defining the limits of resuscitative emergency department thoracotomy: a contemporary Western Trauma Association perspective. *Journal of Trauma*. 2011;70(2):334–339.
34. Paulich S, Lockey D. Resuscitative thoracotomy. *BJA Education*. 2020;20(7):242–248.
35. Luna GK, Pavlin EG, Kirkman T et al. Hemodynamic effects of external cardiac massage in trauma shock. *Journal of Trauma*. 1989;29(10):1430–1433.
36. Watts S, Smith JE, Gwyther R et al. Closed chest compressions reduce survival in an animal model of haemorrhage-induced traumatic cardiac arrest. *Resuscitation*. 2019;140:37–42.
37. Davies GE, Lockey DJ. Thirteen survivors of prehospital thoracotomy for penetrating trauma: a prehospital physician-performed resuscitation procedure that can yield good results. *Journal of Trauma and Acute Care Surgery*. 2011;70(5):E75–E8.
38. Huber-Wagner S, Lefering R, Qvick M et al. Outcome in 757 severely injured patients with traumatic cardiorespiratory arrest. *Resuscitation*. 2007;75(2):276–285.
39. Benhamed A, Mercier E, Freyssenge J et al. Impact of the 2015 European guidelines for resuscitation on traumatic cardiac arrest outcomes and prehospital management: a French nationwide interrupted time-series analysis. *Resuscitation*. 2023;186:109763.
40. Alqudah Z, Nehme Z, Williams B et al. Impact of a trauma-focused resuscitation protocol on survival outcomes after traumatic out-of-hospital cardiac arrest: an interrupted time series analysis. *Resuscitation*. 2021;162:104–111.
41. Alqudah Z, Nehme Z, Williams B et al. Survival outcomes in emergency medical services witnessed traumatic out-of-hospital cardiac arrest after the introduction of a trauma-based resuscitation protocol. *Resuscitation*. 2021;168:65–74.
42. Konesky KL, Guo WA. Revisiting traumatic cardiac arrest: should CPR be initiated? *European Journal of Trauma and Emergency Surgery*. 2018;44(6):903–908.
43. Ryan M, Stella J, Chiu H et al. Injury patterns and preventability in prehospital motor vehicle crash fatalities in Victoria. *Emergency Medicine Australasia*. 2004;16(4):274–279.

44. Beck B, Bray JE, Cameron P et al. Predicting outcomes in traumatic out-of-hospital cardiac arrest: the relevance of Utstein factors. *Emergency Medicine Journal.* 2017;34(12):786–792.
45. Boyle MJ, Smith EC, Archer F. Trauma incidents attended by emergency medical services in Victoria, Australia. *Prehospital and Disaster Medicine.* 2008;23(1):20–28.
46. Boyle MJ, Smith EC, Archer F. A review of patients who suddenly deteriorate in the presence of paramedics. *BMC Emergency Medicine.* 2008;8(1):1–11.
47. Dyson K, Bray J, Smith K et al. Paramedic exposure to out-of-hospital cardiac arrest is rare and declining in Victoria, Australia. *Resuscitation.* 2015;89:93–98.

Cardiac Arrest in Special Circumstances

24

Casey Lewis and Claire Bertenshaw

> **In this chapter you will learn:**
> - In which settings we should modify our typical cardiac arrest management
> - When it is reasonable to suspect hyperkalaemia as a cause for cardiac arrest
> - Which treatment options are typically available to critical care paramedics in hyperkalaemic cardiac arrest
> - Important considerations regarding maternal cardiac arrest management.

Case Details

Dispatch
50-year-old male, cardiac arrest.

History
A 50-year-old male has collapsed at home, witnessed by his wife and son, who have commenced immediate, high-quality CPR and requested an ambulance. Two double-crewed ambulances and a critical care paramedic are dispatched. The response time for the initial resource is six minutes, with the critical care paramedic two minutes behind.

On Arrival of the First Crew
The scene is safe, the patient is supine, lifeless and has effective CPR being provided by family. His primary survey findings and initial vital signs are:

Airway	Patent
Breathing	Absent
Circulation	Pulses absent
Disability	GCS E1, V1, M1 (3)
Environmental	Indoors

The initial responding crews commence effective, high-performance CPR, place a supraglottic airway and establish IV access. They note from the family members that the patient has an arteriovenous fistula with a background of chronic kidney disease, and convey this information to the critical care paramedic.

SECTION 6 Cardiac Arrest

On Your Arrival as the Critical Care Paramedic
Effective CPR is being continued by the initial responding crew. The rhythm remains a broad complex, bizarre PEA rhythm. Both double-clinician crews are on scene and are undertaking high-performance CPR with frequent changes of operator. The supraglottic airway is providing effective ventilations and adrenaline is being prepared.

AMPLE
The patient has a background of renal failure, with haemodialysis three times weekly. He is due for dialysis today. He has no known drug allergies and, although he has some significant health issues, he is independent and still working.

Allergies	NKDA
Medications	Atorvastatin, sevelamer, calcitriol, furosemide, hydralazine, metoprolol
Past history	Hypertension, renal failure, diabetes
Last ins and outs	Normal
Events	Feeling fatigued prior to a sudden collapse

Decision Point
What are your clinical priorities in this situation?
The medical history of advanced renal disease requiring haemodialysis, immediate history of fatigue, which could be suggestive of hyperkalaemia (albeit non-specific), and a broad complex PEA are highly suggestive of hyperkalaemia as a reversible cause of cardiac arrest. While maintaining the fundamentals of effective resuscitation, case-specific hyperkalaemia treatment should also be implemented.

Question 1: In Which Settings Should Paramedics Modify Their Management of Cardiac Arrest?

A core principle of managing cardiac arrest, as outlined in Chapter 21: High-performance CPR, remains relatively unchanged irrespective of the cause of cardiac arrest.[1] This being the case, however, another core principle is identifying and managing any reversible cause. Given that many of these reversible causes are amenable to prehospital treatment (particularly by critical care teams), they require adaptations or additions to our typical management. A useful mnemonic for recalling some of these reversible causes is the four Hs and four Ts:

- Hypoxia
- Hypovolaemia
- Hypo-/hyperkalaemia and other electrolyte disorders
- Hypo-/hyperthermia
- Thrombosis (coronary and pulmonary)
- Tamponade (cardiac)
- Tension pneumothorax
- Toxic agents (poisoning).

CHAPTER 24 Cardiac Arrest in Special Circumstances

Adaptations in cardiac arrest management may also be prudent in certain patient populations, such as pregnant patients, cardiac arrest secondary to asthma or patients with a background of morbid obesity. While many reversible causes were discussed elsewhere, in particular in Chapter 23: Traumatic cardiac arrest, this chapter discusses the rationale and evidence behind some of the other situations in which significant changes in our usual cardiac arrest management are justified.

> **PRACTICE TIP**
>
> While maintaining high-performance CPR:
>
> CONSIDER 4Hs and 4Ts

Question 2: When Should Hyperkalaemia Be Suspected as a Cause of Cardiac Arrest?

As a reversible cause of cardiac arrest, hyperkalaemia requires significant adaptations to typical arrest management beyond high-standard resuscitation and high-performance CPR. Ideally, hyperkalaemia should be confirmed either with formal laboratory results or point-of-care testing, prior to initiating specific treatment. In the prehospital setting, however, this is rarely available for most teams. Where point-of-care testing is available, this should guide care. In its absence, critical care paramedics should be guided by the patient's medical history, symptoms described prior to collapse and any suggestive ECG changes, where performing an ECG has been possible immediately prior to arrest.

The primary tool for diagnosing hyperkalaemia in cardiac arrest will be a thorough and complete history. The primary causes of hyperkalaemia are as follows.

- Renal failure – suspect hyperkalaemia as a cause of cardiac arrest in any patients undergoing haemodialysis, in patients with acute kidney injury or other renal disease.
- Drugs – a range of common medications including ACE inhibitors, angiotensin receptor blockers, mineralocorticoid receptor antagonists, NSAIDs, beta-blockers and suxamethonium.
- Endocrine disorders – such as DKA and Addison's disease.
- Tissue breakdown – rhabdomyolysis (including crush syndrome).
- Diet – high-potassium diets, particularly in patients with chronic renal disease.
- Spurious – although not a cause of cardiac arrest, spurious or pseudo-hyperkalaemia should be considered where a blood test shows elevated potassium despite an absence of signs or symptoms, particularly where the blood draw may have been challenging.

In combination, several of these factors significantly increase the risk of hyperkalaemia. Any pre-collapse symptoms suggestive of hyperkalaemia, such as limb weakness, flaccid paralysis or paraesthesia, should increase suspicion that this may be the cause of arrest.

ECG signs of hyperkalaemia are typically progressive and consist of:

- Tall, tent-shaped 'peaked' T-waves
- Prolonged PR interval
- Decreased amplitude of P-waves

SECTION 6 Cardiac Arrest

- Widening of QRS complex
- Absence of P-wave
- Conduction blocks (fascicular blocks, bundle branch blocks)
- Widening of the QRS complex
- 'Sine-wave' pattern, VF, asystole.[2]

For patients presenting in PEA, those with a wide complex QRS are much more likely to be hyperkalaemic than those with a narrow complex.[3] While this may be helpful, it is important to remember that patients can present with life-threatening hyperkalaemia with a normal, or near normal, ECG. Indeed, the first cardiac manifestation may be cardiac arrest.

> **PRACTICE TIP**
>
> A normal pre-collapse ECG does not exclude hyperkalaemia.

Question 3: What Is the Rationale behind the Various Drugs Used by Paramedics in the Management of Hyperkalaemic Cardiac Arrest?

Five key steps of hyperkalaemic cardiac arrest management are:

- Protect the heart
- Shift potassium into cells
- Remove potassium from the body
- Monitor serum potassium and glucose levels
- Prevent recurrence of hyperkalaemia.

While some of these steps are beyond the scope of prehospital care, others can be offered by critical care paramedics. The evidence supporting drug management in hyperkalaemic cardiac arrest is sparse. Two separate Cochrane reviews from 2005 and 2015 concluded that there was limited evidence supporting the use of any pharmaceutical agent in hyperkalaemia, but what evidence existed favoured salbutamol and combined insulin/dextrose.[4,5] Although there is limited strong evidence in favour of IV calcium salts, Mahoney et al.[5] did suggest that the evidence from anecdotal and animal studies supports IV calcium salts in treating arrhythmias. Wang et al.[6] found limited support for the combination of calcium and sodium bicarbonate in presumed hyperkalaemic cardiac arrest; however, this was a small, retrospective cohort study. Despite the limited evidence, pharmacological interventions remain standard practice.

Calcium, either chloride or gluconate, acts on the first of the five key steps of management, protecting the heart. There is no difference in bioavailability between the two formulations. Calcium gluconate causes less tissue irritation but it contains a third of the calcium ions of calcium chloride. The choice of agent should be driven by local guidelines and availability. Calcium is thought to antagonise the cardiotoxic effects of hyperkalaemia by lowering cardiac threshold potential and restoring the normal electrochemical gradient, thereby diminishing myocardial irritability. It should be noted that calcium has no effect on serum potassium and the effects are short-lived (approximately 30 minutes), so calcium should be used in conjunction with other treatments.

CHAPTER 24 Cardiac Arrest in Special Circumstances

Sodium bicarbonate forms part of the prehospital treatment regimen for hyperkalaemic cardiac arrest through the second of these five key steps, shifting potassium intracellularly. The proposed mechanism is that intracellular hydrogen ions are exchanged for potassium ions, shifting potassium intracellularly, resulting in a transient fall in serum potassium levels. There is, however, limited evidence supporting this mechanism.[4] Despite the lack of strong evidence for sodium bicarbonate, a single dose of between 50 and 100 mL of 8.4% solution is common practice where hyperkalaemia is the suspected cause of cardiac arrest.

The use of nebulised salbutamol (albuterol) in severe hyperkalaemia is common and, like sodium bicarbonate, works by shifting potassium intracellularly. Of the treatment options offered by paramedics, it is perhaps the most grounded in evidence.[4] In the setting of cardiac arrest, however, adrenaline has a similar effect on beta-2 receptors and will likely achieve the same outcome, although this has yet to be tested experimentally. In the peri-arrest setting, or in the event of ROSC, a single, 20 mg nebulised dose of salbutamol is reasonable.

Insulin, in combination with dextrose, while not typically available prehospitally, forms the mainstay of the initial in-hospital management of severe hyperkalaemia. If this pathway has been commenced (in the retrieval setting, for instance), it is critical to closely monitor blood glucose levels, as a secondary hypoglycaemia is common and can be prolonged in patients with renal failure.

The above prehospital treatment options for hyperkalaemia should be considered temporising measures. Transport, ideally to a facility capable of haemodialysis, should be considered early. The use of a mechanical chest compression device as a bridge to either ECMO or emergency dialysis should also be considered, where established pathways exist.

Question 4: What Other Rare Causes of Cardiac Arrest Require Specific Paramedic Management?

Cardiac arrest in pregnancy is a rare but confronting scenario. Paramedics are acutely aware that they have two patients at risk, and the scene can be highly emotive. The goal is to resuscitate the mother to improve outcomes for both her and the foetus. The aetiology of cardiac arrest in pregnancy is diverse but it is important to be aware that pregnant patients are more prone to specific causes of arrest. As practitioners, we must be vigilant to the possible reversible causes of arrest in pregnancy. Pulmonary embolism accounts for 19% and haemorrhage 17% of all pregnancy-related cardiac arrests.[7]

PRACTICE TIP

Although it is true that in maternal cardiac arrest there are two patients:

WHAT'S BEST FOR MOTHER IS BEST FOR BABY

While working through the 4Hs and 4Ts as causes of cardiac arrest, resuscitators should consider rarer causes of arrest in pregnancy, such as placental abruption causing haemorrhage, uterine rupture leading to amniotic fluid embolism, and aortic dissection resulting in pericardial tamponade. Hypertensive disorders in pregnancy, including eclampsia, can also result in cardiac arrest due to hypoxia if left untreated. Amniotic fluid embolism is characterised by a triad of cardiovascular collapse, hypoxia and coagulopathy; it can also be associated with neurological manifestations, including decreased consciousness and seizures (**Table 24.1**).[8]

SECTION 6 Cardiac Arrest

Table 24.1 Obstetric and non-obstetric causes of cardiac arrest in pregnancy[9]

Obstetric causes	Non-obstetric causes
Haemorrhage (17%)	Pulmonary embolism (19%)
Hypertension complications (16%)	Sepsis (13%)
Cardiomyopathy	Stroke (5%)
Complications from anaesthetic	Myocardial infarction
Amniotic fluid embolism	Trauma

Source: Campbell, T. A. and Sanson, T. G. 2009. Cardiac arrest and pregnancy. *Journal of Emergencies, Trauma, and Shock*, 2, 34–42.

If the patient appears to be pregnant, treat them as so. A gravid uterus at the level of the umbilicus is estimated to equate to 20 weeks gestation. The gravid uterus is influenced by the size of the foetus, the number of foetuses, the amount of amniotic fluid and the relative size in comparison to the maternal anatomy.

Modifications to the cardiac arrest algorithm in pregnancy are as follows.

1. Place the patient in the left lateral position to displace the gravid uterus and prevent aortocaval compression. Options include manually pulling the uterus to the left or placing a pillow, towel or wedge under the patient's right hip. If manually displacing the uterus (**Figure 24.1**), stand on the patient's left and pull the gravid uterus towards you with a two-handed technique.[10]
2. Ensure IV/IO access is above the diaphragm to counteract compression of the inferior vena cava and improve medication efficacy through improved drug circulation.

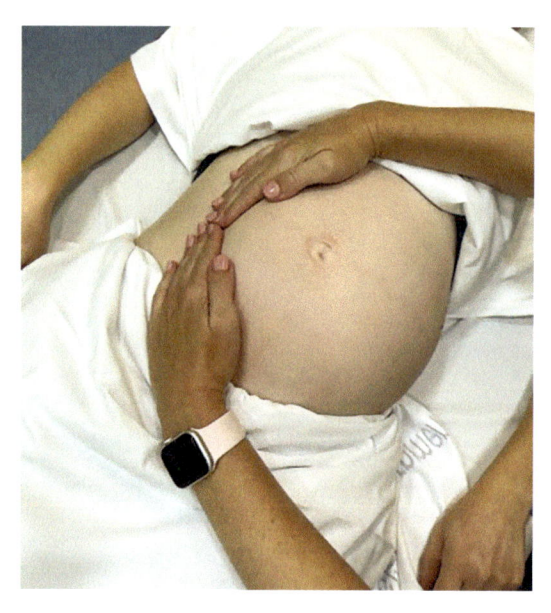

Figure 24.1 Manual displacement of the gravid uterus to the left.
Source: Claire Bertenshaw.

CHAPTER 24   Cardiac Arrest in Special Circumstances

3. In anticipation of a difficult airway, prepare to use a bag-valve-mask, place a laryngeal mask airway and intubate with an endotracheal tube.
    a. Oedema and larger body habitus can have implications for placement of the laryngoscope blade and view. Use a short-handled or stubby laryngoscope.
    b. There is increased risk of emesis and aspiration due to decreased sphincter tone. Maintain head of the bed elevation.
    c. Rapid desaturation may occur.
4. Consider early transport and notification to the receiving hospital emergency department for consideration of extracorporeal CPR (ECPR), if available, or resuscitative hysterotomy, which is aimed to be performed within five minutes of arrest.[11]

Key Evidence

Alfonzo, A., Harrison, A., Baines, R. et al. 2020. Treatment of acute hyperkalaemia in adults. Renal Association Clinical Practice Guidelines. Available at: https://ukkidney.org/sites/renal.org/files/RENAL%20ASSOCIATION%20HYPERKALAEMIA%20GUIDELINE%20-%20JULY%202022%20V2_0.pdf

Batterink, J., Cessford, T. A. and Taylor, R. A. 2015. Pharmacological interventions for the acute management of hyperkalaemia in adults. *Cochrane Database of Systematic Reviews*, 10(10), CD010344.

Deakin, C. D., Soar, J., Davies, R. et al. 2021. UK resuscitation guidelines: Special circumstances guidelines. Resuscitation Council UK. Available at: https://www.resus.org.uk/library/2021-resuscitation-guidelines/special-circumstances-guidelines

Jeejeebhoy, F. M., Zelop, C. M., Lipman, S. et al. 2015. Cardiac arrest in pregnancy, a scientific statement from the American Heart Association. *Circulation*, 132(18), 1747–1773.

Lott, C., Truhlář, A., Alfonzo, A. et al. 2021. European Resuscitation Council Guidelines 2021: Cardiac arrest in special circumstances. *Resuscitation*, 161, 152–219.

Mahoney, B. A., Smith, W. A. D., Lo, D. et al. 2005. Emergency interventions for hyperkalaemia. *Cochrane Database of Systematic Reviews*, 2005(2), CD003235.

Self-Reflection Questions

1. What are the Hs and Ts in the context of reversible cardiac arrest?
2. What would you find in a patient's medical history that would suggest hyperkalaemia?
3. How might you integrate the additional treatment required in a suspected hyperkalaemic cardiac arrest into typical arrest management?
4. What are the pregnancy-specific causes of cardiac arrest a critical care paramedic should be aware of?
5. What special considerations would you have for managing the airway of a pregnant patient?

References

1. Lott, C., Truhlář, A., Alfonzo, A. et al. 2021. European Resuscitation Council Guidelines 2021: Cardiac arrest in special circumstances. *Resuscitation*, 161, 152–219.
2. Mattu, A., Brady, W. J. and Robinson, D. A. 2000. Electrocardiographic manifestations of hyperkalemia. *American Journal of Emergency Medicine,* 18**,** 721–729.
3. Kim, Y. M., Park, J. E., Hwang, S. Y. et al. 2021. Association between wide QRS pulseless electrical activity and hyperkalemia in cardiac arrest patients. *American Journal of Emergency Medicine*, 45, 86–91.
4. Batterink, J., Cessford, T. A. and Taylor, R. A. I. 2015. Pharmacological interventions for the acute management of hyperkalaemia in adults. *Cochrane Database of Systematic Reviews*, 10(10), CD010344.
5. Mahoney, B. A., Smith, W. A. D., Lo, D. et al. 2005. Emergency interventions for hyperkalaemia. *Cochrane Database of Systematic Reviews*, 2005(2), CD003235.

SECTION 6 Cardiac Arrest

6. Wang, C.-H., Huang, C.-H., Chang, W.-T. et al. 2016. The effects of calcium and sodium bicarbonate on severe hyperkalaemia during cardiopulmonary resuscitation: A retrospective cohort study of adult in-hospital cardiac arrest. *Resuscitation*, 98, 105–111.
7. Ducloy-Bouthors AS, Gonzalez-Estevez M, Constans B, Turbelin A, Barre-Drouard C. Cardiovascular emergencies and cardiac arrest in a pregnant woman. *Anaesthesia Critical Care & Pain Medicine*, 2016, 35, S43–50.
8. Soskin, P. N. and Yu, J. 2019. Resuscitation of the pregnant patient. *Emergency Medicine Clinics*, 37, 351–363.
9. Campbell, T. A. and Sanson, T. G. 2009. Cardiac arrest and pregnancy. *Journal of Emergencies, Trauma and Shock*, 2, 34–42.
10. Jeejeebhoy, F. M., Zelop, C. M., Lipman, S. et al. 2015. Cardiac arrest in pregnancy, a scientific statement from the American Heart Association. *Circulation*, 132(18), 1747–1773.
11. Deakin, C. D., Soar, J., Davies, R. et al. 2021. UK resuscitation guidelines: Special circumstances guidelines. Resuscitation Council UK. Available at: https://www.resus.org.uk/library/2021-resuscitation-guidelines/special-circumstances-guidelines

Termination of Resuscitation

25

Natalie Anderson

In this chapter, you will learn:
- The clinical evidence base informing prehospital termination of resuscitation
- The ethical justification for termination of resuscitation
- Resuscitation decision-making considerations beyond prognostication
- Care of family and bystanders in the context of termination of resuscitation.

Case Details

Dispatch
46-year-old male, collapsed, CPR in progress.

History
Sam, a 46-year-old man, has had a cardiac arrest in his backyard while he was undertaking some property maintenance. His wife took him a mid-morning coffee and found him unconscious and pulseless. She had last seen him three hours prior. Sam hadn't eaten much breakfast that morning, and had complained of some reflux and nausea. Sam's wife attributed these symptoms to a hangover, as Sam had consumed 'a few too many beers' with Matthew and Jake – their neighbours – the night before.

On Arrival of the First Crew
The scene is safe, with Sam lying on the lawn, and two men are taking turns providing high-quality chest compression-only CPR. Family members – a woman and two children – are watching nearby. On examination, Sam is generally cyanosed and has no apparent injuries. Once the monitor is connected, initial ECG shows asystole.

On Your Arrival as the Critical Care Paramedic
Your response time is extended (>10 minutes), as you are the only available critical care paramedic in your area. When you arrive, you immediately note that Sam's skin appears waxy and grey. The first ambulance crew are ventilating Sam effectively via a laryngeal mask airway, have successfully gained IV access and administered two doses of adrenaline. The monitor has shown asystole throughout, so no shocks have been given. You introduce yourself and identify that Sam's wife and two daughters are watching, while neighbours Matthew and Jake continue to assist providing excellent chest compressions.

SECTION 6 Cardiac Arrest

AMPLE

Sam has no known medical history or allergies and takes no medications. He works at an investment company and drinks alcohol socially, but doesn't smoke or use other drugs.

Allergies	NKDA
Medications	Nil
Past history	Nil
Last ins and outs	Refused breakfast due to 'reflux' and nausea
Events	Unwitnessed cardiac arrest

Decision Point

What are your clinical priorities in this situation?

You are satisfied that the first crew are providing good basic life support, but your brief patient assessment findings suggest the patient has been in cardiac arrest for a long time. You suspect that further efforts will not successfully resuscitate Sam, and you will need to terminate resuscitation. What are your priorities?

Question 1: What Is the Clinical Evidence Supporting Field Termination of Resuscitation in This Case?

Although there has been a vast investment in strengthening the chain of survival, relatively few people survive out-of-hospital cardiac arrest. Resuscitation efforts – no matter how skilled – will only be successful if basic life support is commenced quickly and the cause of cardiac arrest is reversible. In many OHCA cases (including Sam's), these two key predictors of survival – aetiology and no-flow time – may be difficult to determine.

Validated termination of resuscitation rules and guidelines identify key prognostic factors to predict mortality.[1,2] In Sam's case, prognostic factors associated with non-survival include unwitnessed arrest, non-shockable presenting rhythm, no shocks delivered and no return of spontaneous circulation (ROSC) after >20 minutes of CPR.[3]

More uncertain factors include the initiation of bystander CPR, with an unknown no-flow interval (time elapsed between cardiac arrest and the commencement of effective CPR). Even the most high-quality resuscitation efforts are rendered increasingly ineffective – and eventually futile – as the no-flow interval lengthens.[4] Sam's arrest aetiology is also unclear, although his age, lack of known co-morbidities, and preceding symptoms of nausea and epigastric discomfort could fit with a primary cardiac arrest.

Question 2: Is It Ethical to Terminate Resuscitation in the Field?

Cardiopulmonary resuscitation is one of the few medical procedures where the default position is assumed consent (everyone will want it), and in many countries, clear, current documentation is required to 'opt out'.[5] This is quite remarkable when we consider that everyone goes into cardiac arrest eventually, and for the vast majority of people, this cardiac

CHAPTER 25 Termination of Resuscitation

arrest will coincide with their unavoidable, irreversible death. Although timely CPR is essential to survival from sudden cardiac arrest due to a reversible cause, it will be effective in response to cardiac arrest as part of natural dying or after a lengthy no-flow time. Unfortunately, as discussed above, it can be challenging to differentiate between these circumstances in the emergency context.

Although guidelines (or rules) for field termination of resuscitation vary, there is little evidence to support the transport of patients without ROSC and with ongoing CPR.[6] Survival to discharge outcomes are dire in this patient group and not significantly improved by mechanical CPR devices.[7] Transporting patients with ongoing CPR requires significant resources, including those of the receiving hospital, and increases the risk of injury to providers.

A great deal has been written about the concept of futility, associated clinical factors[8] and its utility (or lack thereof) in the context of resuscitation.[9] In a setting with infinite resources, where no harm could come from resuscitation efforts, an argument could be made for prolonged resuscitation attempts for all. However, every resource in healthcare is limited, and the principle of distributive justice must be considered. While people, spaces and equipment are dedicated to resource-intensive resuscitation efforts for one patient, others may be deteriorating or suffering, awaiting those resources.

Question 3: Should Family Members Be Present during Resuscitation?

The needs of family during and after a cardiac arrest vary depending on the scene, death and family composition. Sam's immediate family members are witnessing an unexpected, sudden event in their own backyard. Resuscitation efforts are resource-intensive, but efforts to acknowledge family and consider their needs should also be a priority.[10,11] In this case, Sam's family members are likely to recall this as one of the worst days of their lives.

A recent systematic review of family presence across all resuscitation settings shows mixed evidence but concludes that organisational guidelines should support family presence.[12] Context is important and excluding someone from an unfamiliar in-hospital resuscitation room is likely different from asking them to leave their own lounge, bedroom or backyard.

In this situation, children are present. Again, facilitating autonomy is important. Older children may strongly desire to stay, watch or leave. In this scenario, Sam's wife might face a conflict if she wants to stay but also allow younger children to leave. Most OHCA resuscitation attempts end in field termination of resuscitation. In many cultures, family presence at the time of death is considered desirable or essential.[13] Sometimes, family members may wish to be nearby but do not want to watch. It is important to support choices, without making assumptions about what is right. Although clinicians can have concerns about family member behaviour impeding resuscitation efforts, it is rare that family presence threatens CPR quality or patient outcomes.[12]

> **PRACTICE TIP**
>
> In the context of unsuccessful resuscitation, transition your attention and resources to the needs of the bereaved, witnesses and others present at the scene.

SECTION 6 Cardiac Arrest

Question 4: How Should Paramedics Break Bad News to Those Present at the Scene of a Death?

In Sam's case, resuscitation efforts are being managed well and the critical care paramedic will need to draw on other skills, including decision making and communication. Paramedics are highly trained in the technical aspects of resuscitation, can demonstrate competency through simulation and can align interventions with clear procedural guidance. By comparison, they feel poorly prepared for the challenging tasks of breaking bad news[14] and supporting bereaved family.[15] This is seldom simulated or assessed,[16] and communication and care after death receive little attention in paramedic clinical guidelines.[17]

One of the reasons for the lack of education and assessment in this important area is its complexity. There is no one best way to break bad news – no checklist or standardised, objective criteria to assess against. As outlined in **Table 25.1**, breaking bad news needs to be tailored to the unique circumstances of each situation.

Existing frameworks for breaking bad news include SPIKES[18] and ABCDE,[19] but these have not been developed for the unique emergency ambulance context, where there is relatively little time to establish rapport and limited control over the setting or the people present.[20,21]

In addition to the above considerations, it is important for paramedics to have high self-awareness when communicating with others at the scene of a death. Past professional and personal experiences with death and bereavement can assist with connection and empathy, but may also contribute to emotional distancing. Experienced, skilled paramedics will seek to quickly build rapport and elicit and provide appropriate information while simultaneously evaluating the expectations and understanding of family members. If family do not appear to

Table 25.1 Tailoring communication and support at the scene of a patient death

Considerations	Actions
Scene	Is the scene safe for all? How can you optimise privacy and comfort? Are key people included? Are other people arriving/expected?
Introductions	Clearly introduce yourself and establish who else is present. What is their relationship to the person who has died? In some cultures, it is important to identify the family spokesperson.
Patient death	Use the words 'death' and 'has died' and avoid euphemisms. Discussion of the sudden death of a young person due to injury or suicide will likely require a different approach to an expected death. Remember, even in the context of known life-limiting illness or advanced age, there are often sudden or unexpected elements of death and dying that can be upsetting for family.
Priorities	Find out what is most important to the family following the death. What are their immediate priorities? Are there cultural, spiritual or traditional needs to consider? Key people to contact? Do they have questions? What comes next?

CHAPTER 25 Termination of Resuscitation

understand that death is a possible outcome, paramedics may fire 'warning shots' – statements that forecast high levels of concern about the patient's survival.

It is also very important to take the opportunity to mentor less experienced colleagues. These sensitive communication skills are usually developed 'in the field' rather than a classroom setting.[22] The evidence for formal debriefing is mixed,[23] but offering an informal opportunity to reflect and ask questions may facilitate professional development and avert misunderstandings.[16]

> **PRACTICE TIP**
>
> Managing the scene of a patient death and breaking bad news are difficult skills to teach in a classroom. Less experienced paramedics may benefit from mentoring, support and opportunities to reflect on these situations.

Question 5: How Can Paramedics Best Support Family and Bystanders Following Termination of Resuscitation?

Family Needs

The medicalisation of death and reduced exposure to death have contributed to an epidemic of death denial and fear of death in many modern western societies. News[24] and entertainment media[25] can depict CPR as a panacea for death, contributing to unrealistic expectations of immediate survival from cardiac arrest. Bereaved family rarely feel 'prepared' for the death of a loved one, even when that person is of very advanced age or known to have a life-limiting illness.[26] Avoid offering false assurances or minimising grief. If you feel a personal emotional response to sad situations, consider your humanity and empathy as strengths, not weaknesses. A paramedic who shows some emotion while authentically stating 'I'm so sorry your Dad has died' may be more able to provide effective support than a paramedic who robotically breaks bad news, then distances themselves.

Bystander Support

Importantly, the nature of relationships at the scene of an emergency can be unclear. Try to avoid making assumptions, instead asking open questions such as 'Who is this person to you?' In this case study, the men providing CPR are not bystanders providing aid to a stranger in the street. They are neighbours and friends of the patient and his family, socialising with him just the night before this event. After termination of resuscitation, they may wish to be absorbed in supporting the dead man's wife and children, but could also have concerns about why their resuscitation efforts were unsuccessful.[27] When in a paramedic leadership role, simple reassuring words to all involved in resuscitation efforts ('You did everything you could') can go a long way.

> **PRACTICE TIP**
>
> Taking a few minutes to provide simple, clear explanations and reassurance that they did everything right can reduce feelings of guilt and confusion sometimes experienced by bystanders and co-responders.

SECTION 6 Cardiac Arrest

Question 6: What Evidence or Guidelines Exist to Support Paramedics with Termination of Resuscitation?

Algorithms and decision-making rules guide many actions in resuscitation. These are based on international consensus statements, which are regularly reviewed and updated in response to the best available evidence. In many settings where there is high concern about medico-legal actions, prehospital providers have adopted termination of resuscitation rules. However, research findings suggest inconsistent application of these algorithmic rules. This may be due to uncertainty around key prognostic factors including time since collapse, patient age, co-morbidities or arrest aetiology. Other barriers to field termination include provider concerns about breaking bad news, family reactions and scene safety.[28] Three criteria for withholding or terminating resuscitation have good international consensus.

1. The patient is obviously, irreversibly dead.
2. Valid, relevant documentation recommends against CPR.
3. The providers' safety is threatened.

However, even the application of these criteria requires some clinical judgement and knowledge of systems. A retrospective review of OHCA terminated without full resuscitation attempts in North America noted high variability in duration of resuscitation efforts, with attempts terminated due to DNR orders or signs of obvious death often being of the same duration as provided to those who survived to discharge from hospital.[29]

In countries where paramedic education and autonomy are greater, resuscitation decision-making is often supported by guidelines rather than rules. Evidence-based decision making using objective, reliable and valid data is highly valued in healthcare. However, even those international organisations tasked with developing consensus guidance based on current evidence synthesis have conceded that the criteria for withholding and terminating resuscitation in OHCA should be locally tailored in response to legal, organisational and cultural factors.

Deciding to terminate resuscitation efforts in the prehospital context can be complex, often involving uncertainty, mixed prognostic factors and cultural, ethical, logistical, interpersonal and emotional challenges.[30,31] It is difficult to measure the impact of non-medical and ethical decision-making factors in decisions to terminate resuscitation, as these are rarely documented.[32] Naturalistic decision-making research suggests that expert complex high-stakes decision making often involves pattern matching developed through experience. Rapid, intuitive decision making is crucial in paramedicine, but cognitive biases can negatively impact these heuristics. Opportunities to critically reflect on resuscitation decisions and discuss these openly with supportive colleagues are essential to professional development.

Key Evidence

Considine J, Eastwood K, Webster H. et al. Family presence during adult resuscitation from cardiac arrest: A systematic review. *Resuscitation*. 2022;180:11–23

Satchell, E., Carey, M., Dicker, B. et al. Family & bystander experiences of emergency ambulance services care: A scoping review. *BMC Emergency Medicine*. 2023;23(1):68

Smyth, M. A., Gunson, I., Coppola, A. et al. Termination of resuscitation rules and survival among patients with out-of-hospital cardiac arrest: A systematic review and meta-analysis. *JAMA Network Open*. 2024;7(7):e2420040–e2420040.

CHAPTER 25 Termination of Resuscitation

Self-Reflection Questions

1. What do you find most challenging when terminating resuscitation in the field? Has this varied across the span of your career?
2. Everyone dies, and most people will have only one cardiac arrest – that which coincides with their death. What is the difference between cardiac arrest and death?
3. Is it important to achieve team consensus before terminating resuscitation?
4. Saving lives is widely regarded as a rewarding part of paramedicine. In your experience, can care in the event of a patient death also be rewarding?

References

1. Nas J, Kleinnibbelink G, Hannink G et al. Diagnostic performance of the basic and advanced life support termination of resuscitation rules: A systematic review and diagnostic meta-analysis. *Resuscitation*. 2020;148:3–13.
2. Smyth, M. A., Gunson, I., Coppola, A., et al. Termination of resuscitation rules and survival among patients with out-of-hospital cardiac arrest: A systematic review and meta-analysis. *JAMA Network Open*. 2024;7(7):e2420040–e2420040.
3. Sasson C, Rogers M, Dahl J et al. Predictors of survival from out-of-hospital cardiac arrest: A systematic review and meta-analysis. *Circulation. Cardiovascular Quality and Outcomes*. 2010;3(1):63–81.
4. Guy A, Kawano T, Besserer F et al. The relationship between no-flow interval and survival with favourable neurological outcome in out-of-hospital cardiac arrest: Implications for outcomes and ECPR eligibility. *Resuscitation*. 2020;155:219–225.
5. Georgiou L, Georgiou A. A critical review of the factors leading to cardiopulmonary resuscitation as the default position of hospitalized patients in the USA regardless of severity of illness. *International Journal of Emergency Medicine*. 2019;12(1):9.
6. Wyckoff MH, Greif R, Morley PT et al. 2022 International Consensus on Cardiopulmonary Resuscitation and Emergency Cardiovascular Care Science With Treatment Recommendations: Summary from the basic life support; advanced life support; pediatric life support; neonatal life support; education, implementation, and teams; and first aid task forces. *Resuscitation*. 2022;181:208–288.
7. Ong MEH, Mackey KE, Zhang ZC et al. Mechanical CPR devices compared to manual CPR during out-of-hospital cardiac arrest and ambulance transport: A systematic review. *Scandinavian Journal of Trauma, Resuscitation and Emergency Medicine*. 2012;20(1):39.
8. Glober NK, Tainter CR, Abramson TM et al. A simple decision rule predicts futile resuscitation of out-of-hospital cardiac arrest. *Resuscitation*. 2019;142:8–13.
9. Ardagh M. Futility has no utility in resuscitation medicine. *Journal of Medical Ethics*. 2000;26(5):396–399.
10. Douma MJ, Graham TAD, Ali S et al. What are the care needs of families experiencing cardiac arrest? A survivor and family led scoping review. *Resuscitation*. 2021;168:119–141.
11. Loch T, Drennan IR, Buick JE et al. Caring for the invisible and forgotten: A qualitative document analysis and experience-based co-design project to improve the care of families experiencing out-of-hospital cardiac arrest. *CJEM*. 2023:1–11.
12. Considine J, Eastwood K, Webster H et al. Family presence during adult resuscitation from cardiac arrest: A systematic review. *Resuscitation*. 2022;180:11–23.
13. Krikorian A, Maldonado C, Pastrana T. Patient's perspectives on the notion of a good death: A systematic review of the literature. *Journal of Pain and Symptom Management*. 2020;59(1):152–164.
14. Mainds MD, Jones C. Breaking bad news and managing family during an out-of-hospital cardiac arrest. *Journal of Paramedic Practice*. 2018;10(7):292–299.
15. Anderson NE, Slark J, Faasse K et al. Paramedic student confidence, concerns, learning and experience with resuscitation decision-making and patient death: A pilot survey. *Australasian Emergency Care*. 2019;22(3):156–161.

16. Anderson NE, Slark J, Gott M. When resuscitation doesn't work: A qualitative study examining ambulance personnel preparation and support for termination of resuscitation and patient death. *International Emergency Nursing*. 2020;49:100827.
17. Juhrmann ML, Anderson NE, Boughey M et al. Palliative paramedicine: Comparing clinical practice through guideline quality appraisal and qualitative content analysis. *Palliative Medicine*. 2022;36(8):1228–1241.
18. Baile WF, Buckman R, Lenzi R et al. SPIKES – A six-step protocol for delivering bad news: Application to the patient with cancer. *Oncologist*. 2000;5(4):302–311.
19. Rabow MW, McPhee SJ. Beyond breaking bad news: Helping patients who suffer. *British Medical Journal*. 2000;320(Suppl S3):000365.
20. Walker E. Death notification delivery and training methods. *Journal of Paramedic Practice*. 2018;10(8):334–341.
21. Campbell I. Paramedic delivery of bad news: A novel dilemma during the COVID-19 crisis. *Journal of Medical Ethics*. 2021;47(1):16–19.
22. Anderson NE, Slark J, Gott M. How are ambulance personnel prepared and supported to withhold or terminate resuscitation and manage patient death in the field? A scoping review. *Australasian Journal of Paramedicine*. 2019;16.
23. Scott Z, O'Curry S, Mastroyannopoulou K. The impact and experience of debriefing for clinical staff following traumatic events in clinical settings: A systematic review. *Journal of Trauma Stress*. 2022;35(1):278–287.
24. Field RA, Soar J, Nolan JP et al. Epidemiology and outcome of cardiac arrests reported in the lay-press: An observational study. *Journal of the Royal Society of Medicine*. 2011;104(12):525–531.
25. Portanova J, Irvine K, Yi JY et al. It isn't like this on TV: Revisiting CPR survival rates depicted on popular TV shows. *Resuscitation*. 2015;96:148–150.
26. Anderson NE, Robinson J, Goodwin H et al. 'Mum, I think we might ring the ambulance, okay?' A qualitative exploration of bereaved family members' experiences of emergency ambulance care at the end of life. *Palliative Medicine*. 2022;36(9):1389–1395.
27. Satchell, E., Carey, M., Dicker, B, et al. Family & bystander experiences of emergency ambulance services care: a scoping review. *BMC Emergency Medicine*. 2023;23(1):68.
28. Tataris KL, Richards CT, Stein-Spencer L et al. EMS provider perceptions on termination of resuscitation in a large, urban EMS system. *Prehospital Emergency Care*. 2017;21(5):610–615.
29. Hutton G, Kawano T, Scheuermeyer FX et al. Out-of-hospital cardiac arrests terminated without full resuscitation attempts: Characteristics and regional variability. *Resuscitation*. 2022;172:47–53.
30. Milling L, Kjaer J, Binderup LG et al. Non-medical factors in prehospital resuscitation decision-making: A mixed-methods systematic review. *Scandinavian Journal of Trauma, Resuscitation and Emergency Medicine*. 2022;30(1):24.
31. Anderson NE, Gott M, Slark J. Commence, continue, withhold or terminate? A systematic review of resuscitation provider decision-making in out-of-hospital cardiac arrest. *European Journal of Emergency Medicine*. 2017;24(2):80–86.
32. Milling L, Binderup LG, de Muckadell CS et al. Documentation of ethically relevant information in out-of-hospital resuscitation is rare: A Danish nationwide observational study of 16,495 out-of-hospital cardiac arrests. *BMC Medical Ethics*. 2021;22(1):82.

SECTION 7

Trauma

The Trapped Patient

26

Tash Adams

> **In this chapter you will learn:**
> - The definition of 'trapped'
> - Morbidity and mortality rates for trapped patients and how this is affected by patient demographics
> - How to use information regarding mechanism and damage to inform the pattern and severity of injuries in the trapped patient
> - How to work with rescue teams toward a common goal
> - How to treat the trapped patient
> - How to communicate effectively with trapped patients.

Case Details

Dispatch
Two-vehicle road traffic collision, multiple patients trapped in vehicles.

History
Two adults and a child are trapped in a saloon after a high-velocity head-on collision with another car. The speed limit of the road is 60 mph (100 kph). Two double-crewed ambulances are dispatched, as well as a critical care paramedic and an operational supervisor. Technical rescue services and police are also attached to the incident.

On Arrival of the First Crew
On the first crew's arrival they find two vehicles with damage consistent with a high-velocity impact. One vehicle is on its side, with moderate damage to the front right side and roof. It is a late-model saloon and all airbags have been deployed. There is no occupant in this vehicle. The other vehicle is 15 years old with no airbags fitted; the passenger side is against the guardrail. This vehicle has severe damage to the driver's side of the car, with intrusion into the driver compartment both from the front and the side. An off-duty nurse is in the back seat of the car providing the patients with reassurance.

On Your Arrival as the Critical Care Paramedic
You are advised from the operational supervisor that there are three patients. The 20-year-old male driver of the rolled car is walking around the scene, with no obvious injuries or concerns. The patients are:

SECTION 7 Trauma

1. An 18-month-old boy in a rear-facing child seat. He is visibly upset; however, no obvious injuries are immediately evident.
2. A 45-year-old female front passenger, with her door against the guardrail, GCS 15 PEARL, able to move all limbs, complaining of neck pain, traumatic chest pain and wrist pain. Her vital signs are grossly normal.
3. A 79-year-old driver, physically trapped by the intrusion into the cabin, GCS E3, V4, M5 (12), respiratory rate 40, SpO_2 89% on air, weak radial pulse 100, BP 90/50, skin cool, pale and diaphoretic.

Decision Point
What are your clinical priorities in this situation?

There are a few different priorities to consider within this situation. Ensuring scene safety is of the utmost importance. This includes for the patients, the paramedics, the bystanders and other emergency services staff. Closed-loop communication should be always utilised to ensure continued safety during the management of the scene.

There are multiple patients and limited resources. As the clinical leader on scene, it will be your responsibility to ensure the right resources are allocated to the right patients.

Consider the priorities with regard to treatment and extrication based on mechanism, patient demographic and presentation.

Question 1: What Is the Definition of 'Trapped'?

The out-of-hospital approach to a road traffic crash is unique as each incident will have different vehicle types, speeds, forces, damage and patient demographics. One important patient type is the patient who is trapped. That is, they remain in their vehicle post collision and require facilitated extrication.[1] The amount of assistance required will vary significantly between patients and is dependent on many factors.

The definition of 'trapped' can be broken down into two separate terms – medically trapped and physically trapped.

- Medically trapped is defined as a patient who is unable to exit the damaged vehicle due to the severity of their condition or injuries. This is due to either painful injury or physiology that prevents their self-extrication.[2]
- Physically trapped is defined as being trapped by the deformity of the vehicle and includes patients who are unable to get out due to entanglement, intrusion or physical barriers such as a bent door or car frame. Out-of-hospital providers should not dismiss the forces that are involved in causing damage to vehicles that prevents the occupant from self-extricating. While modern cars are designed with crumple zones to dissipate forces away from occupants, some of these same forces will be transferred into the patient.[3]

Question 2: Do Trapped Patients have Different Outcomes, and Which Patient Demographics can Influence These Outcomes?

Across the world, road traffic crashes are associated with 1.35 million deaths a year, with tens of millions more who are injured or permanently disabled.[4]

CHAPTER 26 The Trapped Patient

A study in 2021 by Nutbeam et al. examined outcomes and injuries of patients who were trapped following RTCs. These patients have higher rates of morbidity and mortality. They are likely to be more seriously injured, have higher injury severity scores, a greater potential to have spinal injuries and to present with deranged physiology. When compared to non-trapped patients, trapped patients more often have lower blood pressure, lower oxygen saturations and lower Glasgow Coma Scores.[5]

Different demographics have different risk factors in an RTC, and the assessment and risk profile for different age groups is diverse.

Child restraints are highly effective in reducing morbidity and mortality, with a 60% reduction in death if the child is in a properly fitted and age-appropriate child restraint. A higher index of suspicion for serious injury should be considered in children who were not in a child restraint, or in one that is incorrect for their age. Most jurisdictions have enacted laws setting minimum standards for child restraint. In addition, the World Health Organization (WHO) has suggested regulations that are more stringent than many local laws. The WHO regulations suggest that children less than two years old always be restrained in rear-facing car seats, and children less than eight years old be restrained by a harness rather than a seat-belt.[4]

A forward-facing infant has a heavy head, weak neck muscles and poor ability to brace for a crash. They may suffer significant head, neck, chest and internal injuries, without significant external signs. All children trapped in vehicles or involved in RTCs should be transported for further assessment within the hospital system.

Adolescents and young adults are more likely to initially present with normal vital signs despite critical injuries. Continuous monitoring of these patients is required to pick up trends in deterioration.

Elderly persons are more likely to be severely injured with lower mechanisms. A higher index of suspicion should be applied when attending elderly patients who are trapped in vehicles. Their age, co-morbid state and medication status can affect their ability to compensate, as well as mask early signs of deterioration. Elderly patients will have higher base-line blood pressures and may be relatively hypotensive, while their blood pressure remains in the 'normal' parameters. They may also be on heart rate-controlling medications, such as beta-blockers, which may prevent them from mounting a tachycardia in response to shock. Elderly patients may have cerebral atrophy, increasing their risk of intracranial haemorrhage from rapid deceleration, as well as delayed signs of TBI due to more volume for the haemorrhage to fill within the cranium. They have weaker skin, bones and blood vessels, increasing their risk of lacerations, fractures and critical bleeding (see Chapter 36: The older patient). Older adults also have limited physiological reserve and can rapidly deteriorate. Older patients involved in RTCs should be thoroughly assessed and consideration given to transporting directly to a trauma centre, even if they don't meet usual trauma bypass criteria.

The deployment of safety devices, such as pre-tensioned seat-belts and airbags, may also cause injury to the patient. Lap-belts or poorly worn three-point seat-belts may result in thoraco-lumbar hyperflexion spinal injuries and intra-abdominal injuries, and if the lap components of lap-sash belts are not positioned correctly, these may cause damage to intra-abdominal organs or gravid uterus.[6,7] Children sitting in the front passenger seat in cars fitted with airbags may be injured by airbag deployment.[7] Older adults are also more likely to be injured with airbags, with an observational study examining airbag use and c-spine injuries (CSIs) concluding that drivers with CSIs were significantly older than those without CSIs.[8]

SECTION 7 Trauma

Question 3: Can Paramedics Predict Pattern of Injury from Mechanism and Damage?

Road traffic crashes have complex mechanisms; no two crash patterns or mechanisms are is the same. The damage visible to the car is not the only factor that can indicate the forces the body may have been subject to. Injuries in RTCs arise from multiple sources: the primary crash where the vehicle rapidly decelerates, causing external contact in the direction of impact while also leading to potential shearing on internal organs, and other impacts where the occupants are hit by loose items in the car, unrestrained passengers or external debris. All these factors come into play when considering the potential for injury when approaching a scene.

The prehospital description of estimated speed, impact and damage is invaluable to guide prehospital management and in-hospital investigations. The information regarding the mechanism that is provided to doctors by prehospital personnel influences doctor perception of the potential severity of the patient's injuries.[9]

> **PRACTICE TIP**
>
> Use the mechanism of injury to predict the pattern of injury in entrapped patients.

The essential information that needs to be considered when assessing a scene to predict injury patterns includes:

- Crash mechanism
- Impact geometry (where on the vehicle the impact occurred)
- Position of the patient in the car
- Restraint status
- Steering wheel damage
- Windscreen damage
- Compartment intrusion
- Ejection.[10]

Paramedics should use this information to help predict patterns of injury for patients and their subsequent risk of deterioration. This will also guide their decision making around patient priorities and extrication.

For example, in the case study at the start of this chapter, the entrapped driver has experienced both frontal and lateral impact forces. The initial impact and other forces acting upon the patient's body are dependent on crash-related factors, such as deceleration and the combined speeds of the car's impact, external damage and intrusions; patient-specific factors, such as the patient's weight, restraint status and position in the car, can determine patient injury status.

high-energy impacts, such as those seen in RTCs, are known to cause more damage to the head, thorax, pelvis and organs, with RTCs causing approximately 60% of pelvic fractures.[11] Patients involved in these types of incidents often require larger transfusions of blood products. Paramedics have been shown to be able to predict disability outcome from mechanism; this information is important to guide on-scene triage, as well as in-hospital management (**Table 26.1**).[9]

CHAPTER 26   The Trapped Patient

Table 26.1   Relationship of crash-related factors to injury patterns

Crash-related factor	Injury patterns
Dashboard impacting knees	Femur, pelvis and acetabulum fractures
Wheel arch intrusion	Open fractures of lower limbs that may require haemorrhage control
T-bone or broadside	Head, neck, chest, abdominal, lateral compression of the pelvis; multiple long bone fractures on the side of impact
Lap belts	Abdominal and pelvic fractures; chance of fractures to the spine
Unrestrained patients	Axial load from head hitting the windscreen; severe chest, large vessel and abdominal injuries from rapid deceleration and impact into parts of the vehicle
High-speed seat-belt injury	Fractures to clavicles, ribs, sternum; hollow or solid organ injury

PRACTICE TIP

Different ages and sexes will present with different injuries.

Question 4: How Do We Work Best with Rescue Teams?

Attendance at significant RTCs with trapped patients will typically see multiple teams come together to work towards extrication and management of trapped patients. It needs to first be acknowledged that this is when several highly trained teams that are not known to each other are required to operate together with a high level of cohesiveness. To ensure smooth and cohesive interoperability on scene, principles of closed-loop communication and discussion of common goals are vital to ensure the best outcome for the patient.[1,3,12]

Traditionally, non-medical rescue teams, such as fire or volunteer rescue services, have had training and standard operating procedures implemented into their practice based on the principle of the most minimal movement possible to prevent secondary spinal injury.[2,5] Forthright, concise and clear communication of patient priorities with rescue crews is required to ensure that the best access possible is achieved to remove the occupant, as extended time to extrication can cause delays in life-saving care and lead to further harm.[2,3] Self-extrication should be considered as a primary method of extrication for patients who are physically capable and who are still in their vehicles on paramedic arrival, unless it is obviously not a suitable option.[2,12] Self-extrication has been shown to have the least amount of spinal movement, with all other facilitated extrication methods (B-pillar rip off, roof off, rapid) (**Figure 26.1**) showing similar amounts of movement.[12,13] A minimally invasive approach to extrication should be taken for all patients who are not able to self-extricate.

SECTION 7 Trauma

> **PRACTICE TIP**
>
> Clear communication with rescue services is vital to ensure the best extrication method is utilised for the situation.

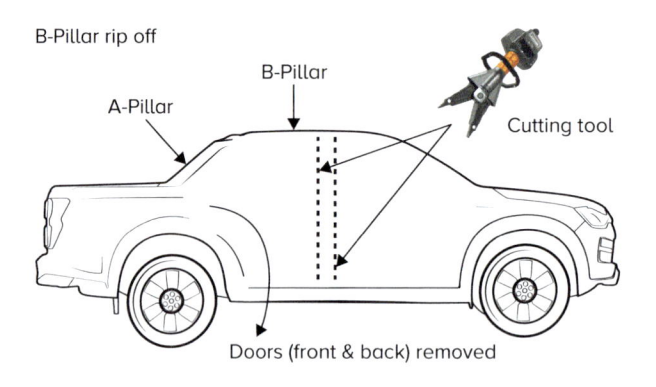

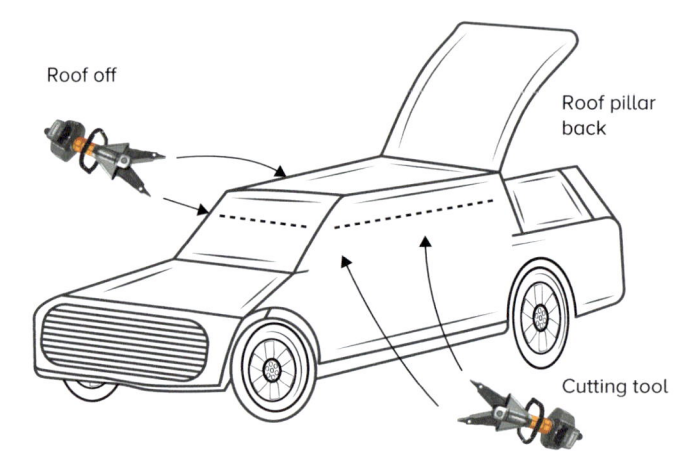

Figure 26.1 Extrication methods.

Question 5: How Do We Best Treat Trapped Patients?

Assessment and treatment of trapped patients is variable and is a dynamic balance between patient accessibility, rapid extrication, performing therapeutic interventions and minimising further injury. Every situation will have a different weighting to these elements, with priorities changing for each incident and at times even for each patient trapped within the same vehicle.

Trapped patients are more likely to die, are more seriously injured and have more deranged physiology than those who are not trapped.[5] The ability to provide initial resuscitation to trapped patients is vital to their care. This allows the initial assessment of the patient's injuries and vital signs and can help determine if a rapid extrication is required versus a

CHAPTER 26 The Trapped Patient

more prolonged extrication method. The initial assessment of the patient's condition should be clearly communicated to the team on scene as well as the rescue team leader to ensure everyone is working towards the same priorities and goals.

The principles of care for severely injured trauma patients also apply to the trapped trauma patient; however, achieving this is more complex. It is difficult to accurately assess and provide high-quality care to a trapped patient in a confined space. Prioritising adequate access and expedited extrication allows for earlier identification of life threats, assessment of patient condition and commencement of meaningful interventions.

The confined environment with potential snag and trip hazards impedes usual care. Restricted space makes it difficult to monitor and treat the patient, with interventions like sedation with ketamine and midazolam becoming more high risk, as airway interventions may be more difficult. Equipment taken into the vehicle may be dropped and become difficult to recover, and similarly IV lines and patient monitoring cables may get snagged and dislodged from the patient upon extrication. As extrication takes time, it is critical to be aware of potential sites of haemorrhage and control them early. Anticipate hypothermia even in moderate temperatures, and provide a warming blanket if possible. Finally continuous monitoring of the patient is essential, as patient deterioration may involve a change in extrication plan.

PRACTICE TIP

Extrication methods should be guided by patient presentation on a case-by-case basis.

Question 6: What Are Some Considerations about the Well-Being of Trapped Patients?

People who are trapped can experience both physical and psychological stressors. The nature of the entrapment can prevent access to the patient for both medical and psychological support. The extrication process can be loud, cause fear and challenge the entrapped patient's sense of safety. Rescuers should be aware of the impact of being trapped on the patient's experience and potential recovery. While extrication and medical management and assessment are at the forefront of rescuers' minds, there needs to be awareness of the importance of communication with the patient to ensure their continued well-being.[14]

A key aspect of the medical management of the trapped patient is the early and appropriate use of analgesia. This not only helps to reduce anxiety in the short term, thereby facilitating extrication and medical management, but early, effective pain management is also associated with decreasing the risk of the patient developing post-traumatic disorder.[15,16]

Communication with patients is vital. Patients report that their experiences were better when a bystander or emergency worker was ever-present in the car with them and continuously explained processes, updated them on their care and the plan for extrication, and reassured them during their period of entrapment.[14]

In contrast, patients who felt that they were not involved in conversation commented that they felt a loss of autonomy. Some reported not being told that their clothes were being cut off and others reported that they felt they were fine to just get out, but no one would listen.[14]

SECTION 7 Trauma

> **PRACTICE TIP**
>
> Ensure clear and open communication with the patient to prevent ongoing distress.

Key Evidence

Nutbeam T, Brandling J, Wallis LA et al. Understanding people's experiences of extrication while being trapped in motor vehicles: a qualitative interview study. *BMJ Open*. 2022;12(9):e063798. Available at: https://pubmed.ncbi.nlm.nih.gov/36127106/.

Nutbeam T, Fenwick R, May B et al. Assessing spinal movement during four extrication methods: a biomechanical study using healthy volunteers. *Scandinavian Journal of Trauma, Resuscitation and Emergency Medicine*. 2022;30(1):7. Available at: https://pubmed.ncbi.nlm.nih.gov/35033160/.

Nutbeam T, Fenwick R, Smith J et al. A comparison of the demographics, injury patterns and outcome data for patients injured in motor vehicle collisions who are trapped compared to those patients who are not trapped. *Scandinavian Journal of Trauma, Resuscitation and Emergency Medicine*. 2021;29(1):17. Available at: https://pubmed.ncbi.nlm.nih.gov/33446210/.

Nutbeam T, Fenwick R, Smith JE et al. A Delphi study of rescue and clinical subject matter experts on the extrication of patients following a motor vehicle collision. *Scandinavian Journal of Trauma, Resuscitation and Emergency Medicine*. 2022;30(1):41. Available at: https://pubmed.ncbi.nlm.nih.gov/35725580/

Nutbeam T, Kehoe A, Fenwick R et al. Do entrapment, injuries, outcomes and potential for self-extrication vary with age? A pre-specified analysis of the UK trauma registry (TARN). *Scandinavian Journal of Trauma, Resuscitation and Emergency Medicine*. 2022;30(1):14. Available at: https://pubmed.ncbi.nlm.nih.gov/35248129/

Self-Reflection Questions

1. What factors will you consider when approaching the scene of an RTC?
2. How will you use your knowledge of risk associated with patient demographics when determining risk of mortality and morbidity?
3. How will you approach working with and directing highly trained rescue teams?
4. What approach will you take to ensure patient psychological welfare?

References

1. Nutbeam T, Fenwick R, Hobson C et al. The stages of extrication: a prospective study. *Emergency Medicine Journal*. 2014;31(12):1006–1008.
2. Nutbeam T, Kehoe A, Fenwick R et al. Do entrapment, injuries, outcomes and potential for self-extrication vary with age? A pre-specified analysis of the UK trauma registry (TARN). *Scandinavian Journal of Trauma, Resuscitation and Emergency Medicine*. 2022;30(1):14.
3. Nutbeam T, Fenwick R, Smith JE et al. A Delphi study of rescue and clinical subject matter experts on the extrication of patients following a motor vehicle collision. *Scandinavian Journal of Trauma, Resuscitation and Emergency Medicine*. 2022;30(1):41.
4. World Health Organization. *Global Status Report on Road Safety, 2018*. Geneva: WHO; 2018.
5. Nutbeam T, Fenwick R, Smith J et al. A comparison of the demographics, injury patterns and outcome data for patients injured in motor vehicle collisions who are trapped compared to those patients who are not trapped. *Scandinavian Journal of Trauma, Resuscitation and Emergency Medicine*. 2021;29(1):17.
6. George I, Stergiannis P. Seat belt syndrome: a global issue. *Health Science Journal*. 2010;4:202.
7. Wallis LA, Greaves I. Injuries associated with airbag deployment. *Emergency Medicine Journal*. 2002;19(6):490.

8. Atkinson P, Bowra J, Milne J et al. International Federation for Emergency Medicine Consensus Statement: Sonography in hypotension and cardiac arrest (SHoC): An international consensus on the use of point of care ultrasound for undifferentiated hypotension and during cardiac arrest. *Canadian Journal of Emergency Medicine*. 2017;19(6):459–470.
9. Vaca FE, Anderson CL, Herrera H et al. Crash injury prediction and vehicle damage reporting by paramedics: a feasibility study. *Western Journal of Emergency Medicine*. 2009;10(2):62–67.
10. Choi YU, Jang SW, Kim SH et al. Correlation between the injury site and trauma mechanism in severely injured patients with blunt trauma. *Emergency Medicine International*. 2022;2022:8372012.
11. Spahn D, Bouillon B, Cerny V et al. The European guideline on management of major bleeding and coagulopathy following trauma: fifth edition. *Critical Care*. 2019;23.
12. Nutbeam T, Fenwick R, May B et al. Assessing spinal movement during four extrication methods: a biomechanical study using healthy volunteers. *Scandinavian Journal of Trauma, Resuscitation and Emergency Medicine*. 2022;30(1):7.
13. Nutbeam T, Fenwick R, May B et al. The role of cervical collars and verbal instructions in minimising spinal movement during self-extrication following a motor vehicle collision – a biomechanical study using healthy volunteers. *Scandinavian Journal of Trauma, Resuscitation and Emergency Medicine*. 2021;29(1):108.
14. Nutbeam T, Brandling J, Wallis LA et al. Understanding people's experiences of extrication while being trapped in motor vehicles: a qualitative interview study. *BMJ Open*. 2022;12(9):e063798.
15. Platts-Mills TF, Nebolisa BC, Flannigan SA et al. Post-traumatic stress disorder among older adults experiencing motor vehicle collision: a multicenter prospective cohort study. *American Journal of Geriatric Psychiatry*. 2017;25(9):953–963.
16. Holbrook TL, Galarneau MR, Dye JL et al. Morphine use after combat injury in Iraq and post-traumatic stress disorder. *New England Journal of Medicine*. 2010;362(2):110–117.

27

Shocked Blunt Trauma

Michael Noonan, Ben Meadley and Alexander Olaussen

> **In this chapter you will learn:**
> - Consolidation of knowledge in prioritisation and complex decision making in shocked trauma resuscitation
> - The complex interaction between evidence and clinical advanced trauma resuscitation practice
> - The evidence base supporting prehospital interventions for traumatic haemorrhagic shock.

Case Details

Dispatch

38-year-old male, motorbike accident (MBA).

History

A motorcyclist was travelling at 70 mph (110 kph) on the motorway. The patient was broadsided by a car. His secondary impact was into the gutter. There is clear deformity to his lower limbs, as well as pelvis and chest pain/bruising.

On Arrival of the First Crew

Traffic is stopped and the scene is made safe. The first paramedic crew to arrive position the patient on his back. His primary survey findings and initial vital signs are:

Airway	Patent
Breathing	Talking in short sentences, RR 28, SpO$_2$ 98% on air
Circulation	Peripheral pulses present, HR 120, regular, BP 80/50, no obvious external haemorrhage
Disability	GCS E4, V5, M6 (15)
Environmental	Outdoors, no specific concerns

The patient's helmet has been removed and is intact with no sign of impact. The secondary survey reveals bilateral lower limb deformity (likely femoral fractures), open fractures to the lower legs, as well as pelvis and chest wall pain, but the rib cage appears to be intact.

CHAPTER 27   Shocked Blunt Trauma

On Your Arrival as the Critical Care Paramedic

The initial paramedic crew is struggling to manage the patient's blood pressure. They have achieved a single point of IV access.

AMPLE

Allergies	NKDA
Medications	Nil
Past history	Nil
Last ins and outs	Normal
Events	MBA

Decision Point
What are your clinical priorities in this situation?

This patient's primary issue is shock. Shock has multiple causes following blunt traumatic injury. The most common causes are bleeding and tension pneumothorax. Less common causes include cardiac tamponade, neurogenic shock and shock secondary to a primary medical event (for example, a primary cardiac event precipitating trauma).

Question 1: How Should I Approach the Patient with Shock Following Blunt Traumatic Injury in the Prehospital Setting?

Traditionally, the 'ABCDE' approach has been taught; however, this approach has been criticised for placing too much emphasis on 'airway' (an uncommon cause of death following traumatic injury) and too little on exsanguination. Contemporary trauma teaching suggests a 'CABc' approach.[1] This practical approach is detailed below.

- Circulation – Seek and manage life-threatening external haemorrhage:
    o Direct wound pressure
    o Tourniquet
    o Haemostatic dressings.
- Airway – Open the airway.
- Breathing – Seek and treat tension pneumothorax.
- Circulation – Seek and treat other forms of bleeding:
    o Long-bone splinting
    o Pelvic binder application
    o Wide-bore IV access (+/- blood component resuscitation).

A helpful table to consider treatable causes and subsequent management is provided below (**Table 27.1**).

SECTION 7 Trauma

Table 27.1 Treatable causes and subsequent management of blunt traumatic injury

SEEK (life threat)	TREAT (life-saving intervention)
External bleeding	• Direct pressure • Tourniquets • Haemostatic dressing
Tension pneumothorax	• Bilateral pleural decompression
Cardiac tamponade	• Resuscitative thoracotomy (where available)
Pelvic fractures	• Pelvic binder
Long-bone fractures	• Splinting

Question 2: What Devices and Equipment Can Help Manage Bleeding in the Prehospital Setting?

There are numerous commercially available devices to assist in the management of the shocked trauma patient. The evidence basis behind most of these devices is weak.

Devices and equipment to consider include:

- Haemostatic dressings (for example, Quickclot)
- Long-bone splints (for example, KTD traction splint) (**Figure 27.1A**)
- Pelvic binder (for example, SAM pelvic splint) (**Figure 27.1B**)
- Tourniquet (for example, CAT) (**Figure 27.1C**)
- Simple IV lines.

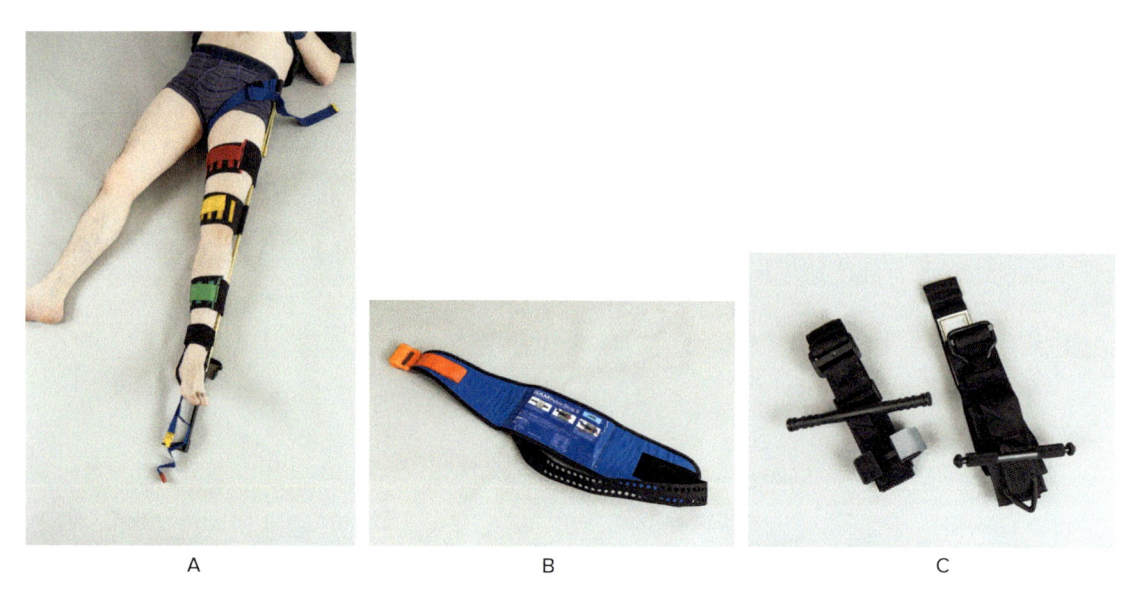

Figure 27.1 Devices to assist in the management of the shocked trauma patient: (A) KTD traction splint; (B) SAM pelvic binder; (C) CAT tourniquet.

CHAPTER 27 Shocked Blunt Trauma

Question 3: What Is the Role of Tourniquets in the Prehospital Setting for Patients in Traumatic Haemorrhagic Shock?

The use of tourniquets has up - commonplace place since the conflicts in the Middle East in the 1990s and 2000s, where improvised explosive devices led to severe limb trauma. This military practice has evolved such that the widespread use of tourniquets has demonstrated improvements in survivability for these soldiers.[2] Although there is an absence of prospective randomised studies, similar outcomes have been seen in the civilian environment.[3]

Tourniquets seem to be an intuitive management strategy for bleeds that are open and compressible. They are readily available and are not limited by cost. However, concerns over their use exist. These include the potential side-effects of tourniquet clots, myonecrosis, rigor, pain, palsies, renal failure, amputation and compartment syndrome. However, prospective studies have failed to identify significant morbidity. A study of 232 patients with 428 tourniquets applied, in a combat support hospital in Baghdad, found that four patients (1.7%) sustained transient nerve palsy at the level of the tourniquet, whereas six patients had palsies at the wound level.[4] The study did not find any association between tourniquet time and morbidity. Nonetheless, it is vital to note the application time by writing on the tourniquet or limb in permanent or surgical ink. If prolonged application time is likely (≥4 hours), clinicians should advise the receiving trauma centre early to ensure an adequate plan for a 'tourniquet down' plan.

There is no high-quality evidence to guide the use of prophylactic tourniquets for the patient with haemorrhagic shock. A 2021 systematic review of four studies with a total of 1762 trauma patients found that the evidence base was weak and the impact on mortality was non-significant, with an adjusted odds ratio (aOR) of 0.47 (95% confidence interval (CI) 0.19-1.16; three studies; 377 patients) for overall mortality.[5]

Question 4: Now That Reversible Haemorrhage Has Been Addressed, What Must Be Done about the Hypotension? What Is the Evidence Base behind Permissive Hypotension?

Wide-bore IV access and blood component resuscitation remain mainstay treatment for traumatic haemorrhagic shock. Permissive hypotension may have a role in penetrating trauma. The concerns around giving too much fluid, and thus raising mean arterial pressure and furthering bleeding, have been debated among clinician-scientists for more than a century.[6] The landmark article by Bickell et al. in 1994,[7] which was a prospective trial comparing immediate and delayed fluid resuscitation in 598 adults with penetrating torso injuries and shock (SBP ≤90 mmHg), found 70% of delayed fluid resuscitation patients survived, compared to 62% in the immediate fluid resuscitation arm (P = 0.04). This pioneering study propagated the concept of permissive hypotension.

While permissive hypotension is supported by animal and human studies in penetrating trauma, in developed nations the majority of trauma is blunt (97% in Australia and 92% in the US). However, there are limited data to support permissive hypotension in this cohort. Moreover, in blunt trauma there may be competing priorities for patients with concurrent head and spinal cord injuries, which require maintenance of adequate mean arterial pressure to maintain vital organ perfusion. Thus, target blood pressure should be tailored to individual clinical circumstances.

Question 5: If Giving Fluids and Medications for Shock, Which Should They Be?

The primary infusion in the setting of trauma is blood or blood components, where available, and this is supported by numerous studies.[8] Decompensated shock may be responsive to second-line options, such as the vasopressors adrenaline and noradrenaline, for optimising mean arterial pressure. Third, and last, are intravenous crystalloid fluids, such as normal saline 0.9%, although high-volume crystalloid infusion has been associated with harmful side-effects by worsening trauma-induced coagulopathy and furthering bleeding.[9]

Question 6: What Is the Role of Prehospital Blood Transfusion? What Additional Products Should Be Considered?

Blood and blood component resuscitation is now the standard of care for bleeding patients following traumatic injury. Prehospital blood transfusion can help to rapidly replace lost blood volume; however, access is not universal in all jurisdictions and may carry logistical challenges, financial cost and potential risk. Systems set up to administer prehospital blood transfusions to major trauma patients have established specific governance and training frameworks to mitigate these factors. In general, the decision to administer a transfusion should only be made by an experienced clinician who is familiar with the procedure and its risks.

Military studies investigating whole blood suggest this is best option when available. As this is rare, there is a reliance on blood components instead, such as red cells and plasma (fresh or freeze-dried). Other components, such as fibrinogen concentrate, have been trialled but are not yet common practice.

The evidence base for prehospital blood transfusions has so far been mixed and is expanding. There are only a handful of well-conducted trials answering the question of blood transfusion in prehospital haemorrhage. The PAMPER trial, a multicentre, cluster-randomised, superiority trial, which compared the administration of thawed plasma with standard care resuscitation during air medical transport, showed that of a total of 501 enrolled patients, mortality at 30 days was significantly lower in the plasma group compared to the standard care group (23.2% versus 33.0%; difference, −9.8 percentage points; 95% CI, −18.6 to −1.0%; $P = 0.03$).[10] On the other hand, the COMBAT trial showed no benefit.[11] However, a post hoc analysis of both the COMBAT trial and the PAMPER trials,[12] comparing patients who got two units of prehospital plasma with crystalloid-based resuscitation, demonstrated that patients with haemorrhagic shock following trauma showed a significant overall survival benefit for plasma (hazard ratio [HR], 0.65; 95% CI, 0.47–0.90; $P = 0.01$) after adjustment for injury severity, age and clinical trial cohort. Notably, a significant association with prehospital transport time was detected. Increased mortality was observed in patients in the standard care group when prehospital transport was longer than 20 minutes (HR 2.12; 95% CI 1.05–4.30; $P = 0.04$)

The recent RePHILL trial, which studied whether lyophilised plasma (LyoPlas) was superior to use of placebo (normal saline) in trauma-related haemorrhagic shock, was a multicentre open-label, randomised, controlled trial undertaken in four civilian prehospital critical care services in the UK. Of the 432 participants enrolled, the composite primary outcome (of mortality or impaired lactate clearance or both) occurred in 64% of patients given PRBC-LyoPlas and 65% of patients given 0.9% sodium chloride (P = 0.996).[13] This trial suggested that there was no benefit to prehospital administration of lyophilised plasma, although it must be noted that the transport times in this trial were relatively short, so it may also support the findings of COMBAT and PAMPER and suggest that there may still be a role for prehospital plasma administration where transport times are longer.

Another adjunct to blood transfusions, particularly after many units of delivery, is calcium. Hypocalcaemia commonly occurs in the shocked trauma patient, and association between hypocalcaemia and mortality has been identified.[14] Well-designed prospective trials are essential to explore this association further.

Question 7: What Treatment Options Are on the Horizon for the Bleeding Shock Trauma Patient?

Other techniques and procedures (beyond blood products and splinting) are on the horizon and will soon be part of a prehospital treatment protocol for shocked trauma patients. Some procedures are already being undertaken in certain jurisdictions by prehospital medical personnel, while others are currently only performed in hospital but will likely move to the prehospital arena in coming years for certain patient presentations.

Resuscitative endovascular balloon occlusion of the aorta (REBOA) is one such therapy. It involves the placement of a balloon inside the aorta for patients with non-compressible torso injuries and uncontrolled haemorrhagic shock. A systematic review with studies up until June 2020, from the in-hospital setting, found that eleven studies with 5,866 participants concluded that REBOA was associated with lower mortality when compared to resuscitative thoracotomy (aOR 0.38; 95% CI 0.20–0.74), but was not different from cases that were treated without REBOA (aOR 1.40; 95% CI 0.79–2.46).[15] The interest and feasibility testing for prehospital REBOA in light of these findings are growing.[16,17]

A multicentre RCT, the UK-REBOA trial, randomised adults with exsanguinating haemorrhage (97% of whom had blunt trauma) to REBOA versus standard care and unexpectedly showed an increase in mortality in the REBOA group compared with the standard care group (54% versus 42%).[18] This finding places a question mark over the use of REBOA, although it should be noted that in this trial it was performed in the ED; there may still be the opportunity to evaluate prehospital use of REBOA, although only in the context of a trial. Perhaps the UK-REBOA trial highlights the vitally important message that the key factor affecting survival in the shocked trauma patient is time to definitive control of bleeding.

PRACTICE TIP

There are a limited number of useful interventions that can be employed in the prehospital setting. Early institution of these and rapid transport to an appropriate level trauma centre should be undertaken.

SECTION 7 Trauma

Question 8: Is It Better to 'Scoop and Run' or 'Stay and Play'?

The best approach for the shocked patient is 'scoop and play'. Any prehospital intervention in the shocked trauma patients needs to be rapid and must be aimed at stopping bleeding as a primary intervention and providing resuscitation. However, definitive diagnosis and management will only occur in hospital, and as such transport times need to be shortened and not unnecessarily prolonged.

Intubation in many cases leads to worsening of shocked states, and should only be undertaken where patient and provider safety demands it (for example, if a patient is in a helicopter and needs to be controlled, or if the patient is hypoxic).

> **PRACTICE TIP**
>
> 'Scoop and play'
> Time to definitive care is key in shocked trauma.

Question 9: Should Prehospital Pleural Decompression Take Place in the Shocked Trauma Patient?

Thoracic injury is the third most common cause of death (after abdominal and head injury) in blunt mechanism multi-trauma patients.[19] Attention to pleural drainage is therefore paramount. Patients in shock following chest injuries may be suffering haemothorax, tension pneumothorax or both (i.e. haemo-pneumothorax). For details on pleural decompression the reader is referred to the chapter on chest trauma (Chapter 29: Severe chest injury).

Should the patient with undifferentiated shock be treated with both types of chest decompression? While there are a number of factors that will influence this decision, on balance there are probably more risks associated with not treating a tension haemo-pneumothorax swiftly compared with the risks of finger or needle thoracostomy in the patient without the injury.

Key Evidence

Systematic Review/Meta-Analysis

Latina R, Iacorossi L, Fauci AJ et al. Effectiveness of pre-hospital tourniquet in emergency patients with major trauma and uncontrolled haemorrhage: a systematic review and meta-analysis. *International Journal of Environmental Research and Public Health*, 2021, *18*(23), p. 12861.

Randomised Controlled Trials

CRASH-2 trial collaborators et al. (2010) 'Effects of tranexamic acid on death, vascular occlusive events, and blood transfusion in trauma patients with significant haemorrhage (CRASH-2): a randomised, placebo-controlled trial', *Lancet*, 376(9734), pp. 23–32. Available at: https://doi.org/10.1016/S0140-6736(10)60835-5.

Crombie N, Doughty HA, Bishop JRB et al. Resuscitation with blood products in patients with trauma-related haemorrhagic shock receiving prehospital care (RePHILL): a multicentre, open-label, randomised, controlled, phase 3 trial. *Lancet Haematology*, 2022, 9(4), pp. 250–261.

Moore HB, Moore EE, Chapman MP et al. Plasma-first resuscitation to treat haemorrhagic shock during emergency ground transportation in an urban area: a randomised trial. *Lancet*, 2018, 392(10144), pp. 283–291.

Sperry JL, Guyette FX, Brown JB et al. Prehospital plasma during air medical transport in trauma patients at risk for hemorrhagic shock. *New England Journal of Medicine*, 2018;379(4):315–326.

Self-Reflection Questions

1. What is the role of a paramedic in the management of the shocked trauma patient?
2. Reflecting on your own jurisdiction, what extended scope or management exists for blood and blood product delivery, as well as the use of devices such as tourniquets?
3. Do you think the evidence supports the use of prehospital blood?
4. These complex patients require a detailed handover when you arrive at hospital. Using the table below, prepare a handover of the patient described using the IMIST AMBO format.

Introduction
Mechanism
Injuries
Symptoms
Treatment
Allergies
Medications
Background history
Other information

References

1. Ferrada, P., Callcut, R.A., Skarupa, D.J. et al. (2018) 'Circulation first – the time has come to question the sequencing of care in the ABCs of trauma; an American Association for the Surgery of Trauma multicenter trial', *World Journal of Emergency Surgery*, 13(1), p. 8. Available at: https://doi.org/10.1186/s13017-018-0168-3.
2. Kragh, J.F.Jr., Dubick, M.A., Aden, J.K. et al. (2015) 'U.S. military use of tourniquets from 2001 to 2010', *Prehospital Emergency Care*, 19(2), pp. 184–190. Available at: https://doi.org/10.3109/10903127.2014.964892.
3. Eilertsen, K., Winberg, M., Jeppesen, E. et al. (2021) 'Prehospital tourniquets in civilians: a systematic review', *Prehospital and Disaster Medicine*, 36(1), pp. 86–94. Available at: https://doi.org/10.1017/S1049023X20001284.
4. Kragh, J.F. Jr., Walters, T.J., Baer, D.G. et al. (2008) 'Practical use of emergency tourniquets to stop bleeding in major limb trauma'. *Journal of Trauma*, 64(2 Suppl), pp. S38–49; discussion S49–50. https://doi.org/10.1097/TA.0b013e31816086b1. PMID: 18376170.
5. Latina, R., Iacorossi, L., Fauci, A.J. et al. (2021) 'Effectiveness of pre-hospital tourniquet in emergency patients with major trauma and uncontrolled haemorrhage: a systematic review and meta-analysis', *International Journal of Environmental Research and Public Health*, 18(23), p. 12861. Available at: https://doi.org/10.3390/ijerph182312861.
6. Gurd, F.B. (1918) 'The nature and treatment of wound shock and allied conditions', *Journal of the American Medical Association*, 70(9), pp. 607–621. Available at: https://doi.org/10.1001/jama.1918.02600090027013.

SECTION 7 Trauma

7. Bickell, W.H., Wall, M.J.Jr., Pepe, P.E. et al. (1994) 'Immediate versus delayed fluid resuscitation for hypotensive patients with penetrating torso injuries', *New England Journal of Medicine*, 331(17), pp. 1105–1109. Available at: https://doi.org/10.1056/NEJM199410273311701.

8. Meneses, E., Boneva, D., McKenny, M. et al. (2020) 'Massive transfusion protocol in adult trauma population', *American Journal of Emergency Medicine*, 38(12), pp. 2661–2666. Available at: https://doi.org/10.1016/j.ajem.2020.07.041.

9. Sheppard, F.R., Schaub, L.J., Cap, A.P. et al. (2018) 'Whole blood mitigates the acute coagulopathy of trauma and avoids the coagulopathy of crystalloid resuscitation', *Journal of Trauma and Acute Care Surgery*, 85(6), pp. 1055–1062. Available at: https://doi.org/10.1097/TA.0000000000002046.

10. Sperry, J.L., Guyette, F.X., Brown, J.B. et al. (2018) 'Prehospital plasma during air medical transport in trauma patients at risk for hemorrhagic shock', *New England Journal of Medicine*, 379(4), pp. 315–326. Available at: https://doi.org/10.1056/NEJMoa1802345.

11. Moore, H.B., Moore, E.E., Chapman, M.P. et al. (2018) 'Plasma-first resuscitation to treat haemorrhagic shock during emergency ground transportation in an urban area: a randomised trial', *Lancet*, 392(10144), pp. 283–291. Available at: https://doi.org/10.1016/S0140-6736(18)31553-8.

12. Pusateri, A.E., Moore, E.E., Moore, H.B. et al. (2020) 'Association of prehospital plasma transfusion with survival in trauma patients with hemorrhagic shock when transport times are longer than 20 minutes: a post hoc analysis of the PAMPer and COMBAT clinical trials', *JAMA Surgery*, 155(2), p. e195085. Available at: https://doi.org/10.1001/jamasurg.2019.5085.

13. Crombie, N., Doughty, H.A., Bishop, J.R.B. et al. (2022) 'Resuscitation with blood products in patients with trauma-related haemorrhagic shock receiving prehospital care (RePHILL): a multicentre, open-label, randomised, controlled, phase 3 trial', *Lancet. Haematology*, 9(4), pp. e250–e261. Available at: https://doi.org/10.1016/S2352-3026(22)00040-0.

14. Vasudeva, M., Mathew, J.K., Groombridge, C. et al. (2021) 'Hypocalcemia in trauma patients: a systematic review', *Journal of Trauma and Acute Care Surgery*, 90(2), pp. 396–402. Available at: https://doi.org/10.1097/TA.0000000000003027.

15. Castellini, G., Gianola, S., Biffi, A. et al. (2021) 'Resuscitative endovascular balloon occlusion of the aorta (REBOA) in patients with major trauma and uncontrolled haemorrhagic shock: a systematic review with meta-analysis', *World Journal of Emergency Surgery*, 16(1), p. 41. Available at: https://doi.org/10.1186/s13017-021-00386-9.

16. Brede, J.R., Lafrenz, T., Klepstad, P. et al. (2019) 'Feasibility of pre-hospital resuscitative endovascular balloon occlusion of the aorta in non-traumatic out-of-hospital cardiac arrest', *Journal of the American Heart Association*, 8(22), p. e014394. Available at: https://doi.org/10.1161/JAHA.119.014394.

17. Lendrum, R., Perkins, Z., Chana, M. et al. (2019) 'Pre-hospital resuscitative endovascular balloon occlusion of the aorta (REBOA) for exsanguinating pelvic haemorrhage', *Resuscitation*, 135, pp. 6–13. Available at: https://doi.org/10.1016/j.resuscitation.2018.12.018.

18. Jansen, J.O., Hudson, J., Cochran, C. et al. (2023) 'Emergency department resuscitative endovascular balloon occlusion of the aorta in trauma patients with exsanguinating hemorrhage: the UK-REBOA randomized clinical trial', *Journal of the American Medical Association*, 330(19), pp. 1862–1871. Available at: https://doi:10.1001/jama.2023.20850

19. Beshay, M., Mertzlufft, F., Kottkamp, H.W. et al. (2020) 'Analysis of risk factors in thoracic trauma patients with a comparison of a modern trauma centre: a mono-centre study', *World Journal of Emergency Surgery*, 15(1), p. 45. Available at: https://doi.org/10.1186/s13017-020-00324-1.

Penetrating Trauma

28

Kat Baird, Peter Sherren and Scott Wallman

In this chapter you will learn:

- How to assess a patient with penetrating trauma
- The importance of acute traumatic coagulopathy (ATC)
- What the priorities and management options are for a patient with penetrating trauma
- The considerations when triaging patients with penetrating trauma
- The principles of damage control resuscitation.

Case Details

Dispatch

16-year-old male, stab wounds, police already on scene.

History

A 16-year-old male has been stabbed in the right buttock following an altercation on the way home from school. He ran back into his home, alerting his mother, who quickly called for an ambulance. She reported that she could see blood on the rear of his jeans, and believed he may have been stabbed. The patient was reported to be awake but diaphoretic and agitated at the time of the initial call to emergency services.

Multiple resources including a critical care paramedic (CCP) are dispatched, and an ambulance with a paramedic and emergency medical technician arrive on scene eight minutes after the initial emergency call.

On Arrival of the First Crew

Police have deemed the scene safe for emergency personnel to approach. On arrival, the patient is found in the downstairs living room in blood-soaked jeans, with a degree of agitation, diaphoresis and breathlessness. A number of highly emotional family members are also present.

Given the penetrating trauma and potential haemorrhage, the patient is rapidly assisted to the ambulance outside for further assessment and management. Following a 'stab/wound check' on the ambulance stretcher, only a single 2 cm incised wound is identified on the right buttock, 10 cm lateral to the midline, with moderate ongoing external bleeding. The patient's primary survey findings and initial vital signs are:

SECTION 7 Trauma

Catastrophic haemorrhage	Nil
Airway	Patent and maintained
Breathing	Effortless tachypnoea at 45 bpm, good equal air entry and a poor pulse oximetry trace intermittently picking up SpO$_2$ 96% on room air
Circulation	Ashen, cool peripherally, HR 90, difficult to palpate radial but strong carotid pulse and poor venous tone, BP repeatedly cycled out and then finally gave a value of 150/130
Disability	GCS E3, V5, M6 (14), moving all limbs, pupils equal and reactive, complaining of thirst
Environmental	Single incised wound

The patient is administered supplemental oxygen via a non-rebreather mask, and direct pressure is applied to the wound with a basic trauma dressing before the paramedics proceed to peripheral intravenous (PIV) access, which fails just before your arrival.

On Your Arrival as the Critical Care Paramedic

You arrive on scene and take a handover. You establish a rapid rapport with the patient prior to the removal of his clothes so as to comprehensively exclude any further wounds, provide wound care and facilitate ongoing attempts at PIV access. The patient is successfully cannulated after two further attempts, but due to poor venous tone, only a 20-gauge cannula in the left antecubital fossa is possible. A haemostatic dressing is packed tightly into the wound and expedited transport to definitive care is then prioritised.

Decision Point: Triage

The nearest major trauma centre (MTC) is 40 minutes away by road, and you elect to bypass the local community hospital given the patient's signs of shock and potential need for resuscitative surgery. During transfer the patient becomes increasingly difficult to rouse, with worsening tachypnoea, and it is difficult to palpate his central pulses. In addition to 1 g of tranexamic acid, volume resuscitation is initiated as per local protocol for penetrating trauma. Due to difficulty maintaining flow rates through the small-gauge PIV access, only 200 ml of crystalloid and one unit of packed red blood cells are administered prior to arrival at the MTC.

On Arrival At Hospital

At handover to the multidisciplinary team, the patient is obtunded and in peri-arrest. A large-bore sheath introducer is placed in the left subclavian vein, through which ongoing haemostatic resuscitation is delivered. A concurrent focused assessment sonography trauma (FAST) scan identifies free fluid in the pelvis, and a decision for damage control laparotomy is made. Despite an ongoing massive transfusion, the patient continues to rapidly deteriorate and suffers a cardiac arrest prior to departing the emergency department. A resuscitative thoracotomy is undertaken for aortic control prior to proceeding to laparotomy. Significant

CHAPTER 28   Penetrating Trauma

retroperitoneal and peritoneal blood is noted but the exact bleeding point is difficult to identify and control surgically. Temporary packing is undertaken, and the patient is transitioned to interventional radiology, where an internal iliac artery injury is embolised. Sadly, despite aggressive damage-control resuscitation and multi-organ support, the patient succumbs 24 hours later to the inflammatory and cardiometabolic sequelae of the multiple insults.

Question 1: How Should Penetrating Injuries Be Assessed?

Scene safety is paramount when approaching a patient who is the victim of any penetrating injury. Liaison with law enforcement personnel and consideration of appropriate personal protective equipment are essential for team and personal safety. Once involved with patient management, a continued awareness of scene safety is required, as these are often very dynamic situations.

The range of injury and sequelae from penetrating injury can be vast. Some patients may have superficial wounds with limited need for emergency management, while others experience exsanguinating haemorrhage and death. Identifying those with significant pathology, then managing that pathology and rapid triage to definitive care, is an essential skill in the prehospital field.

Patients with penetrating trauma can have one of two main patterns of shock: obstructive or haemorrhagic shock.

Obstructive Shock

There are two key pathological processes that generate obstructive shock in those who have suffered penetrating trauma:

- Tension pneumothorax
- Cardiac tamponade.

Haemorrhagic Shock

Patient assessment begins with the scene approach. The information you gather in these first few moments will prove invaluable in shaping a global overview. Assessment of the scene can provide considerable amounts of information. If the patient is seen where the assault occurred there may be evidence of blood loss patterns and spread. Spending time trying to estimate volume of blood loss is not advised. Prehospital estimations of blood loss are known to often be inaccurate due to variable absorbance of different surfaces and clothing; a recognition of significant blood loss will suffice.[1] While some blood loss is external to the patient's body, large volumes can be lost internally at the chest, abdomen, pelvis, long bones (predominantly femurs) and retroperitoneal space. A high index of suspicion can help identify these 'hidden' sources of bleeding. In addition to potentially underappreciating the volume of external blood loss, the specificity of some physiological signs may be limited by a significant exertional period prior to clinical assessment if a patient has fled the scene of the assault, for example. Visualising the weapon used can be informative but is not essential, as 'small-bladed' weapons or even short screwdrivers can result in life-threatening injuries.

Visual inspection of a patient can be undertaken rapidly and can ensure early identification of a patient who is shocked. Many of the physiological subtleties of exsanguinating trauma can be gleaned without even touching the patient, and the value of initial visual inspection should not be underestimated. This inspection should ideally be done with the patient fully undressed. This allows for a full inspection looking for wounds or a full 'stab check'. This comprehensive examination should be completed as soon as possible, even before the primary survey. Close inspection of axilla, neck, buttocks and groin should be completed, as these are known regions where wounds can be readily missed. If it is not possible to fully expose the patient immediately (environment or patient compliance), this should be achieved as soon as practicably possible or documented and handed over to the receiving hospital team.

While the classic advanced trauma life support (ATLS) classification of hypovolaemic shock is well known, the real-world physiological decline with exsanguinating trauma can be a little more complex and occasionally idiosyncratic.[2] Rather than focus on linear progression of vital signs, it may be more appropriate to identify the common clinical features associated with progressive shock. These are:

- Pulse: tachycardia
- Pressure: hypotension
- Poor peripheral perfusion: cold hands and feet
- Poor cerebral perfusion: confusion or agitation
- Panting: Kussmaul breathing due to lactic acidosis.

Classic quantitative vital signs, such as narrowed pulse pressure or blood pressure, can add information but can be difficult to obtain reliably with non-invasive techniques in critically ill patients and the dynamic prehospital environment.

PRACTICE TIP

Before progressing further with assessment, it is worth considering that victims of penetrating trauma are often young and fit, with otherwise good cardiovascular reserve. This, combined with any recreational drugs and sympathetic surges, means they compensate well but can deteriorate rapidly and unpredictably.

The patient may be in pain and frightened, so exemplary communication and reassurance are key skills. Patients who feel cared for, respected and not judged are more likely to co-operate with the prehospital team as concurrent work is undertaken. Delegation of tasks to the wider team enables rapid assessment and concurrent management of the scene and patient.

Many of the features above can be related to the hypoperfusion associated with significant blood loss. 'Air hunger' is a well-recognised feature of hypovolaemic shock associated with significant bleeding. It may also be a brain starved of essential substrate sending altered messages to the respiratory centres in the medulla oblongata and pons. The relative hypoperfusion of the brain may also account for the altered level of consciousness seen in patients with significant haemorrhage.

Tachycardia is a recognised feature of shock; however, this is not always the case. Heart rates can be high, low or normal. This concept of non-tachycardia in hypovolaemic shock is important as a 'normal' heart rate taken in isolation without this background knowledge may be falsely reassuring.

CHAPTER 28 Penetrating Trauma

Question 2: What Is Acute Traumatic Coagulopathy?

Hypothermia, acidaemia and coagulopathy form a well-recognised lethal triad, which carries with it a significant mortality implication.[3] The tissue hypoperfusion associated with bleeding results in decreased oxygen delivery, a shift to anaerobic metabolism, lactate production and a metabolic acidosis. Hypothermia is frequently found in haemorrhagic shock due to a combination of exposure, massive cold fluid administration and impaired endogenous heat production. Early coagulation dysfunction has been found in 25% of severely injured trauma patients with a significant mortality implication that is unrelated to fluid administration and temperature.[4] This entity has been termed acute trauma coagulopathy (ATC) or acute coagulopathy of trauma shock (ACoTS). It is an impairment of homeostasis of coagulation that is initiated immediately after an injury, and it appears to be driven primarily by the combination of tissue injury and hypoperfusion. Damage control resuscitation (DCR) is a package of care that can be initiated in the prehospital phase to target the ATC and lethal triad. DCR is composed of rapid haemorrhage control/damage control surgery, haemostatic resuscitation and permissive hypotension. While the importance of ATC management in major trauma continues, there is an increasing interest in a move away from these traditional constituents of the lethal triad to a more contemporary one involving coagulopathy, hypocalcaemia and hyperkalaemia.

Haemostatic or damage control resuscitation describes the approach to fluid management and adjunctive haemostatic therapies in the haemorrhaging trauma patient. Excess volume resuscitation of any sort may be injurious in trauma, and a permissive approach outlined below is preferable. While a recent prehospital randomised control trial[5] suggested that packed red blood cells (PRBC) with lyophilised plasma was not superior to low-volume crystalloid fluid resuscitation, the standard of care in most evolved trauma systems for massive haemorrhage is balanced transfusions. Excess cold crystalloid resuscitation may not only negatively affect patient's temperature but will also dilute essential clotting factors. Early, balanced use of PRBCs, clotting products (plasma, platelets and fibrinogen) and coagulation adjuncts (tranexamic acid, calcium) to mitigate the effects of the ATC and tissue hypoperfusion is increasingly becoming a gold standard for major haemorrhage policies worldwide. The future prehospital roles of whole blood and plasma-only resuscitation are particularly interesting, with potential mortality benefits being seen in recent trials; however, further studies are both urgently needed and eagerly awaited. When cold blood products are available and utilised, they should be warmed during administration. There is significant international variability in the availability of prehospital blood and blood products, and clinicians should be familiar with what local enhanced care teams can provide.

Permissive hypotension involves titrated volume resuscitation, which targets a subnormal end point that maintains organ viability until haemorrhage is definitively controlled. By avoiding overzealous fluid/blood resuscitation that targets normotension, the hope is to preserve the first, and often best, clot. Although permissive hypotension is frequently employed in traumatic haemorrhage, there is only robust evidence that it is advantageous in penetrating trauma in the urban environment. The end point for resuscitation will depend on age, pre-morbid autoregulation, acute pathology, timeline and clinical judgement. Time to hospital destination should also be considered. 'Rule of thumb' end point in penetrating trauma is a blood pressure sufficient to maintain cerebral perfusion or a central pulse. Appropriate verbal contact and interaction are reflective of this. Some services will have recommended blood pressure values to guide therapy. Beyond 60 minutes after injury, the ongoing perceived benefits of permissive hypotension may be outweighed by the detrimental effects of hypoperfusion on coagulation integrity. Under such circumstances, novel hybrid resuscitation might be appropriate to normalise perfusion following an initial permissive approach.

Question 3: What Are the Priorities and Management Options for a Patient with Penetrating Trauma?

The immediate aid provided for the bleeding patient can significantly influence patient trajectory. The hierarchy of management priorities in the exsanguinating penetrating trauma is illustrated in **Figure 28.1**.

Immediate haemorrhage control
Expedited scene time
Haemostatic resuscitation
Permissive hypotension
Multi-disciplinary centre

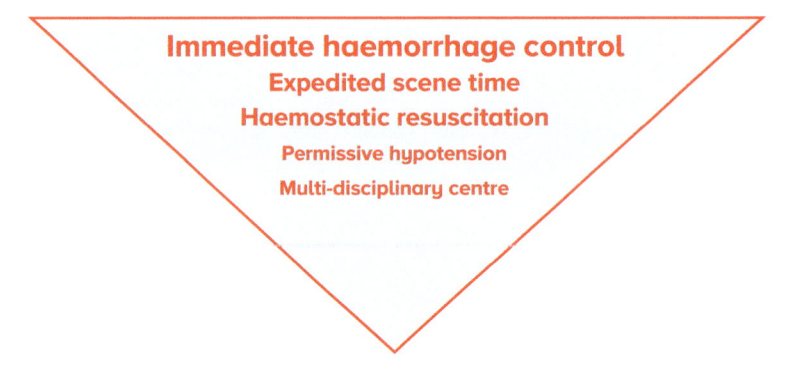

Figure 28.1 Hierarchy of management priorities in exsanguinating penetrating trauma.

The control of blood loss should be a primary action with adherence to the C-ABC approach. Catastrophic haemorrhage should be managed rapidly and ideally in conjunction with a primary patient survey. Direct pressure over a wound with a trauma dressing or gauze is a suitable initial approach. Wounds, if large enough, can be packed with haemostatic agents or gauze, with a specialised trauma dressing applied over the top. Direct physical pressure can then be superimposed with a digit, fist or even a knee if required. If this is unsuccessful, the deployment of a tourniquet can be utilised if the position of the wound is amenable to tourniquet management. These should be placed proximal to the wound but as close as possible to avoid excess ischaemic tissue injury. If a tourniquet and dressing have been applied prior to your arrival, note the time of application and check they are still tight and efficacious.

There are many specialised dressings available on the market to help manage haemorrhage. Many of them are impregnated with pro-coagulant material. It is worth having a good knowledge of the dressing types carried by the local service. Allergic reactions to these types of dressings have not been recorded in the literature. A full review of all types of pro-coagulant dressings is beyond the scope of this chapter.

Junctional wounds, such as those in the neck and groin, can be more difficult to manage. Beyond good basic wound care as described above, there may be some occasions where a foley catheter can be introduced into the wound and gently inflated with saline and then clamped, and this may help tamponade bleeding. Exsanguinating non-compressible truncal trauma, such as in the case described, can be a hugely challenging group to manage. Beyond expediting transport and limiting time to definitive haemorrhage control, there are limited other options available to most prehospital services. Resuscitative endovascular balloon occlusion of the aorta (REBOA) for a highly select group of exsanguinating cases may have a function within a high-volume and tightly governed prehospital critical care service. The UK-REBOA trial did not demonstrate any significant improvement with the use of REBOA compared to standard care amongst trauma patients (n=90) in the emergency department with exsanguinating shock. Ninety-day all-cause mortality was statistically non-significantly higher in the REBOA group compared to the standard care (54% versus 42%; odds ratio (OR) 1.58; 95% confidence interval 0.72-3.52).[6] More evidence and targeted patient selection may be needed. The role for more novel intra-abdominal haemostatic agents is awaited with great interest, but human data is currently lacking.

Intravenous access is both a critical and occasionally challenging component of penetrating trauma management. It can often be delegated on scene to clinicians with appropriate skills as concurrent activity is managed. As patients bleed and lose their vascular tone, this procedure can become increasingly challenging. The larger the cannula, the better; ideally, patients should have two large-bore cannulas placed proximal and preferably contra-lateral to any penetrating thoracic wounds with likely vascular injury. Intra-osseous access is an alternative option that is commonly available with reasonable success rates but requires pressure to drive higher flow rates. Some specialist services carry larger 'trauma lines', designed for central venous cannulation. These tend to be wide calibre and short in length to facilitate rapid infusion of volume and blood products. Intravenous access generally can be established in transit to hospital to limit scene times; however, given the difficulties related to worsening venous tone and movement en route, it might be sensible to have one rapid 'best attempt' to ensure working access prior to leaving the scene.

Permissive hypotension has been well described for the management of penetrating trauma in the absence of traumatic brain injury. The underlying principle of permissive hypotension is to keep the blood pressure high enough to just perfuse the brain, but low enough to avoid disruption of newly formed blood clots at the site of injury. Targets for fluid resuscitation vary, but common targets include presence of a radial pulse, ability to mentate normally, or a systolic BP >70 mmHg.

Penetrating trauma that has led to significant bleeding will require definitive imaging and management. In all cases, but particularly in non-compressible haemorrhage, short scene times are essential. Once suitable efforts have been made to control the bleeding, any additional time at the scene is wasted. Some of the measures above can be delivered during transit to hospital, such as second access, warming, analgesia and ongoing resuscitation. Patient comfort and reassurance should always be addressed. Nuanced use of analgesic medication is necessitated by its potential effects on blood pressure.

Patients with penetrating major trauma should ideally be taken to a centre that has all the necessary specialists and capabilities on a single site. As such, triage destination should be considered along with initial management of the patient. A good local knowledge of service provision is essential to this end. If transfer distances are long, a risk–benefit decision is required when considering bypassing local hospitals. These are often difficult decisions to make with myriad factors to consider; seeking advice from senior personnel within the region may be of use for difficult cases.

SECTION 7 Trauma

Question 4: What Is the Role of Tranexamic Acid in the Bleeding Trauma Patient?

Tranexamic acid (TXA) is an anti-fibrinolytic drug with immunomodulatory effects that attenuates the hyperfibrinolysis observed in ATC. It may help preserve earlier clot formation in major trauma. Tranexamic acid has been used for many years in the operating room to reduce bleeding, particularly in obstetrics and cardiac surgery. CRASH-2 – a very large international multicentre study in 2010 – showed a survival benefit in major trauma, particularly if TXA was administered within three hours of injury.[7] This trial was carried out in a mixture of high- and low-income countries with varying EMS capabilities. More recently, a trial of prehospital TXA (PATCH) was carried out in Australia, New Zealand and Germany.[8] This trial showed the same survival benefit as CRASH-2, but this was only a secondary outcome. The primary outcome of the trial was functional outcome at six months, and it found no difference.

A meta-analysis including the PATCH trial results confirms that there is a significant improvement in mortality when TXA is administered, particularly in the prehospital environment.[9]

TXA is administered as a bolus of 1 g (administered over ten minutes) followed by an infusion administered over one hour. The PATCH trial suggests that there are minimal adverse effects of prehospital TXA administration. In particular, there is no increased incidence of thromboembolic disease, such as pulmonary embolism. (See Question 6 in Chapter 27: Shocked blunt trauma, for more on TXA.)

Key Evidence

Brohi K, Cohen MJ, Ganter MT et al. Acute coagulopathy of trauma: hypoperfusion induces systemic anticoagulation and hyperfibrinolysis. *Journal of Trauma*. 2008;64(5):1211–1217. Available at: https://pubmed.ncbi.nlm.nih.gov/18469643/

CRASH-2 Trial Collaborators. Effects of tranexamic acid on death, vascular occlusive events, and blood transfusion in trauma patients with significant haemorrhage (CRASH-2): a randomised, placebo-controlled trial. *Lancet*. 2010 Jul 3;376(9734):23–32. Available at: https://pubmed.ncbi.nlm.nih.gov/20554319/

Howells M, Jones B. Acute traumatic coagulopathy: the lethal triad of trauma. *Journal of Paramedic Practice*. 2018;10:12:510–516. Available at: https://www.magonlinelibrary.com/doi/abs/10.12968/jpar.2018.10.12.510?journalCode=jpar

Little RA, Kirkman E, Driscoll P et al. Preventable deaths after injury: why are the traditional 'vital' signs poor indicators of blood loss? *Journal of Accident and Emergency Medicine*. 1995 Mar;12(1):1–14. Available at: https://pubmed.ncbi.nlm.nih.gov/7640820/

Velez DR. The history of hemorrhagic shock and damage control resuscitation. *American Surgeon*. 2022 Nov;88(11):2656–2659. Available at: https://pubmed.ncbi.nlm.nih.gov/33856934/

Self-Reflection Questions

1. What clinical features would support a diagnosis of obstructive shock?
2. What reasons might explain why patients with penetrating injuries compensate well?
3. How can you prevent acute traumatic coagulopathy in the prehospital setting?
4. In your service, is tranexamic acid used and what are the pros and cons of its use?
5. What is your understanding of the permissive hypotensive resuscitation approach, and do you think this will change with increasing use of prehospital blood products?

References

1. Townend ML, Byers S. Visual estimation of blood loss by UK pre-hospital clinicians: an observational study. *British Paramedic Journal*. 2018 Jun 1;3(1):16–22. Available at: https://pubmed.ncbi.nlm.nih.gov/33328801/
2. Mutschler M, Hoffmann M, Wölfl C et al. Is the ATLS classification of hypovolaemic shock appreciated in daily trauma care? An online-survey among 383 ATLS course directors and instructors. *Emergency Medicine Journal*. 2015;32:134–137. Available at: https://pubmed.ncbi.nlm.nih.gov/24071947/
3. Howells M, Jones B. Acute traumatic coagulopathy: the lethal triad of trauma. *Journal of Paramedic Practice*. 2018;10:12:510–516. Available at: https://www.magonlinelibrary.com/doi/abs/10.12968/jpar.2018.10.12.510?journalCode=jpar
4. Brohi K, Cohen MJ, Ganter MT et al. Acute coagulopathy of trauma: hypoperfusion induces systemic anticoagulation and hyperfibrinolysis. *Journal of Trauma*. 2008;64(5):1211–1217. Available at: https://pubmed.ncbi.nlm.nih.gov/18469643/
5. Crombie N, Doughty HA, Bishop JRB et al. Resuscitation with blood products in patients with trauma-related haemorrhagic shock receiving prehospital care (RePHILL): a multicentre, open-label, randomised, controlled, phase 3 trial. *Lancet. Haematology* 2022;9(4):e250–e261. Available at: https://doi.org/10.1016/S2352-3026(22)00040-0.
6. Jansen JO, Hudson J, Cochran C, et al. Emergency department resuscitative endovascular balloon occlusion of the aorta in trauma patients with exsanguinating hemorrhage: the UK-REBOA randomized clinical trial. *JAMA*. 2023;330(19):1862–1871. doi:10.1001/jama.2023.20850
7. CRASH-2 Trial Collaborators. Effects of tranexamic acid on death, vascular occlusive events, and blood transfusion in trauma patients with significant haemorrhage (CRASH-2): a randomised, placebo-controlled trial. *Lancet*. 2010 Jul 3;376(9734):23–32. Available at: https://pubmed.ncbi.nlm.nih.gov/20554319/
8. PATCH-Trauma Investigators and the ANZICS Clinical Trials Group et al. Prehospital tranexamic acid for severe trauma. *New England Journal of Medicine*. 2023 Jul 13;389(2):127–136. Available at: https://pubmed.ncbi.nlm.nih.gov/37314244/
9. Fouche PF, Stein C, Nichols M et al. Doi SA. Tranexamic acid for traumatic injury in the emergency setting: a systematic review and bias-adjusted meta-analysis of randomized controlled trials. *Annals of Emergency Medicine*. 2024 May;83(5):435–445. doi: 10.1016/j.annemergmed.2023.10.004.

29

Severe Chest Injury: Tension Pneumothorax

Mark Fitzgerald and Toby St Clair

> **In this chapter you will learn:**
> - The potential anatomical site for needle thoracocentesis
> - The role of blunt thoracostomy in prehospital practice
> - The value of lung ultrasound in identifying a pneumothorax
> - The 'mid-ARM approach' as a reliable/recommended tool for landmarking the thoracostomy site
> - An overview of the procedural steps in a safe prehospital thoracostomy.

Case Details

Dispatch

35-year-old male, blunt chest injury, conscious with severe respiratory distress and traumatic chest pain.

History

A 35-year-old male was working at a horse-racing stable. He was kicked by a horse in the right anterior chest wall. It was an isolated mechanism with immediate and progressively worsening difficulty breathing. Staff witnessed the incident and moved the patient to safety and then called for an ambulance. He remains conscious and in severe pain. A double-crewed ambulance, an in-field manager and a critical care paramedic are dispatched.

On Arrival of the First Crew

The patient has been relocated to outside the horse stable and is seated on the ground, leaning against the stable wall. The scene is safe. His primary survey findings and initial vital signs are:

Airway	Patent
Breathing	RR 32, shallow, SpO_2 83% on air
Circulation	Peripheral pulses present, HR 121, BP 119/81, cool peripheries
Disability	GCS E3, V5, M6 (14), BGL 7.1 mmol/L
Environmental	Temp 36.5 °C

CHAPTER 29   Severe Chest Injury: Tension Pneumothorax

The first paramedics initiate oxygen therapy via a non-rebreather mask at 15 L/min, establish IV access and provide intravenous analgesia with aliquots of fentanyl. Their secondary survey rules out any palpable subcutaneous emphysema and confirms unequal breath sounds on auscultation and painful crepitus to right anterior/lateral wall, with noticeable shallow respirations.

On Your Arrival as the Critical Care Paramedic

The patient presents with increased WOB and pain on inspiration rated as severe, despite 300 mcg IV fentanyl. His SpO_2 has improved to 89% on high-flow oxygen, his heart rate remains tachycardic at 112, and currently his blood pressure is 103/74. An anterior lung ultrasound clearly identifies lung slide on the left-hand side of the chest wall, but there are no lung slide signs on the right, which is indicative of pneumothorax. With further analgesia the patient's tidal volumes have increased, revealing a large antero-lateral flail segment involving four ribs over 8 cm with paradoxical chest wall movement.

AMPLE

The patient has no past medical history of note; however, he has suffered previous long-bone fractures secondary to work-related falls and injuries. He has undergone surgical repair in the past with no reported anaesthetic complications.

Allergies	NKDA
Medications	Nil
History	Fractured femur and humerus (separate incidents)
Last ins and outs	Nil orally since breakfast five hours prior, normal voiding
Events prior	Kicked in the chest by a horse

Decision Point 1

You have evidence of likely pneumothorax both clinically with vital signs deterioration and diagnostically with the assistance of a lung ultrasound. Furthermore, there is now ongoing hypoxia despite adequate analgesia and high-flow oxygen. Decompression of a tension pneumothorax may be warranted if vital signs continue to deteriorate.

Decision Point 2

Despite anterior needle pleural decompression, adequate analgesia and ongoing oxygen therapy via non-rebreather mask at 15 L/min, the patient's hypoxia persists. Intubation for mechanical ventilation and support of the ongoing respiratory failure is performed. Post intubation, the patient's vital signs worsen, with a reduction in blood pressure to 78/43 and a heart rate of 131 beats per minute. Lung ultrasound confirms isolated pneumothorax on the right-hand side. The pneumocath in situ is flushed with normal saline; however, the deranged parameters remain. Should the anterior needle decompression be escalated to a lateral blunt (finger) thoracostomy?

SECTION 7 Trauma

Question 1: Is There a Role for Prehospital Point-of-Care Ultrasound (POCUS) for Pneumothorax Diagnosis?

Expert opinion recognises the clinical value of prehospital point-of-care ultrasound (POCUS) in a variety of assessments. The evidence is rapidly evolving on several key aspects of the validity of the widespread introduction of POCUS use by paramedics to help guide clinical decision making.[1,2]

Further research into the capacity for quality assessment and interpretation in the hands of novice users, in addition to the impact the technology may have on clinical interventions, decision making and ultimately patient outcomes, is needed.

Quality of initial training, along with the frequency of subsequent refresher training, is yet to be validated, and the challenges of prehospital real-time supervised practice limit the progression from novice to competent practitioner. The advent of remote decision support with live transmission of prehospital ultrasonography to the receiving trauma facility to guide both interpretation and clinical implications may be one novel method to progress this technology more broadly, with further focused research required.[3]

Lung ultrasound is known to produce higher sensitivity than anteroposterior x-ray of the chest when diagnosing pneumothorax, and it is recognised that the use of prehospital ultrasound of the lungs for pneumothorax assessment also has a high diagnostic accuracy.[4–6] The probability that a patient with a positive (abnormal – absence of lung-slide sign) lung ultrasound in fact has a pneumothorax has a positive predictive value as high as 90%. This means that, as a diagnostic tool in the field, when endeavouring to differentiate a pneumothorax, this assessment provides a confirmation with reasonable confidence; however, this must be applied within the clinical context.

Several studies looking at the capability of prehospital providers with varied levels of clinical experience to learn and retain knowledge in lung ultrasound for identification of lung slide have shown high levels of accuracy.

Recognising that the literature demonstrates a high failure rate of anterior chest needle decompression and associated iatrogenic complications, improved patient selection and diagnostics are imperative.[7] Appropriately implemented prehospital lung ultrasound may not only reduce the number of unnecessary anterior needle placements but may guide decisions around successful pleural decompression of a pneumothorax and inform repeat efforts to decompress the pleura. A need for further targeted research of the value in this setting remains.

Question 2: What Are the Landmarks for Needle Decompression of Pneumothorax?

A multitude of studies have demonstrated a range of limitations and unreliability of catheter over needle thoracocentesis (NT) in the setting of suspected pneumothorax.[8,9] Limitations include extrapleural placement, lung biopsies, inaccurate surface anatomical landmark identification and insufficient catheter length, along with a number of significant iatrogenic injuries. As a result, failure to successfully and safely decompress the pleural is widely reported in the literature (**Figure 29.1**).

CHAPTER 29 Severe Chest Injury: Tension Pneumothorax

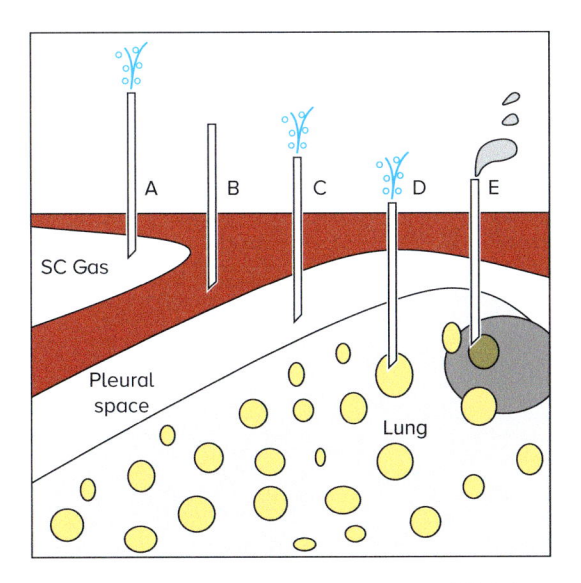

Figure 29.1 Possible positions of needle thoracocentesis: (A) false positive – as needle decompresses subcutaneous emphysema; (B) false negative – as needle does not reach pleural space; (C) correct position of NT with decompression of tension pneumothorax; (D) false positive – with needle intrapulmonary in bulla or bronchial tree (if the tension pneumothorax is loculated due to pulmonary adhesions and missed by NT a false negative result may occur with intra-pulmonary placement); (E) true negative – with needle in a major vessel or the heart (this may be misinterpreted as a false positive for haemothorax). Only C will decompress a tension pneumothorax. A, B, D and E have all been associated with failure to decompress the pleural space and fatal outcomes.

In an effort to reduce the rate of failure and subsequent patient harm, several studies have investigated optimal landmarks for catheter-over-needle decompression, in conjunction with optimal minimal catheter length.[10]

Some international trauma recommendations switched in 2018 from recommending the second intercostal space in the mid-clavicular line (2-ICS-MCL) to either the fourth or fifth intercostal space in the mid-axillae line (4/5-ICS-MAL) or the fourth or fifth intercostal space in the anterior axillae line (4/5-ICS-AAL) (**Figure 29.2**). Several studies, including a meta-analysis, suggested that the chest wall thickness of the mid- and anterior axillae sites were likely to be thinner and therefore enhance the likelihood of successful penetration of the skin, subcutaneous tissues and muscular structures of the chest wall. However, a recent ultrasonography assessment of healthy volunteers did not replicate the findings suggesting no statistical difference in chest wall thickness. Further identifying that in obese subjects, the chest wall was thicker in 4/5-ICS-AAL than in 2-ICS-MCL, theorising that the successful needle decompression of a tension pneumothorax is significantly higher in 2-ICS-MCL compared to 4/5-ICS-AAL.

SECTION 7 Trauma

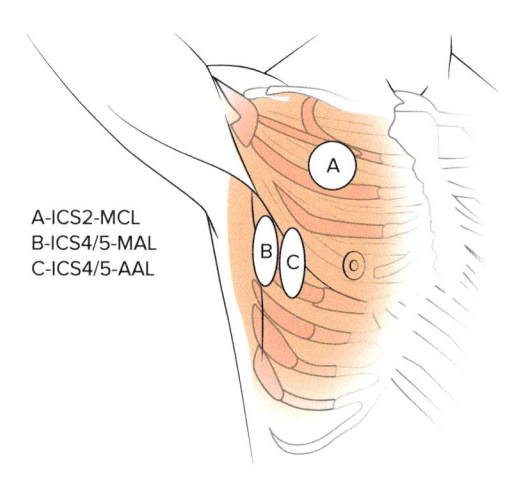

Figure 29.2 Anatomical locations for needle thoracostomy decompression: (A) currently recommended second intercostal space mid-clavicular line (2-ICS-MCL); (B) the fourth and fifth intercostal spaces mid-axillary line (4/5-ICS-MAL); (C) the fourth and fifth intercostal spaces anterior axillary line (4/5-ICS-AAL).

> **PRACTICE TIP**
>
> When performing catheter-over-needle thoracocentesis, know all the possible alternative sites and anatomical landmarks.

The evidence does not demonstrate one particular site as definitively more likely to successfully decompress the pleura with a statistically significant reduction in iatrogenic injury in all patient groups.[11,12] The critical care paramedic should understand the variety of potential sites and the limitations and consequences of catheter-over-needle decompression. The limitations relate not only to identifying a pneumothorax under tension with clinical assessment alone, but also to the challenges in recognising subtle clinical improvement following a catheter placement.

Equally as important as site selection is the technique for placing the pneumocath or catheter over the trocar device. The placement of the needle into the chest wall should be perpendicular to the chest wall (90 degrees) and angled towards the spine, immediately superior to the rib below, avoiding any contact with the neurovascular bundle situated in the inferior aspect of each rib.

When performing the thoracentesis at the 2-ICS-MCL, ensuring accurate anatomical landmarks are identified is key to procedural safety. Note that the clavicle extends from its articulation with the manubrium of the sternum trochanter to the sternoclavicular joint – there, the acromion wraps the end of the clavicle. This important distinction is highlighted, as all too frequently the MCL is poorly located, resulting in too medial an entry into the chest wall, which significantly increases the risk of damaging major vessels and organs within the thorax (**Figure 29.3**).

CHAPTER 29 Severe Chest Injury: Tension Pneumothorax

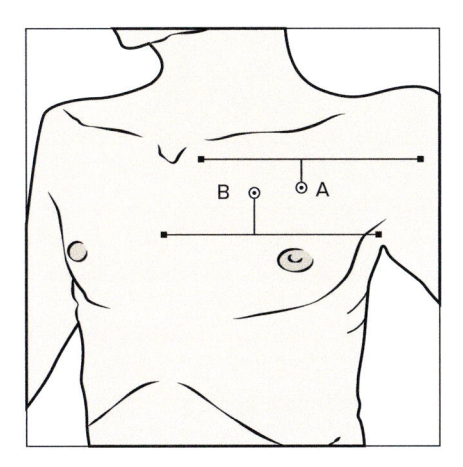

Figure 29.3 Identification of the mid-clavicular line. The recommended insertion point (A) in the second intercostal space in the mid-clavicular line is more lateral to the point commonly identified, which is half-way between the midline and the lateral chest wall (B).

Ensuring sufficient catheter length is paramount. A 2015 meta-analysis concluded that the needle decompression catheter should be at least 6.5 cm in length to ensure that 95% of patients would have penetration into the pleural space.[13] Alternatively an 8 cm catheter would be capable of entering the pleural space 100% of the time in an anterior approach. This is a critical decision point, as some cadaveric studies placing 5 cm angiocaths showed a failure to penetrate the pleural cavity in up to 50% of samples.

However, simply increasing the length of the catheter is not without risk. Some studies found that, when increasing the catheter length to 8 cm, the rate of injury to underlying structures increased from 9% to 32% with shallow angles at the 4/5-ICS-AAL, calling into question the safety of using longer catheters at alternative sites.

The prehospital critical care provider must consider a variety of factors when selecting the optimal approach, tailored for the individual patient's needs. Factors to consider include the accident mechanism and patient access, adequacy of patient assessment and competing multi-trauma causes for deterioration in vital signs. Once decompression of a potential tension pneumothorax is indicated, the optimal approach will be guided by patient habitus, physical access and the effectiveness of prior thoracentesis attempts with persistently deteriorating vital signs. The critical care paramedic should be familiar with each alternative anatomical site and recognise the limitations and risks associated with each.

Question 3: Is There Superiority for Prehospital Blunt (Finger) Thoracostomy over Needle Decompression in Tension Pneumothorax by Paramedics?

The efficacy of anterior needle decompression remains variable and must be considered in the context of the environment, patient clinical conditions, practitioner capability and competing urgent clinical interventions. Finger thoracostomy has recently been introduced in the prehospital setting as an alternative method of pleural decompression.

SECTION 7 Trauma

The technique for finger thoracostomy performed by paramedics has been described in the literature as follows. Under sterile conditions, a 20–30 mm scalpel incision is made over the 4/5-ICS-MAL on the affected side of the chest.[14] Next, a blunt dissection into the pleural space is performed using forceps, and subsequent dilation with a sterile, gloved finger utilising a sweeping motion to free adhesions, enabling expulsion of intra-pleural gas and allowing reinflation of the affected lung.

The literature has associated an increased likelihood of definitive pleural decompression, which is essential for clinical improvement among pneumothorax patients with tension physiology.

While no definitive evidence supports finger thoracostomy over needle thoracentesis in the prehospital environment, expert opinion supports a preference for blunt lateral finger thoracostomy for positive-pressure ventilation in the prehospital setting; however, this stops short of extending the recommendation to the spontaneously breathing patient. With the procedure and prehospital research into its outcomes still in their infancy, there exists no sufficiently powered study establishing superiority of either technique.

The diagnosis of tension pneumothorax in the prehospital environment remains difficult, and as such there is a need to provide decision support tools to moderate the balance between omission of treating a life-threatening injury and performing an unnecessary high-risk procedure.

PRACTICE TIP

When performing a blunt finger thoracostomy, use the 'mid-arm approach' to safely and reliably identify the correct anatomical location for the thoracostomy incision.

Some data suggests that up to 25% of major trauma patients eventually require tube thoracostomy.[15] Prehospital data is far more challenging to accurately research, given the difficulty in diagnosing tension pneumothorax in the field, and despite subsequent in-hospital imaging, it is not possible to ascertain the pre-existence of the imaged pneumothorax prior to placement of either thoracentesis or thoracostomy.

Regardless of which technique is employed, the effectiveness is not simply defined by the selection of a particular procedure but is more about the precision and technical proficiency of the provider. The concept that thoracentesis, blindly placed to the hilt of the needle, will not biopsy the pneumothorax or lung tissue is unrealistic, and as such the iatrogenic injury incidence can be mitigated by very precise procedural proficiency.

A recent systematic review of prehospital paramedic pleural decompression concluded that despite finger thoracostomy having a lower rate of procedural complications, improved pleural cavity access and improved vital signs post procedure, there is lack of high-quality evidence to confer procedural superiority.[7]

Practically speaking, the blunt finger thoracostomy is not a technically challenging procure, and it affords the practitioner immediate tactile confirmation of plural penetration and subsequent decompression and lung inflation. Furthermore, the capacity to rapidly identify or rule out a pneumothorax when managing a shocked poly-trauma patient is advantageous when considering alternative interventions to address deteriorating vital signs.

The aforementioned systematic review further stated that, while there is no definitive evidence to support one pleural decompression method over another in the prehospital setting, the findings suggest finger thoracostomy can be both safe and effective and may confer advantage over needle decompression in some prehospital situations.

The critical care paramedic must consider the advantages and disadvantages of both techniques and should be competent in each, tailoring care to each individual patient's needs. Considerations such as suitable access to the patient, concurrent procedures, capability to maintain a sterile field and proximity to a receiving trauma centre should all influence the paramedic's approach. Where suitably qualified, the critical care paramedic should consider that an anterior needle thoracentesis is a temporising method for urgent pleural decompression of pressure differential, and therefore in the setting of a patient receiving positive-pressure ventilation escalation to blunt thoracostomy, it should be considered at the earliest opportunity.

PRACTICE TIP

> When performing a blunt finger thoracostomy, finger lacerations from fractured rib edges are a procedural safety risk. Wear a double layer of sterile gloves and employ a delicate, deliberate approach.

Question 4: Is There an Optimal Procedural Technique for Safe Prehospital Finger Thoracostomy?

Several small studies looking at both effectiveness and safety have demonstrated prehospital finger thoracostomy to be a reliable and retainable skill by prehospital providers, with the rate of complications reported comparable to that within the in-hospital environment.

Several factors ensure this efficacy and safety, including the reliable identification of the 'safe zone'. This safe zone aims to identify the fourth, fifth and sixth intercostal spaces in an inverse triangle demarcated by the lateral border of the pectoralis major, anterior border of latissimus dorsi and the base of the axilla. Additionally, adherence to establishing and maintaining a sterile field and ensuring that the procedure impacts minimally on prehospital scene times are the keys to the broader safety of the procedure.

The utilisation of the 'mid-arm point' (MAP) to identify the safe zone is a technique that increases the reliability of landmark identification.[16] The MAP approach uses the relationship with the arm's skeletal anatomy and the thoracic anatomy to act as a marker for identifying the safe zone. The mid-point of the humerus is identified, transposed to the correlating point on the chest wall and then with abduction of the arm, the site is reliably consistent in locating either the fourth, fifth or sixth ICS. Note that the 5ICS in the AAL is often reported as the optimal location for the thoracostomy in the literature. This technique works for both adults and paediatrics, with only slight modification for the paediatric population, requiring the practitioner to then move 'up' one intercostal space.[17]

Infection control remains a priority when undertaking the procedure in the prehospital environment. The use of a sterile solution such as chlorhexidine or iodine solution along with a sterile fenestrated drape with adhesive is essential. The use of sterile gloves and the maintenance of the sterile field for not only the initial procedure but any subsequent 're-sweeps' of the ostomy are required to reduce the patient's risk of infection. Finger thoracostomy does pose an increased risk to the paramedic, particularly in the form of finger lacerations from fractured rib edges; as such, it is paramount to use a double gloving technique and employ a delicate, deliberate and safe approach.

A number of small studies have reported that, when employing such techniques, there are similar rates of post-procedure infection to those within the emergency trauma centre. The use of routine prophylactic antibiotics for thoracostomy performed prehospitally remains an area for further investigation. In situations where the thoracostomy site cannot adequately be cleansed and prepared to a sterile standard, the procedure must be avoided at all costs.

In-hospital intercostal catheter (ICC)-related complications have been reported to be as high as 37%, predominantly associated with incorrect insertion sites and poor tube positioning. The additional scene time, in conjunction with the potential for false passage and iatrogenic injury, support the notion of deferring ICC until arrival in the trauma centre. As such 're-sweeping' of the ostomy as required, based on clinical and ventilation parameters, may be required in transit.

Key Evidence

Bing F, Fitzgerald M, Olaussen A et al. Identifying a safe site for intercostal catheter insertion using the mid-arm point (MAP). *Journal of Emergency Medicine, Trauma and Acute Care*. 2017;2017:3.

Meadley B, Olaussen A, Delorenzo A et al. Educational standards for training paramedics in ultrasound: a scoping review. *BMC Emergency Medicine*. 2017;17(1):18.

Sharrock MK, Shannon B, Garcia Gonzalez C et al. Prehospital paramedic pleural decompression: a systematic review. *Injury*. 2021;52(10):2778–2786.

Self-Reflection Questions

1. Do you know all the anatomical landmarks to help identify thoracentesis and thoracostomy sites?
2. Do you think the evidence supports the use of prehospital lung ultrasound when diagnosing potential pneumothorax?
3. Which patients are likely to benefit from a prehospital blunt finger thoracotomy?
4. What are the risks associated with needle thoracentesis in the field?
5. What measures must be taken to ensure a prehospital blunt finger thoracotomy is safe for both the practitioner and the patient?

References

1. Amaral CB, Ralston DC, Becker TK. Prehospital point-of-care ultrasound: a transformative technology. *SAGE Open Medicine*. 2020;8:2050312120932706.
2. Bøtker MT, Jacobsen L, Rudolph SS et al. The role of point of care ultrasound in prehospital critical care: a systematic review. *Scandinavian Journal of Trauma, Resuscitation and Emergency Medicine*. 2018; 26(1):51.
3. Meadley B, Olaussen A, Delorenzo A et al. Educational standards for training paramedics in ultrasound: a scoping review. *BMC Emergency Medicine*. 2017;17(1):18.
4. Bhat SR, Johnson DA, Pierog JE et al. Prehospital evaluation of effusion, pneumothorax, and standstill (PEEPS): point-of-care ultrasound in emergency medical services. *Western Journal of Emergency Medicine*. 2015;16(4):503–509.

CHAPTER 29 Severe Chest Injury: Tension Pneumothorax

5. Khalil PA, Merelman A, Riccio J et al. Randomized controlled trial of point-of-care ultrasound education for the recognition of tension pneumothorax by paramedics in prehospital simulation. *Prehospital and Disaster Medicine*. 2021;36(1):74–78.
6. Husain LF, Hagopian L, Wayman D et al. Sonographic diagnosis of pneumothorax. *Journal of Emergencies, Trauma and Shock*. 2012;5(1):76–81.
7. Sharrock MK, Shannon B, Garcia Gonzalez C et al. Prehospital paramedic pleural decompression: a systematic review. *Injury*. 2021;52(10):2778–2786.
8. Aylwin CJ, Brohi K, Davies GD et al. Pre-hospital and in-hospital thoracostomy: indications and complications. *Annals of the Royal College of Surgeons*. 2008;90(1):54–57.
9. Fitzgerald M, Mackenzie CF, Marasco S et al. Pleural decompression and drainage during trauma reception and resuscitation. *Injury*. 2008;39(1):9–20.
10. Laan DV, Vu TDN, Thiels CA et al. Chest wall thickness and decompression failure: a systematic review and meta-analysis comparing anatomic locations in needle thoracostomy. *Injury*. 2016;47(4):797–804.
11. Azizi N, ter Avest E, Hoek AE et al. Optimal anatomical location for needle chest decompression for tension pneumothorax: a multicenter prospective cohort study. *Injury*. 2021;52(2):213–218.
12. Henry R, Ghafil C, Golden A et al. Prehospital needle decompression improves clinical outcomes in helicopter evacuation patients with multisystem trauma: a multicenter study. *Journal of Special Operations Medicine*. 2021;21:49–54.
13. Clemency BM, Tanski CT, Rosenberg M et al. Sufficient catheter length for pneumothorax needle decompression: a meta-analysis. *Prehospital and Disaster Medicine*. 2015;30(3):249–253.
14. Hannon L, St Clair T, Smith K et al. Finger thoracostomy in patients with chest trauma performed by paramedics on a helicopter emergency medical service. *Emergency Medicine Australasia*. 2020;32(4):650–656.
15. Mohrsen S, McMahon N, Corfield A et al. Complications associated with pre-hospital open thoracostomies: a rapid review. *Scandinavian Journal of Trauma, Resuscitation and Emergency Medicine*. 2021;29(1):166.
16. Bing F, Fitzgerald M, Olaussen A et al. Identifying a safe site for intercostal catheter insertion using the mid-arm point (MAP). *Journal of Emergency Medicine, Trauma and Acute Care*. 2017;2017:3.
17. Quinn N, Ward G, Ong C et al. Mid-arm point in paediatrics (MAPPAED): an effective procedural aid for safe pleural decompression in trauma. *Emergency Medicine Australasia*. 2023;35(3):412–419.

SECTION 8

Toxicology

Tricyclic Antidepressant Toxicity

30

Ben Fitzgerald and Michael Mann

In this chapter you will learn:

- The framework for developing a differential diagnosis in a patient presenting with a toxic ingestion
- The clinical presentation of a tricyclic antidepressant (TCA) overdose
- Typical ECG findings in TCA overdose
- Treatment options for tricyclic antidepressant toxicity.

Case Details

Dispatch
18-year-old female, suicidal ideation, possible OD, second-hand call.

History
An 18-year-old female had an argument with family members and stated that she didn't want to live any more. The patient locked herself in her room and called a friend, stating that she had taken a lot of pills, then hung up the phone. The friend tried to return the call but there was no answer, so she called emergency services.

On Arrival of the First Crew
The initial crew is met at the front door of the house by the mother of the patient. The mother had an argument with the daughter approximately two hours ago, after which the patient went to her bedroom and locked the door. According to the mother, arguments are fairly common, and on occasion the patient will make threats of self-harm, although she has never followed through. After determining that it was safe to enter the bedroom, the crew made access and found the patient supine on the bed. Her primary survey findings and initial vital signs are:

Airway	Patent
Breathing	RR 26, SpO$_2$ 97% on room air
Circulation	Peripheral pulses present, HR 120, BP 102/66, cool peripheries
Disability	GCS E3, V4, M6 (13), BGL 5.4 mmol/L
Environmental	Temp 37.1 °C

SECTION 8 Toxicology

The first attending crew made the determination that the patient was critically ill and requested a critical care paramedic response.

On Your Arrival as the Critical Care Paramedic

The updated report on your arrival is that the patient appears to have a declining mental status. She is not quite as responsive to verbal commands, and her speech has become a little more garbled. Her vital signs remain consistent from the initial findings.

AMPLE

The patient has a past medical history of depression and ADHD. She is a college student locally.

Allergies	NKDA
Medications	Amitriptyline, Adderall, Nexplanon
Past history	Depression, ADHD, eating disorder
Last ins and outs	Unknown
Events	Overdose

Decision Point

A witnessed decrease in mentation in the face of a potential tricyclic overdose is concerning. The concurrent priorities in this case are to closely monitor changes in vital signs and mental status, begin to build a differential diagnosis list, and rapidly identify and mitigate potentially life-threatening conditions. It is critical to aggressively identify potential root causes, such as medication, alcohol, drug use and/or potential sources of trauma. The physical examination should prioritise a physical survey for trauma, a neurological examination, and a 12-lead ECG.

Question 1: What Early Assessments Should Be Undertaken in a Patient with Altered Mental Status? How Should You Approach Assessment of a Toxicity Patient and Build a Differential?

The initial priorities for any incident in the field are scene control and a determination of whether there are sufficient resources to manage the incident. Scene control includes the security/stability of the scene, identification of the incident perimeter and ingress/egress routes, and body substance isolation. Responses to self-harm have the potential to be unstable and care should be taken to prioritise scene control. Additionally, patients who are medically complex or difficult to manage may require additional resources with regard to staffing and/or expertise. Early requests for additional resources are particularly important in volatile situations or in remote areas with extended response times.

Tricyclic antidepressant (TCA) overdoses commonly present with altered mental status (AMS). In the case of a patient with AMS that is a suspected overdose, scenes may occasionally

CHAPTER 30 Tricyclic Antidepressant Toxicity

be confusing, unstable and/or chaotic. To help organise the scene, it is useful to identify the scope of the problem by answering the 5Ws and 1H.

Who?	Who is overdosed? Depending on the circumstances, it may be a challenge to identify the patient or if there are actually multiple patients.
What?	What substance(s) was taken?
When?	How long ago was the substance(s) taken?
Where?	Where are the substance(s)? In the case of medications, how many are missing?
Why?	Was the overdose intentional or accidental?
How?	How was the substance taken (for example, IV, IM, ingestion, IN)?

Patient Assessment Priorities

First, when evaluating any patient, it is critical for the paramedic to move forward through the assessment and treatment phases while, at the same time, avoiding early diagnostic closure. Investing in early assumptions on aetiology can heavily bias the examination and it is best practice, while moving forward with treatment modalities, to continue to consider alternative aetiologies throughout the management course of the patient.

Once assured that there are no immediately life-threatening conditions, move on to gathering historical information and performing the physical examination. The top three tools of clinical evaluation to determine the aetiology of AMS are a history of a similar event in the past, past medical history and the physical examination.

EMS providers frequently have an opportunity to obtain direct, pertinent information from the family, bystanders and the incident scene. There are many potential causes of AMS (**Figure 30.1**); therefore, the information provided by this initial historical and environmental survey can be very useful in rapidly identifying underlying causes. If the underlying cause is not clear, a thorough physical examination should help. If the aetiology remains elusive, the acronym AEIOU-TIPS can be a useful tool to develop a differential diagnosis.

The differential diagnosis for AMS can be large. **Figure 30.1** identifies AMS aetiologies identified in the emergency room and not in the field. It is reasonable to assume that the majority of AMS patients seen in the field will end up in the emergency room and that these ratios could reasonably be projected to the field experience. Point-of-care testing can provide a useful tool for the focused examination in assessing aetiology.

Recommendations[1]

- Mitigate any immediately life-threatening conditions.
- Determine any history of similar events in the past.
- Identify past medical history.
- Perform a thorough physical examination.
- Examine the scene for evidence of potential causes for AMS.
- Consider the use of the acronym AEIOU-TIPS if the AMS cause is not obvious.
- Point-of-care testing should include:

SECTION 8 Toxicology

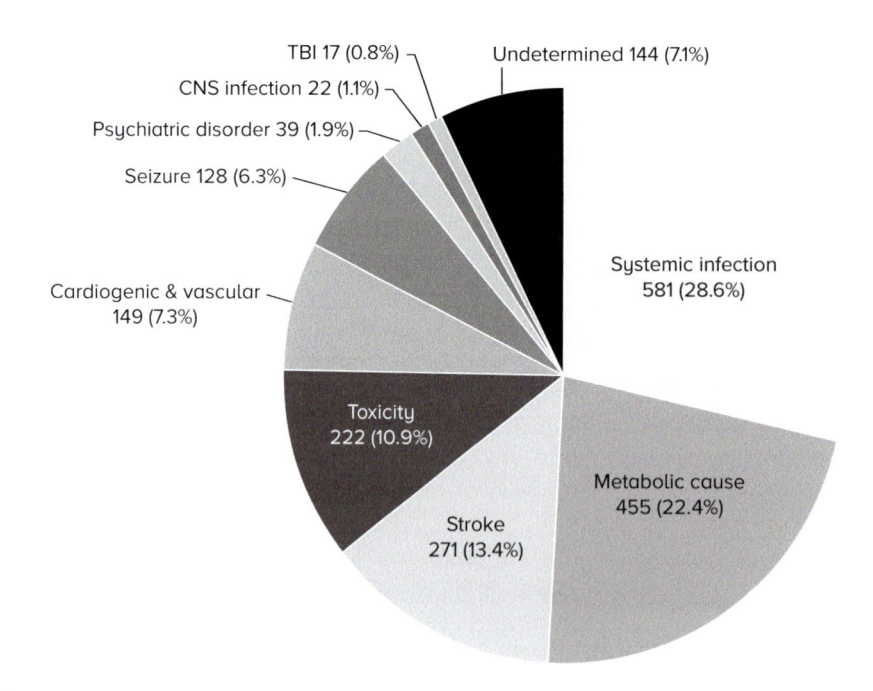

Figure 30.1 Aetiologies of altered level of consciousness in the emergency department.
Source: Kim KT, Jeon JC, Jung CG et al. Etiologies of altered level of consciousness in the emergency room. *Science Reports*. 2022;12:4972. Available at: https://doi.org/10.1038/s41598-022-09110-2. (Creative Commons Attribution 4.0 International License.)

- ECG monitor
- Pulse oximetry
- Blood glucose
- If age >65, consider evaluating for cardiac causes
- 12-lead ECG (if possible ingestion, OD, intoxication or abnormal ECG finding).

Question 2: What Are the Possible Clinical Effects/Toxidromes in Tricyclic Antidepressant Overdose?

Tricyclic antidepressants have been used to treat depression since the mid-twentieth century. Because of newer medications with broader safety profiles, tricyclic antidepressants have largely fallen out of the common practice for treatment of depression but are still used for the treatment of other conditions such as chronic pain, obsessive-compulsive disorder and sleep disorders. Common names of TCAs include amitriptyline, clomipramine, dothiepin, doxepin, imipramine, nortriptyline and trimipramine.

They are rapidly absorbed in the gastrointestinal tract, though absorption may be slowed due to diminished GI motility in cases of massive overdose. Toxic doses are recognised as ingestions of greater than 10 mg/kg in adults, but toxicity may be seen in overdoses as low as 5 mg/kg in children. They are thus recognised as a 'one-pill-can-kill' medication due to

CHAPTER 30 Tricyclic Antidepressant Toxicity

toxicity in paediatric patients. Toxicity can occur in both an acute overdose, as well as via chronic ingestion, and these present similarly.

TCA toxicity typically presents as a combination of cardiac and neurological findings, clinically manifesting as arrhythmias, hypotension, altered mental status and seizures. However, TCAs act on many receptors, and can thus present with a range of clinical characteristics.[2]

At therapeutic levels, TCAs inhibit reuptake of noradrenaline and serotonin, leading to their antidepressant effects, and we may thus see sympathomimetic/serotonergic signs and symptoms in overdose, such as tachycardia, hypertension, agitation, delirium and muscle rigidity. They inhibit muscarinic acetylcholine receptors, which can manifest as an anticholinergic toxidrome including tachycardia, fever, dry mucous membranes and altered mental status. Inhibition of histamine receptors and GABA chloride channels can also cause altered mental status. Potassium channel blockade may predispose to arrhythmias.

Inhibition of the fast sodium channel is perhaps the most implicated for characteristic ECG findings and cardiovascular effects and is the basis for treatment with sodium bicarbonate. This is discussed in further detail below. Ventricular dysrhythmias may also be seen, such as wide-complex tachycardia, ventricular tachycardia or torsade de pointes. Hypotension occurs as a result of direct myocardial dysfunction from sodium channel inhibition as well as blockade of peripheral alpha-1 receptors causing vasodilation.

Altered mental status is the most common neurological finding in TCA toxicity. This can range from agitation, delirium or psychosis to lethargy and coma. It is important to recall that altered mental status is not a specific finding for TCA overdose, so index of suspicion for alternative diagnosis or co-ingestion must remain high.

Seizures may occur in up to a quarter of cases of severe toxicity. The mechanism for seizures in cases of toxicity is not well known, but may be due in part to effects from multiple channels above, particularly inhibition of both sodium channels and GABA chloride channels.

Table 30.1 Tricyclic antidepressant interactions with endogenous channels and their clinical effects

Interaction	Effect
Fast-gated sodium channel inhibition	Prolonged QRS/PR/QT intervals, ventricular arrhythmias, myocardial depression, hypotension, seizures
Alpha-1 receptor inhibition	Peripheral vasodilation, hypotension
GABA-A receptor inhibition	Somnolence, seizures
Noradrenaline and serotonin reuptake inhibition	Tachycardia, hypertension, agitation, delirium, muscle rigidity
Histamine channel inhibition	Somnolence, delirium
Muscarinic acetylcholine receptor inhibition	Tachycardia, hypertension
Potassium channel inhibition	Prolonged QRS, arrhythmias

SECTION 8 Toxicology

Question 3: What ECG Findings Can Aid in Diagnosis of Tricyclic Antidepressant Toxicity?

Beyond a good history and physical examination, the ECG is the mainstay of diagnostic testing in the prehospital setting, as findings are critical to predicting toxicity, recognising life-threatening arrhythmias and evaluating response to treatment.[3]

Sinus tachycardia is the most common finding in TCA toxicity and is present in essentially all clinically significant overdoses.[4]

A blockade of inactivated fast sodium channels results in several ECG changes. QRS prolongation is a highly sensitive predictor of toxicity. Sodium channels are responsible for the phase 0 depolarisation of an action potential. When these channels are inhibited, it slows the rate of depolarisation, thus resulting in a prolonged action potential. Potassium channel blockade also prolongs the QRS complex through delayed repolarisation. Thus, for a QRS duration of greater than 100 ms, the clinician should be highly suspicious of TCA toxicity.[5]

The terminal R-wave in aVR is also a specific indicator of sodium channel blockade. Look for a terminal R-wave in aVR of (1) greater than 3 mm height or (2) R/S ratio of greater than 0.7 (**Figure 30.2**).

Right-axis deviation and right bundle branch block morphology are common and are due to increased sensitivity of the right bundle of His to the sodium channel blockade. PR and QT prolongation can also be seen.

The expert clinician must put these ECG findings in the context of the clinical presentation of the patient. TCA overdose/sodium channel blockade should be considered when these findings are present.[6]

> **PRACTICE TIP**
>
> ECG is the main diagnostic modality to predict toxicity, and serial ECGs should be performed to evaluate for response to treatment.

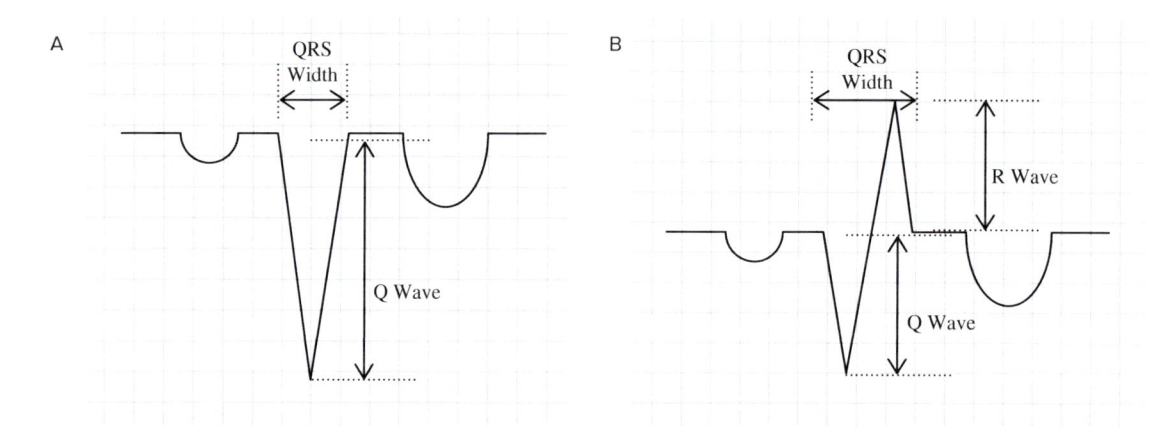

Figure 30.2   A: Normal aVR. B: aVR with R-wave >3 mm and Q/R ratio >0.7.

CHAPTER 30 Tricyclic Antidepressant Toxicity

Question 4: How Is Cardiovascular and Neurological Toxicity Recognised and Managed?

Cardiovascular Toxicity

In addition to the characteristic ECG findings above, sodium channel blockade also directly depresses myocardial function and alpha-1 blocking properties can cause peripheral vasodilation. This can clinically present as a mixture of cardiogenic and distributive shock. Thus, therapy should focus on reversing the effects of this inhibition.[7]

It is important to recognise the role of serum pH and TCA activity. TCAs are weakly basic, which means they exist in their ionised form more in an acidic environment. This ionised form is the active form of the molecule, so they will have greater affinity for the receptors that cause toxicological effects if the serum remains acidic.

Sodium bicarbonate is the mainstay of treatment of cardiac toxicity, and it works through two mechanisms.

1. Serum sodium load: This sodium load directly competes with the sodium channel blocking effects of the TCAs, thus reversing dysrhythmias and cardiac depression.[8]
2. Alkalinisation of serum: As discussed above, TCAs are weakly acidic. The bicarbonate causes the serum to become basic, thus causing more of the TCA molecules to become de-ionised (inactive).[9]

Prophylactic use of sodium bicarbonate is not supported by the literature. Thus, treatment is recommended if cardiovascular toxicity is present (QRS duration >100 ms, ventricular dysrhythmias or hypotension). Dosing is in the range of 1–2 mEq/kg as a bolus over several minutes. This dose can be repeated as needed every 3–5 minutes until the QRS narrows. If blood gas data is available, pH should be titrated to a level of 7.50–7.55. Serial ECG monitoring should be performed.

Once treated with sodium bicarbonate, this will lead to accumulation of CO_2 within the body, which will need to be exhaled. The patient should be hyperventilated if intubated.

For treatment of ventricular dysrhythmias refractory to sodium bicarbonate, lidocaine is the recommended antiarrhythmic, though robust human clinical studies supporting its efficacy are lacking. This may be counterintuitive as lidocaine also inhibits sodium channels; however, the Class 1B antiarrhythmic kinetics are favourable for treating toxicity. Class 1A (quinidine, procainamide and disopyramide) and Class 1C (flecainide, propafenone) antiarrhythmics are contraindicated, as are beta blockers and amiodarone.

> **PRACTICE TIP**
>
> Sodium bicarbonate is the mainstay of initial treatment of toxicity.

If the patient is hypotensive, a fluid bolus should be initiated to ensure adequate volume as the patient may be vasodilated. However, most crystalloid solutions are mildly acidic, which may increase TCA activity if given in large volumes. If the patient remains hypotensive refractory to fluid bolus, pressors should be initiated. Noradrenaline should be used as a first line given both alpha and beta adrenergic agonism. Adrenaline may also be considered, but will have less alpha activity. Phenylephrine is a pure alpha agonist.

SECTION 8   Toxicology

> **PRACTICE TIP**
>
> NaHCO$_3$ has limited alkalising effects if the lungs do not adjust to the increase in CO$_2$. Sufficient ventilation is critical to the effective reduction in TCA induced acidosis.

Neurological Toxicity

As discussed above, altered mental status can present as agitation, delirium, psychosis, lethargy or coma. Treatment of altered mental status involves supportive care. Early airway securement with intubation should be used in cases of declining mental status and concern for airway compromise.

Seizures occur in cases of severe toxicity. The mechanism of the development of seizures is not well understood, but they are probably due in part to inhibition of both sodium channels and GABA chloride channels.

Benzodiazepines (such as lorazepam and diazepam) are used as a first-line therapy to treat these seizures. There is a theoretical benefit that treatment with sodium bicarbonate may be therapeutic for seizures, as seizures may be due in part to CNS sodium channel blockade. Cardiovascular findings of QRS duration >100 ms, terminal R-wave in aVR, dysrhythmias and hypotension are predictive of severe toxicity and are associated with seizures. Thus, treatment with sodium bicarbonate should be initiated in these cases.

Hypotension may occur immediately after a seizure, so the clinician must anticipate and recognise this. The mechanism is thought to be due to a metabolic acidosis that increases activity of TCAs on cardiac sodium channels.[10]

Other Treatment Considerations

If you evaluate a patient with a recent ingestion, consider activated charcoal to prevent absorption if presentation is within two hours and no contraindications exist.

Additional therapies may be considered in the hospital that are less common in the prehospital setting, such as whole bowel irrigation, intralipid emulsion or extracorporeal membrane oxygenation in refractory cases. TCAs cannot be dialysed, and gastric lavage has not been proven to be useful. Thus, rapid transport should be prioritised in cases of toxicity.

Figure 30.3 provides a summary of the management priorities and options available to critical care paramedics in the prehospital setting.

Key Evidence

Callaham M, Kassel D. Epidemiology of fatal tricyclic antidepressant ingestion: implications for management. *Annals of Emergency Medicine*. 1985 Jan;14(1):1–9. Available at: https://pubmed.ncbi.nlm.nih.gov/3964996/

Caravati EM, Bossart PJ. Demographic and electrocardiographic factors associated with severe tricyclic antidepressant toxicity. *Journal of Toxicology. Clinical Toxicology*. 1991;29(1):31–43. Available at: https://pubmed.ncbi.nlm.nih.gov/2005664/

Foulke GE. Identifying toxicity risk early after antidepressant overdose. *American Journal of Emergency Medicine*. 1995 Mar;13(2):123–126. https://pubmed.ncbi.nlm.nih.gov/7893291/

Hoffman JR, Votey SR, Bayer M et al. Effect of hypertonic sodium bicarbonate in the treatment of moderate-to-severe cyclic antidepressant overdose. *American Journal of Emergency Medicine*. 1993 Jul;11(4): 336–341. Available at: https://pubmed.ncbi.nlm.nih.gov/8216512/

CHAPTER 30 Tricyclic Antidepressant Toxicity

I. Management priorities
1. **Limit absorption**: Activated charcoal may be considered if available.
2. **Enhance elimination**: There are no useful tools in the field to enhance elimination of TCAs.
3. **Antidotes**: There are no true antidotes for TCAs.
4. **Decrease the amount of free drug**: Sodium bicarbonate decreases the ionised (active) form of the drug.

II. Supportive care
The dangers of TCAs and the concomitant supportive care are:
1. **Acidosis**: Treat with sodium bicarbonate and hyperventilation.
2. **Arrhythmias/myocardial depression**: For arrhythmias/myocardial depression refractory to sodium bicarbonate boluses and hyperventilation, lidocaine is the preferred antiarrhythmic. In severe cases, consider transportation to a facility that can implement ECMO.
3. **Hypotension**: Treat initially with crystalloid fluid bolus; however, do not delay initiating pressors for hypotension refractory to fluids.
4. **Hypoxia**: Consider early endotracheal intubation as hypoxia exacerbates systemic acidosis.
5. **Airway compromise due to coma**: Perform endotracheal intubation if needed.
6. **Seizure**: Treat with benzodiazepines.

Figure 30.3 Summary of toxicity management priorities and options.

Kanich W, Brady WJ, Huff JS et al. Altered mental status: evaluation and etiology in the ED. *American Journal of Emergency Medicine*. 2002 Nov;20(7):613–617. Available at: https://pubmed.ncbi.nlm.nih.gov/12442240/

Woolf AD, Erdman AR, Nelson LS et al. Tricyclic antidepressant poisoning: an evidence-based consensus guideline for out-of-hospital management. *Clinical Toxicology*. 2007;45(3):203–233. Available at: https://pubmed.ncbi.nlm.nih.gov/17453872/

Self-Reflection Questions

1. What are the top clinical tools that can aid in identifying the causes of AMS?
2. What are the main point-of-care tests used when assessing AMS?
3. What are the typical signs and symptoms of a TCA overdose?
4. Which point-of-care test is the most useful in determining the level of TCA toxicity and the potential for seizure?
5. Why is acidosis harmful in a patient with a TCA overdose and how do we prevent this?
6. When trying to manage acidosis in a TCA overdose, what must be considered in addition to the administration of sodium bicarbonate?

References

1. Sanello A, Gausche-Hill M, Mulkerin W et al. Altered mental status: current evidence-based recommendations for prehospital care. *Western Journal of Emergency Medicine*. 2018 May;19(3): 527–541. Available at: https://pubmed.ncbi.nlm.nih.gov/29760852/
2. Foulke GE. Identifying toxicity risk early after antidepressant overdose. *American Journal of Emergency Medicine*. 1995 Mar;13(2):123–126. Available at: https://pubmed.ncbi.nlm.nih.gov/7893291/
3. Fasoli RA, Glauser FL. Cardiac arrhythmias and ECG abnormalities in tricyclic antidepressant overdose. *Clinical Toxicology*. 1981 Feb;18(2):155–163. Available at: https://pubmed.ncbi.nlm.nih.gov/7226729/
4. Caravati EM, Bossart PJ. Demographic and electrocardiographic factors associated with severe tricyclic antidepressant toxicity. *Journal of Toxicology. Clinical Toxicology*. 1991;29(1):31–43. Available at: https://pubmed.ncbi.nlm.nih.gov/2005664/

5. Boehnert MT, Lovejoy FH Jr. Value of the QRS duration versus the serum drug level in predicting seizures and ventricular arrhythmias after an acute overdose of tricyclic antidepressants. *New England Journal of Medicine*. 1985 Aug 22;313(8):474–479. Available at: https://pubmed.ncbi.nlm.nih.gov/4022081/
6. Liebelt EL, Ulrich A, Francis PD et al. Serial electrocardiogram changes in acute tricyclic antidepressant overdoses. *Critical Care Medicine*. 1997 Oct;25(10):1721–1726. Available at: https://pubmed.ncbi.nlm.nih.gov/9377889/
7. Thanacoody HK, Thomas SH. Tricyclic antidepressant poisoning: cardiovascular toxicity. *Toxicology Review*. 2005;24(3):205–214. Available at: https://pubmed.ncbi.nlm.nih.gov/16390222/
8. Hoffman JR, Votey SR, Bayer M et al. Effect of hypertonic sodium bicarbonate in the treatment of moderate-to-severe cyclic antidepressant overdose. *American Journal of Emergency Medicine*. 1993 Jul;11(4):336–341. Available at: https://pubmed.ncbi.nlm.nih.gov/8216512/
9. Blackman K, Brown SG, Wilkes GJ. Plasma alkalinization for tricyclic antidepressant toxicity: a systematic review. *Emergency Medicine*. 2001 Jun;13(2):204–210. Available at: https://pubmed.ncbi.nlm.nih.gov/11482860/
10. Lipper B, Bell A, Gaynor B. Recurrent hypotension immediately after seizures in nortriptyline overdose. *American Journal of Emergency Medicine*. 1994 Jul;12(4):452–453. Available at: https://pubmed.ncbi.nlm.nih.gov/8031432/

Acute Behavioural Disturbance: Emergency Pharmacological Sedation

31

Claire Bertenshaw and Lachlan Parker

> **In this chapter you will learn:**
> - The definition of acute behavioural disturbance (ABD)
> - The common causes of ABD
> - The assessment and management principles of a patient exhibiting ABD
> - Indications and considerations for the administration of emergency pharmacological sedation
> - The medications that are commonly administered to facilitate emergency pharmacological sedation
> - The adverse events commonly associated with emergency pharmacological sedation.

Case Details

Dispatch
26-year-old male, acute behavioural disturbance.

History
A 26-year-old male, heavily intoxicated, is currently restrained by police due to severe agitation and aggression. A double-crewed ambulance and a single critical care paramedic are dispatched.

On Arrival of the First Crew
The scene is considered safe, the patient is handcuffed (behind the back) and positioned left lateral with two police officers providing reasonable and appropriate force.

Prolonged de-escalation attempts by police have been ineffective with the patient presenting with a sedation assessment tool[1] score of +2 (previously +3).

The first ambulance crew builds rapport and attempts de-escalation strategies without success.

The patient's primary survey findings and initial vital signs are:

SECTION 8   Toxicology

Airway	Patent
Breathing	RR 30, SpO$_2$ 98% on air
Circulation	HR 136, regular, BP unable to be obtained
Disability	Agitated, moving all 4 limbs, BGL unable to be obtained
Environmental	Temp 37.8 °C

On Your Arrival as the Critical Care Paramedic

The initial ambulance crew and police have been unable to de-escalate the situation. The patient remains moderately agitated and is considered by the on-scene paramedics and police to be at imminent risk of serious harm to themselves and/or others.

AMPLE

The following information was obtained from the patient (and friends) on scene:

Allergies	NKDA
Medications	Nil
Past history	Usually fit and well, occasional recreational drug user
Last ins and outs	Normal
Events prior	ABD secondary to suspected alcohol/substance toxicity

Decision Point

What are your clinical priorities in this situation?

This patient is agitated and aggressive. What is your plan to ensure safety for the patient, the paramedics, police and bystanders?

Question 1: What Is ABD?

ABD is a constellation of displayed behaviours and actions, both verbal and physical, that place the patient or others at immediate risk of serious harm. This may include highly threatening and aggressive behaviour that leads to a major injury or death.

> **PRACTICE TIP**
>
> All paramedics involved in managing patients with ABD must be trained in the safe and effective delivery of de-escalation strategies and emergency pharmacological sedation.

Question 2: What Are the Common Causes of ABD?

There are several potential causes of ABD, and in some cases the cause is multifactorial. The five general categories are:[2–5]

CHAPTER 31 Acute Behavioural Disturbance: Emergency Pharmacological Sedation

1. Substance toxicity/withdrawal, for example, alcohol, psychostimulants, opioids, lysergic acid diethylamide, benzodiazepines
2. General medical conditions, for example, hypoxia, hypoglycaemia, infections, electrolyte disorders, toxins, head injuries, seizures or postictal, dementia, pain
3. Acute mental health conditions, for example, schizophrenia, bipolar disorder, psychotic disorders, personality disorders
4. Situational crisis, for example, overwhelming stress
5. Existing behavioural disorders, for example, exacerbation of an existing intellectual disability, autism, impulse control disorders.

Recent prospective studies have identified that the most common causes of ABD attended by ambulance clinicians in the out-of-hospital environment are:

- Paediatrics (<16 years) – self-harm and/or harm to others[6]
- Adults (17–64 years) – substance toxicity[7]
- Elderly (>65 years) – dementia.[8]

It is essential that patients presenting with ABD receive a comprehensive assessment to determine and manage the likely cause(s). The paramedic's priority should be the early identification and treatment of any reversible cause (for example, hypoxia or hypoglycaemia) prior to the administration of any sedative agent.

Question 3: What Are the Assessment and Management Principles for a Patient Exhibiting ABD?

A detailed assessment of the patient exhibiting ABD may not be immediately possible due to the level of patient agitation and/or aggression. Safe patient assessment may only be achieved following the commencement of de-escalation strategies, and in some cases the cautious administration of emergency pharmacological sedation.

The patient assessment, when safe to conduct, should include:

- A detailed VSS – HR, RR, BP, temperature, SpO_2 and BGL
- Sedation assessment tool (SAT) score[1]
- Head-to-toe examination
- Information relating to recent alcohol and/or drug consumption or withdrawal
- Any pertinent collateral history from family/friends/bystanders.

The sedation assessment tool (SAT)[1] is a simplified version of the altered mental status score, which is commonly used by paramedics and emergency department clinicians to measure the degree of agitation, and the response to pharmacological sedation, in the ABD patient.

Scores are allocated from a seven-point scale by objectively determining the highest-ranking descriptors based on the patient's current responsiveness and speech (**Table 31.1**).

A SAT score of +2 or +3 is a good predictor to consider the administration of emergency pharmacological sedation. Comprehensive SAT scores should be assessed and recorded prior to, and at regular intervals following, the administration of any pharmacological sedative. An effective response to sedation can be defined as a reduction of two levels in the SAT, or a return to a score of 0.

SECTION 8 Toxicology

Table 31.1 Sedation assessment tool

Score	Responsiveness	Speech
+3	Combative, violent, out of control	Continual loud outbursts
+2	Very anxious	Loud outbursts
+1	Anxious/restless	Normal/talkative
0	Awake and calm/co-operative	Speaks normally
-1	Asleep but rouses if name is called	Slurring or prominent slowing
-2	Responds to physical stimulation	Few recognisable words
-3	No response to stimulation	Nil

Source: Calver, L. A., Stokes, B. and Isbister, G. K. 2011. Sedation assessment tool to score acute behavioural disturbance in the emergency department. *Emergency Medicine Australasia*, 23, 732–740.

> **PRACTICE TIP**
>
> Always embrace a patient-focused stepwise and considered approach.

> **PRACTICE TIP**
>
> A SAT score assessment should be calculated for ABD patients prior to, and at regular intervals following, the administration of any pharmacological sedative.

The initial approach to managing any patient exhibiting ABD should focus on a combination of patient-centred, non-pharmacological de-escalation strategies and techniques. Only when these have been unsuccessful should paramedics consider the use of emergency pharmacological sedation.

Commonly used de-escalation strategies include a combination of verbal and non-verbal techniques,[9] specifically the following.

- Use a calm, confident, empathic, non-threatening and respectful approach to the patient.
- Avoid sudden movements, intrusion into the patient's personal space, prolonged eye contact, provocation or confronting or intimidating behaviour.
- Introduce yourself – use both your own name and the patient's name to personalise the interaction.
- Involve carers and/or family members if available.
- Explain your role and wishes to help them; be clear and concise.

CHAPTER 31 Acute Behavioural Disturbance: Emergency Pharmacological Sedation

- Offer the patient time to state their concerns and needs in a non-judgemental and empathic atmosphere. Listen closely – this may encourage them to engage in calmer discussion.
- If possible, identify the trigger for their behaviour (for example, unmet needs, pain, communication difficulties).
- Offer support, such as food, drink (for example, a cup of lukewarm tea or coffee), toileting, access to a telephone or analgesia if indicated.
- Offer options and optimism, but set clear limits.
- Negotiate with, and debrief, the patient when it is appropriate to do so.

At all times, actions undertaken for the management ABD patients must be in the best interest of the patient, while using the least restrictive method possible. It is useful to consider the patient journey; what is the goal of the sedation? Usually, it is for safe transfer and assessment at hospital. It may also be to prevent the sequalae of prolonged psycho-motor stimulation, which can be seen in stimulant drug use. Provide as much information to the hospital staff as possible, as the transported patient's condition will not be reflective of the prehospital scene, and key aspects may be lost.

Once the patient is sedated, there is a risk for the prehospital clinician to not remain vigilant as the scene de-escalates, but conversely this is the time when potential complications can arise. Immediately following effective sedation, the patient should be positioned in left lateral position, with full monitoring, including nasal capnography. Once safe to do so, all mechanical restraint should be immediately removed, with handcuffs placed at the front of the patient. The patient should never be positioned prone or transported without close observation and continuous monitoring. Once sedated, closely assess for any indication of the cause for the ABD or complications from the behaviour, including trauma or signs of infection or drug use.

Question 4: What Are the Indications and Considerations for Emergency Pharmacological Sedation?

Emergency pharmacological sedation is high risk and should only be performed after careful consideration of the alternatives and acceptance of the risk. Paramedics should ensure appropriate resources are available to optimise safety and safeguard against any potential adverse events.

> **PRACTICE TIP**
>
> Incorporation of the SAT into paramedic practice improves patient care.

The intramuscular (IM) route is preferred over intravenous (IV) for all parenteral ABD emergency medication administration. This also applies for the administration of subsequent or rescue sedation when first-line pharmacological treatment has failed. IV administration should be reserved for experienced senior clinicians with the necessary skills and equipment to manage potential adverse events and ensure continuous monitoring of the patient.[9]

SECTION 8 Toxicology

Indications:

- Patient SAT score of two (2) or greater; and
- Patient's behaviour indicates imminent risk of serious harm to themselves and/or others; and
- Non-pharmacological de-escalation strategies have failed to appropriately reduce the risk of harm.

Considerations:

- Known contraindication to the emergency pharmacological sedation available
- Consider the patient's age, weight, co-morbidities and current VSS to create a detailed risk assessment.

> **PRACTICE TIP**
>
> Pharmacological sedation is high risk; preparation and close patient monitoring are paramount.

Question 5: What Medications Are Commonly Administered to Facilitate Emergency Pharmacological Sedation?

ABD is a common occurrence in the out-of-hospital environment, with paramedics often required to manage this group of challenging patients. Traditional pharmacological management includes benzodiazepines (for example, midazolam), typical antipsychotics (for example, droperidol), atypical antipsychotics (for example, olanzapine) and, in very severe cases, a dissociative anaesthetic (for example, ketamine) (**Table 31.2**).

Ensuring patients receive the most appropriate and least restrictive agent is crucial to optimising safety and sedation effectiveness in this vulnerable patient group.

> **PRACTICE TIP**
>
> Moderate sedation (SAT -1) will be optimal in most situations. Deep sedation (SAT -3) should be avoided in the out-of-hospital environment, due to the increased risks of adverse events.

In the rare situation when immediate control is required and first-line emergency pharmacological sedation has failed, intramuscular rescue sedation using alternative second-line pharmacology may be considered. Always follow local guidelines or advice from an appropriate senior clinician.

> **PRACTICE TIP**
>
> Don't underestimate the benefits of IM medication administration.

CHAPTER 31 Acute Behavioural Disturbance: Emergency Pharmacological Sedation

Table 31.2 Commonly administered medications to facilitate emergency pharmacological sedation

Medication	Route	Dose[9]	Specific ABD indications	Considerations
Droperidol	IM (preferred) / IV	Adult – 10 mg; if required, repeat after at least 15 minutes. Total maximum dose 20 mg. Older people (>65 years), frail or cachectic – 5 mg; if required, repeat dose at 15 minutes. Total maximum dose 10 mg.	All causes of ABD	Parkinson's disease Lewy body dementia Previous dystonic reaction Neuroleptic malignant syndrome Care in sepsis Preservation of respiratory drive
Midazolam	IM (preferred) / IV	Adult – 5–10 mg; if required, repeat after at least 15 minutes. Total maximum dose 20 mg. Older people (>65 years), frail or cachectic – 2.5 mg; if required, repeat after at least 15 minutes. Total maximum dose 10 mg.	Serotonin syndrome Drug and alcohol-associated seizures Ketamine emergence	Respiratory depression Airway compromise Benefits of amnesia
Ketamine	IM (preferred) / IV	Adult – 4–6 mg/kg; single dose of 200–400 mg. Adhere to local guidelines for maximum dose.	Patient requiring rapid sequence induction for management of ABD, especially in high-risk situations, such as aeromedical retrieval, dangerous environment	Uncontrolled hypertension Emergence Laryngospasm Hypersalivation Preservation of respiratory drive

SECTION 8 Toxicology

Question 6: What Are the Common Adverse Events Associated With Emergency Pharmacological Sedation?

Adverse events following emergency pharmacological sedation are common. However, with early and prompt recognition, the majority of cases can safely be managed with supportive care (**Table 31.3**).

Table 31.3 Managing common adverse events associated with emergency pharmacological sedation

Adverse event	Medication association	Management
Airway obstruction	All – especially if the patient is in a poor position	Patient position – left lateral, head up. Commence basic airway manoeuvres and consider use of basic airway adjuncts – oropharyngeal/nasopharyngeal airways. Utilise nasal CO_2 monitoring.
Hypoxia	All	Administration of oxygen and/or ventilatory support.
Hypoventilation	All Can be marked with midazolam	Gentle tactile stimulation to encourage respiratory drive. Support breathing with bag-valve-mask (BVM) ventilation if required, being mindful of aspiration risk.
Extrapyramidal/dystonic reaction	Droperidol Olanzapine	Benzatropine 1–2 mg IV/IM.
Laryngospasm	Ketamine	Maintain positive end expiratory pressure (PEEP) via BVM. Deepen sedation. Paralysis as part of rapid sequence induction.
Hypersalivation	Ketamine	Atropine 20 mcg/kg, maximum 600 mcg (IV, IM, IO). Suction as required.
Hypotension	All	IV fluid bolus. Gentle tactile stimulation.
Excessive sedation	All	Gentle tactile stimulation. Supportive care as per above for adverse reactions.

CHAPTER 31 Acute Behavioural Disturbance: Emergency Pharmacological Sedation

Adverse events include:

- Airway obstruction requiring support
- Hypoxia
- Hypoventilation
- Hypotension
- Over/excessive sedation
- Laryngospasm and hypersalivation
- Extrapyramidal reactions (droperidol)

PRACTICE TIP

All clinicians undertaking emergency sedation must have the knowledge and skills to recognise and manage adverse events.

Key Evidence

Isbister, G. K., Calver, L. A., Page, C. B. et al. 2010. Randomized controlled trial of intramuscular droperidol versus midazolam for violence and acute behavioral disturbance: the DORM study. *Annals of Emergency Medicine*, 56, 392–401.

Page, C. B., Parker, L. E., Rashford, S. J. et al. 2018. A prospective before and after study of droperidol for prehospital acute behavioral disturbance. *Prehospital Emergency Care*, 22, 713–721.

Self-Reflection Questions

1. What are the risks associated with emergency pharmacological sedation?
2. Which patient populations are high risk for sedation?
3. What medication would you choose for emergency pharmacological sedation, and does it depend on the patient's SAT and suspected cause of ABD?
4. How can you maximise patient safety during emergency pharmacological sedition?

References

1. Calver, L. A., Stokes, B., Isbister, G. K. 2011. Sedation assessment tool to score acute behavioural disturbance in the emergency department. *Emergency Medicine Australasia*, 23, 732–740.
2. McCarthy, S. 2016. Complex acute severe behavioural disturbance – impact and issues [Online]. NSW Health, Whole of Health Program. Available at: https://www.health.nsw.gov.au/wohp/Documents/mc8-mccarthy-asbd-data.pdf
3. Queensland Health. 2017. Management of patients with acute severe behavioural disturbance in emergency departments [Online]. Available at: https://www.health.qld.gov.au/__data/assets/pdf_file/0031/629491/qh-gdl-438.pdf
4. New South Wales Health. 2015. Management of patients with acute severe behavioural disturbance in emergency departments [Online]. Available at: https://www1.health.nsw.gov.au/pds/ActivePDSDocuments/GL2015_007.pdf
5. Safer Care Victoria. 2021. Caring for people displaying acute behavioural disturbance: Clinical guidance to improve care in emergency settings [Online]. Available at: https://www.safercare.vic.gov.au/sites/default/files/2020-04/Guidance_Acute%20behavioural%20disturbance.pdf
6. Page, C. B., Parker, L. E., Rashford, S. J. et al. 2019. A prospective study of the safety and effectiveness of droperidol in children for prehospital acute behavioral disturbance. *Prehospital Emergency Care*, 23, 519–526.

7. Page, C. B., Parker, L. E., Rashford, S. J. et al. 2018. A prospective before and after study of droperidol for prehospital acute behavioral disturbance. *Prehospital Emergency Care*, 22, 713–721.
8. Page, C. B., Parker, L. E., Rashford, S. J. et al. 2020. Prospective study of the safety and effectiveness of droperidol in elderly patients for pre–hospital acute behavioural disturbance. *Emergency Medicine Australasia*, 32, 731–736.
9. Judd, F., Burkett, E., Chan, B. et al. 2021. Approach to managing acute behavioural disturbance [Online]. *Therapeutic Guidelines*.

Severe Metabolic Acidosis

32

Tash Adams and John Glasheen

In this chapter you will learn:

- The physiology of metabolic acidosis
- Causes of metabolic acidosis
- Clinical clues to the presence of severe metabolic acidosis
- Modifications to standard patient management.

Case Details

Dispatch
24-year-old female, altered level of consciousness, abnormal breathing.

History
A 24-year-old female, with a past medical history of type 1 diabetes mellitus. She has been unwell for 2–3 days with lower abdominal and bilateral flank pain, polyuria and dysuria. She was drowsy when found by her partner this morning.

On Arrival of the First Crew
The patient is located in bed upstairs, complaining of lower abdominal and flank pain with dysuria and urinary frequency. She has been drinking more fluid than usual, feeling unwell and having cold chills.

Airway	Patent
Breathing	RR 28, SpO_2 97% on room air
Circulation	Peripheral pulses present, HR 120, BP 103/71, cool peripheries
Disability	GCS E4, V4, M6 (14), BGL 'HI'
Environmental	Temp 38.4 °C

On Your Arrival as the Critical Care Paramedic
The first crew has achieved a 20-gauge IV access in the antecubital fossa after multiple attempts, and 1 L NaCl 0.9% has been commenced. There is ongoing evidence of poor perfusion, including pale, cool peripheries. The patient's trunk feels hot and clammy. She is

SECTION 8 Toxicology

co-operative but slightly confused and is complaining of thirst. Further investigation measures capillary ketones at 3.8 mmol/L. An ECG shows a sinus tachycardia with normal axis and normal intervals. There is no history or evidence to suggest deliberate toxic ingestion. The primary crew have made an extrication plan involving the carry chair to move the patient downstairs to the ambulance.

AMPLE

Allergies	NKDA
Medications	Long-acting insulin, short-acting insulin, escitalopram, oral contraceptive pill
Past history	T1DM, depression, recurrent urinary tract infections
Last ins and outs	Has been eating intermittently over the past 2–3 days, only fluids for previous 18 hours; large volume of clear urine
Events	Gradual onset lower abdominal and flank pain with dysuria and urinary frequency; has been drinking more fluid than usual, feeling unwell and having cold chills

Decision Point

This patient is critically ill. The differential diagnosis includes diabetic ketoacidosis, severe sepsis and toxic ingestion. The patient is likely to have a metabolic acidosis. Management of this case involves cardiovascular supportive care and maintenance of respiratory compensation during extrication, with a plan to manage deterioration at all stages of the extrication. Destination planning should consider that this patient is likely to require an intensive care level of support.

Question 1: What Are the Causes of Severe Metabolic Acidosis?

Homeostatic mechanisms maintain a serum pH in the normal 7.35–7.45 range. Alteration in this results in acidaemia (pH <7.35) or alkalaemia (pH >7.45). Multiple acid–base abnormalities (metabolic or respiratory acidosis/alkalosis) may be simultaneously present contributing to a net acidaemia or alkalaemia.

Metabolic acidosis results from conditions causing increased production of acid, decreased acid excretion, abnormal renal or gastrointestinal loss of bicarbonate or exogenous acid ingestion. Severe metabolic acidosis is defined as pH ≤7.20, $PaCO_2$ ≤45 mmHg and bicarbonate concentration ≤20 mmol/L.[1] Metabolic acidosis is associated with a high mortality, reported to be up to 48% in some studies.[2] Common causes of metabolic acidosis include the following.

- **Lactic acidosis**, which occurs in critical illness when there is a mismatch between oxygen delivery (DO_2) and oxygen consumption (VO_2). Lactataemia is not a condition in itself, but a consequence of another pathological process. Multiple subtypes of lactic acidosis may co-exist:
  o **Type A** lactic acidosis results from decreased oxygen delivery secondary to hypoxia or poor tissue perfusion.

CHAPTER 32 Severe Metabolic Acidosis

- o **Type B1** lactic acidosis is due to impaired cellular oxygen utilisation secondary to organ dysfunction (for example, sepsis, hepatic failure, renal failure, mitochondrial dysfunction).
- o **Type B2** lactic acidosis results from drug toxicity, including alcohols, paracetamol, aspirin, metformin, lactulose, cyanide. Type B2 lactic acidosis may also be iatrogenic from adrenaline, salbutamol or propofol administration.
- **Diabetic ketoacidosis (DKA)** occurs when a lack of insulin results in production of hydroxybutyrate and acetoacetate as a result of hepatic metabolism of fat.
- **Hyperchloraemic metabolic acidosis** is an iatrogenic condition most commonly seen following isotonic fluid administration and is unlikely to be encountered in a primary prehospital setting but should be considered as a contributor to acidaemia in healthcare settings, including interhospital transfers.
- **Loss of bicarbonate** is seen in patients with severe diarrhoea, renal tubular acidosis, enteric or pancreatic fistulas and in Addison's disease.

PRACTICE TIP

With all critically ill or injured patients, consider metabolic acidosis as an element of the presentation.

Question 2: What Is the Clinical Presentation of Severe Metabolic Acidosis?

Patients with metabolic acidosis present with the features of the condition that are the underlying cause of the acidosis, and the acidosis can contribute to a progressive deterioration. Clinical assessment is focused on identifying the cause of the metabolic acidosis; for example, diabetic ketoacidosis will manifest with hyperglycaemia and hyperketonaemia, while septic patients will often have fever and a septic source. Any shocked patient should be expected to have a degree of metabolic acidosis. The clinician should also predict metabolic acidosis from any presentation with increased metabolic demand and/or poor perfusion, for example, in patients who are physically restrained following acute behavioural disturbance.[3,4]

Severe metabolic acidaemia causes myocardial depression and reduced cardiac output resulting in reduced perfusion.[5] The patient may present with a progressive shocked state. Primary compensation for metabolic acidosis is by hyperventilation (Kussmaul respiration).[6] This generates a respiratory alkalosis, thus reducing the magnitude of the acidaemia. Respiratory compensation is limited and never overcompensates for metabolic acidosis. Achieving and maintaining hypocapnia causes significant respiratory fatigue. Accurate and continuous respiratory assessment with monitoring of respiratory rate and depth is vital, particularly in the setting of predicted respiratory muscle fatigue or pharmacological respiratory depression. Any decrease in minute ventilation (respiratory rate x tidal volume) is concerning and may indicate imminent decompensation.

PRACTICE TIP

Respiratory function should be closely monitored clinically and with $EtCO_2$. Avoid pharmacological or physical suppression of ventilation.

Question 3: Are Any Prehospital Tests Useful in Severe Metabolic Acidosis?

The combination of a suggestive clinical history, hyperventilation and cardiovascular compromise should prompt consideration of the diagnosis of severe metabolic acidosis in critical illness. Identification of the likelihood of severe metabolic acidosis is vital, as these patients are at a considerable risk of deterioration.

A cornerstone of the emergency department assessment of these patients is the blood gas. As well as measuring the degree of acidaemia, further evaluation of the blood gas including lactate values and the presence or absence of an anion gap is useful in identification of the underlying cause of the acidosis. This in turn will guide the investigation and treatment plan. Venous blood gas measurement combined with SpO_2 is comparable to arterial blood gas measurements, and this avoids the requirement for arterial sampling in the initial stages of assessment and management.[7]

Blood gas measurement can be performed in the prehospital environment, but evidence of improvement in diagnostic accuracy is lacking, and resultant change in management is limited.[8] Prehospital management of severe metabolic acidosis is largely resuscitative and supportive, with avoidance of suppression of physiological compensation mechanisms. Recognition of the likelihood of acidaemia is sufficient to inform the immediate management in the prehospital phase of care.

Performing a blood gas measurement (pH, lactate, electrolytes) may add extra time on scene for limited clinical benefit. As always in prehospital care, there is an efficiency–thoroughness trade-off – further information is obtained at the cost of potential delay to extrication and distraction from the priorities of clinical management. Capillary lactate measurement has the advantage of being rapid and minimally invasive; however, there is conflicting evidence on the accuracy of the measurement.[9,10]

The value of blood gas testing in the prehospital environment remains unclear. There may be a role for serial blood gas monitoring to guide ventilation strategy post intubation, and to assess response to therapy as the clinical course progresses, particularly during extended field care or interhospital transfer missions.

End-tidal carbon dioxide ($EtCO_2$) is a readily available, non-invasive and inexpensive investigation. Hyperventilation in severe metabolic acidosis produces hypocarbia, and $EtCO_2$ values correlate directly with serum bicarbonate in severe metabolic acidosis. This could be used as a surrogate of bicarbonate, aiding in the diagnosis of severe metabolic acidosis. Monitoring of trends in the $EtCO_2$ may predict the onset of respiratory fatigue and may therefore be useful in planning escalation of care, for example, intubation. In those patients who proceed to intubation, targeting a similar (or lower) post-intubation $EtCO_2$ is vital in ensuring appropriate post-intubation management.

Question 4: What Is the Prehospital Management of Severe Metabolic Acidosis?

Management of severe metabolic acidosis centres on treating the underlying condition that led to the acidosis. Accurate scene assessment, clinical history and patient examination are key to identification of the cause of acidosis.

CHAPTER 32 Severe Metabolic Acidosis

Management includes fluid resuscitation and optimisation of cardiac output to reverse any ongoing shock state.[11] This may require haemodynamic support with inotropic or vasopressor agents. Catecholamine resistance has been reported in severe metabolic acidosis, and these patients may require high doses of adrenaline and/or noradrenaline to achieve the desired effect.[12] When a specific cause has been identified, the appropriate treatment can be instituted, for example, insulin infusion to treat diabetic ketoacidosis.

Maintenance of respiratory compensation is vital. A reduction in minute ventilation may result in a critical decrease in pH precipitating sudden deterioration.[13] If respiratory fatigue is identified, bi-level non-invasive ventilation can be commenced to help maintain compensation. Administration of sedative or respiratory depressive agents should be avoided where possible. Prehospital emergency anaesthesia is a high-risk procedure in this clinical situation. In patients requiring intubation, recognition of a physiologically difficult airway should prompt consideration of apnoeic ventilation,[14] or the use of ventilator-assisted preoxygenation.[15] Post-intubation ventilation strategy should match the patient's intrinsic minute ventilation, with a focus on maintaining appropriate hypocapnia.

> **PRACTICE TIP**
>
> Many patients with metabolic acidosis are haemodynamically compromised and may be susceptible to orthostatic hypotension. Change in patient position (for example, sitting in a carry chair for extrication) resulting in syncope may lead to an apnoeic period, which could in turn precipitate worsening of acidosis, resulting in cardiac arrest.

Question 5: What Is the Role of Bicarbonate?

Resolution of the metabolic acidosis is a key part of overall clinical management. This includes treatment of the underlying cause of acidosis to limit ongoing acid production, as well as optimising excretion of the excess (H+). The underlying pathological process often causes gradual onset of the metabolic acidosis, and resolution of the acidosis is also gradual. Administration of bicarbonate (usually in the form of sodium bicarbonate) can be used to treat acidaemia, with the aim to improve cardiac function and perfusion in the short term.[16] Bicarbonate administration increases arterial pH, serum bicarbonate sodium and $PaCO_2$, and decreases anion gap and serum potassium concentration.

Despite these biochemical and physiological effects, early sodium bicarbonate administration is not associated with improved outcomes in ICU patients with severe metabolic acidosis.[17] Evidence of improvement in haemodynamic function is also lacking,[18] although there may be some benefit in vasopressor-dependent patients.[14] Bicarbonate administration has the potential negative effect of increased CO_2 production, which requires further ventilatory compensation. Bicarbonate may also cause a deterioration of intracellular pH, possibly due to increased intracellular CO_2.

There are some specific clinical situations where bicarbonate may be recommended for management of severe metabolic acidosis in an intensive care unit setting, for example, acidosis secondary to gastrointestinal or renal losses, metabolic acidaemia in patients with moderate to severe renal insufficiency or following salicylate poisoning.[19] The Surviving Sepsis campaign has made a 'weak recommendation' for the use of sodium bicarbonate

SECTION 8 Toxicology

in the subset of patients with a combination of septic shock, severe metabolic acidosis and acute kidney injury.[20]

With the exception of out-of-hospital cardiac arrest management (cardiac arrest produces a profound metabolic acidosis), there is currently no primary evidence investigating the role or efficacy of bicarbonate for severe metabolic acidosis in the prehospital setting.

Key Evidence

Jaber S, Paugam C, Futier E et al. Sodium bicarbonate therapy for patients with severe metabolic acidaemia in the intensive care unit (BICAR-ICU): a multicentre, open-label, randomised controlled, phase 3 trial. *Lancet*. 2018 Jul 7;392(10141):31–40. Available at: https://pubmed.ncbi.nlm.nih.gov/29910040/. Erratum in: Lancet. 2018 Dec 8;392(10163):2440.

Lentz S, Grossman A, Koyfman A et al. High-risk airway management in the emergency department. Part I: diseases and approaches. *Journal of Emergency Medicine*. 2020 Jul;59(1):84–95. Available at: https://pubmed.ncbi.nlm.nih.gov/32563613/

Matyukhin I, Patschan S, Ritter O et al. Etiology and management of acute metabolic acidosis: an update. *Kidney and Blood Pressure Research*. 2020;45(4):523–531. Available at: https://pubmed.ncbi.nlm.nih.gov/32663831/

Zwisler ST, Zincuk Y, Bering CB et al. Diagnostic value of prehospital arterial blood gas measurements – a randomised controlled trial. *Scandinavian Journal of Trauma, Resuscitation and Emergency Medicine*. 2019;27:32. Available at: https://sjtrem.biomedcentral.com/articles/10.1186/s13049-019-0612-8

Self-Reflection Questions

1. Which patients are at the highest risk of developing severe metabolic acidosis?
2. What are the foundational principles of resuscitation for patients presenting with suspected severe metabolic acidosis?
3. Would a blood gas change your diagnosis or management in the prehospital environment?
4. How would you optimise prehospital emergency anaesthesia and intubation in the setting of severe metabolic acidosis?
5. Should sodium bicarbonate be administered to all patients with suspected metabolic acidosis?

References

1. Jaber S, Paugam C, Futier E et al. Sodium bicarbonate therapy for patients with severe metabolic acidaemia in the intensive care unit (BICAR-ICU): a multicentre, open-label, randomised controlled, phase 3 trial. *Lancet*. 2018 Jul 7;392(10141):31–40. Available at: https://pubmed.ncbi.nlm.nih.gov/29910040/. Erratum in: *Lancet*. 2018 Dec 8;392(10163):2440.
2. Jaber S, Paugam C, Futier E, et al. Sodium bicarbonate therapy for patients with severe metabolic acidaemia in the intensive care unit (BICAR-ICU): a multicentre, open-label, randomised controlled, phase 3 trial. *Lancet*. 2018 Jul 7;392(10141):31–40.
3. Weedn V, Steinberg A, Speth P. Prone restraint cardiac arrest in in-custody and arrest-related deaths. *Journal of Forensic Science*. 2022 Sep;67(5):1899–1914. Available at: https://pubmed.ncbi.nlm.nih.gov/35869602/
4. Hick JL, Smith SW, Lynch MT. Metabolic acidosis in restraint-associated cardiac arrest: a case series. *Academic Emergency Medicine*. 1999 Mar;6(3):239–243. Available at: https://pubmed.ncbi.nlm.nih.gov/10192677/
5. Wildenthal K, Mierzwiak DS, Myers RW et al. Effects of acute lactic acidosis on left ventricular performance. *American Journal of Physiology*. 1968 Jun;214(6):1352–1359. Available at: https://pubmed.ncbi.nlm.nih.gov/5649491/

6. Kapitan KS. Ventilatory failure: can you sustain what you need? *Annals of the American Thoracic Society*. 2013;10:396–399. Available at: https://pubmed.ncbi.nlm.nih.gov/23952866/
7. Zeserson E, Goodgame B, Hess JD et al. Correlation of venous blood gas and pulse oximetry with arterial blood gas in the undifferentiated critically ill patient. *Journal of Intensive Care Medicine*. 2018 Mar;33(3):176–181. Available at: https://pubmed.ncbi.nlm.nih.gov/27283009/
8. Zwisler ST, Zincuk Y, Bering CB et al. Diagnostic value of prehospital arterial blood gas measurements – a randomised controlled trial. *Scandinavian Journal of Trauma, Resuscitation and Emergency Medicine*. 2019;27:32. Available at: https://sjtrem.biomedcentral.com/articles/10.1186/s13049-019-0612-8
9. Raa A, Sunde GA, Bolann B et al. Validation of a point-of-care capillary lactate measuring device (Lactate Pro 2). *Scandinavian Journal of Trauma, Resuscitation and Emergency Medicine*. 2020 Aug 18;28(1):83. Available at: https://pubmed.ncbi.nlm.nih.gov/32811544/
10. Collot V, Malinverni S, Haltout J et al. Agreement between arterial and capillary pH, pCO_2, and lactate in patients in the emergency department. *Emergency Medicine International*. 2021 Jul 6;2021:7820041. Available at: https://pubmed.ncbi.nlm.nih.gov/34306758/
11. Matyukhin I, Patschan S, Ritter O et al. Etiology and management of acute metabolic acidosis: an update. *Kidney and Blood Pressure Research*. 2020;45(4):523–531. Available at: https://pubmed.ncbi.nlm.nih.gov/32663831/
12. Yagi K, Fujii T. Management of acute metabolic acidosis in the ICU: sodium bicarbonate and renal replacement therapy. *Critical Care*. 2021 Aug 31;25(1):314. Available at: https://pubmed.ncbi.nlm.nih.gov/34461963/
13. Lentz S, Grossman A, Koyfman A et al. High-risk airway management in the emergency department. Part I: diseases and approaches. *Journal of Emergency Medicine*. 2020 Jul;59(1):84–95. Available at: https://pubmed.ncbi.nlm.nih.gov/32563613/
14. Casey JD, Janz DR, Russell DW et al. Bag-mask ventilation during tracheal intubation of critically ill adults. *New England Journal of Medicine*. 2019 Feb 28;380(9):811–821. Available at: https://pubmed.ncbi.nlm.nih.gov/30779528/
15. Grant S, Khan F, Keijzers G et al. Ventilator-assisted preoxygenation: protocol for combining non-invasive ventilation and apnoeic oxygenation using a portable ventilator. *Emergency Medicine Australasia*. 2016;28:67–72. Available at: https://pubmed.ncbi.nlm.nih.gov/26764895/
16. Adrogué HJ, Madias NE. Management of life-threatening acid-base disorders. First of two parts. *New England Journal of Medicine*. 1998 Jan 1;338(1):26-34. Available at: https://pubmed.ncbi.nlm.nih.gov/9414329/
17. Fujii T, Udy AA, Nichol A et al. Incidence and management of metabolic acidosis with sodium bicarbonate in the ICU: an international observational study. *Critical Care*. 2021 Feb 2;25(1):45. Available at: https://pubmed.ncbi.nlm.nih.gov/33531020/
18. Cooper DJ, Walley KR, Wiggs BR et al. Bicarbonate does not improve hemodynamics in critically ill patients who have lactic acidosis. A prospective, controlled clinical study. *Annals of Internal Medicine*. 1990;112(7):492–498. Available at: https://pubmed.ncbi.nlm.nih.gov/2156475/
19. Jung B, Martinez M, Claessens YE et al. Diagnosis and management of metabolic acidosis: guidelines from a French expert panel. *Annals of Intensive Care*. 2019;9:92. Available at: https://pubmed.ncbi.nlm.nih.gov/31418093/
20. Evans L, Rhodes A, Alhazzani W et al. Surviving sepsis campaign: international guidelines for management of sepsis and septic shock 2021. *Intensive Care Medicine*. 2021 Nov;47(11):1181–1247. Available at: https://pubmed.ncbi.nlm.nih.gov/34599691/

SECTION 9

Paediatrics, Obstetrics and Gynaecology

Croup and Epiglottitis

33

Brad Gander and Claire Wilkin

In this chapter you will learn:
- What croup is
- About croup severity assessment
- Differential diagnoses
- How to identify croup versus epiglottitis
- Prehospital management of croup and epiglottitis.

Case Details

Dispatch
3-year-old male, respiratory distress, stridor, high temperature.

History
The parents of a 3-year-old child have called emergency services. They report the child has woken suddenly in the night and appears to be having difficulty breathing. The call-taker can hear a loud barking cough in the background. The patient has a 2-day history of coryzal symptoms and a mild temperature. A paramedic crew and critical care paramedic have been dispatched.

On Arrival of the First Crew
The mother is holding the child, who is distressed but consolable and has an audible inspiratory stridor.

His initial vital signs are:

Airway	Patent
Breathing	RR 36, SpO$_2$ 97% on room air
Circulation	HR 145
Disability	GCS E4, V5, M6 (15)
Environmental	Temp 38.7 °C

The paramedic crew choose to move the patient into the ambulance with the mother. They remove the child's clothing and administer 180 mg oral paracetamol to manage his elevated temperature.

SECTION 9 Paediatrics, Obstetrics and Gynaecology

On Your Arrival as the Critical Care Paramedic

On arrival at the ambulance, the crew and mother are attempting to console the child, who has become distressed. You can hear a clear inspiratory stridor and notice intercostal recession. You conduct your own primary survey.

Airway	Clear and self-maintained, slight drooling
Breathing	Respiratory rate now 40, SpO$_2$ 97% on room air, inspiratory stridor, intercostal recession
Circulation	Warm to touch, HR 150, strong brachial pulse, unable to assess BP as patient distressed and not tolerating cuff
Disability	GCS 15, distressed but appears to be tiring
Environmental	Flushed cheeks, no rash

AMPLE

The patient has no known allergies. They are up to date on all immunisations and take no regular medications. They have no previous medical history. Over the past few days they have had a reduced appetite. Two days ago, the child developed cold symptoms and has complained of a sore throat throughout the day today.

Allergies	NKDA
Medications	Nil
Past history	Nil
Last ins and outs	Reduced appetite for several days
Events prior	Cold symptoms for 2 days, sore throat today

Decision Point

What is the most likely cause of respiratory distress in this patient and how is this best managed?

Question 1: What Is Croup?

The clinical diagnosis of croup refers to upper airway signs and symptoms that may be caused by laryngotracheitis, laryngotracheobronchitis or laryngotracheobronchopneumonitis.[1] Croup is a common paediatric respiratory illness, affecting around 3% of children between 6 months and 3 years of age per year.[2] It is uncommon in children aged older than 6,[3] although rare cases occur in adolescents.[4] Boys are more frequently affected than girls, at a ratio of 1.5:1.[1,3] Several retrospective reviews of emergency department attendances have found croup was responsible for 1.3%–5.1% of all attendances to emergency departments by children.[5,6]

CHAPTER 33   Croup and Epiglottitis

Croup occurs most frequently in the autumn months but may present at any time throughout the year. Viral infections are the most common precipitating cause, with parainfluenza types 1, 2 and 3 responsible for over 40% of cases.[7] Other viral causes include respiratory syncytial virus, adenovirus, influenza A and B and COVID-19.[4] The aetiology of viral croup does not affect the prognosis or treatment principles. Patients may also develop croup symptoms without a viral trigger, known as spasmodic croup. This subtype of croup is thought to have an allergic or reflux-initiated trigger. Symptom duration is usually shorter than viral croup but may recur.[8] Bacterial causes are rare, but may include *Corynebacterium diphtheriae*, *Staphylococcus aureus*, *Streptococcus pneumoniae*, *Haemophilus influenzae* or *Moraxella catarrhalis*.[9] This is often referred to as bacterial tracheitis. More recently, several case reports have emerged highlighting cases of croup caused by COVID-19.[10]

A diagnosis of croup can be made by physical examination and history taking. The clinical presentation of this condition is characterised by a sudden onset of a barking cough, often described as a 'seal bark', accompanied by inspiratory stridor, hoarse voice and respiratory distress.[1,4] Prior to presenting with the classical signs and symptoms of croup, patients often have between 12 and 72 hours of mild upper respiratory tract symptoms, including coryza, cough, rhinorrhoea, nasal congestion and a low-grade fever.[1,3,4] The clinical features of stridor and respiratory distress occur due to progressive subglottic or laryngeal inflammation in response to infection by one of the aforementioned pathogens.[11] In comparison to adults, children have narrower subglottic airway regions. Inflammation within the upper airway mucosa can disrupt airflow and produce related symptoms, such as stridor, a barking cough and intercostal recession. The severity of symptoms is dependent on several factors, including individual anatomy and the immunocompetence of the affected patient.

Croup symptoms frequently manifest nocturnally and may be exacerbated by agitation and distress, which can also increase parental concern. The reasons for the frequent nocturnal presentation of croup are not fully known, but it has been postulated to be linked to increased tissue inflammation due to reduced serum cortisol levels.[12] Symptoms usually resolve within 48 hours, and less than 6% of patients attending emergency departments require admission.[6] Of those admitted to hospital, only between 1% and 3% require intubation, and mortality remains low at a rate of less than 0.5%,[1] or about 1 in 30,000 cases.[12] Complications following croup are rare but include pneumonia, dehydration, otitis media, pulmonary oedema and bacterial tracheitis.[2,8]

Question 2: How Is Croup Severity Assessed?

Several scoring systems have been developed to assess the severity of croup. These are often utilised in clinical research to stratify patients who may benefit from a specific treatment regime and assess outcomes. The most commonly utilised croup scoring system is the Westley Croup Severity Score,[13] which evaluates the level of consciousness, cyanosis, stridor, air entry and retractions (**Table 33.1**).

In clinical practice, croup scoring systems are of limited value and may be prone to interobserver variability.[14] However, utilising the elements contained within these may be helpful for clinicians to gauge the severity of croup during clinical assessment and guide subsequent management.[15] Croup is traditionally categorised as mild, moderate, severe or 'impending respiratory failure'. The clinical features of these categories are shown in **Table 33.2**. Mild

SECTION 9 Paediatrics, Obstetrics and Gynaecology

Table 33.1 Westley Croup Severity Score

Clinical findings	Points
Level of consciousness	
Normal (including sleep)	0
Disoriented	5
Cyanosis	
None	0
Cyanosis with agitation	4
Cyanosis at rest	5
Stridor	
None	0
When agitated	1
At rest	2
Air entry	
Normal	0
Decreased	1
Markedly decreased	2
Retractions	
None	0
Mild (alar flaring)	1
Moderate (suprasternal and intercostal)	2
Severe (all accessory muscles used)	3
Maximum total points	**17**

Level of severity	Westley Croup Score
Mild	0–2
Moderate	3–5
Severe	6–11
Impending respiratory failure	12–17

Source: Westley, C.R., Cotton, E.K. and Brooks, J.G., 1978. Nebulized racemic epinephrine by IPPB for the treatment of croup: a double-blind study. *American Journal of Diseases of Children*, *132*(5), pp. 484–487.

croup is defined as an isolated seal-bark cough and no stridor or recession. Moderate croup involves the presence of stridor and sternal recession at rest, with no or minimal agitation. Patients with severe croup display prominent stridor and recession associated with agitation or lethargy. Patients presenting with signs of impending respiratory failure, such as cyanosis, respiratory fatigue and a decreased level of consciousness, are at high risk of cardiac or respiratory arrest. Stridor may appear to decrease at this point, or be less prominent, due to a reduction in tidal volumes because of respiratory fatigue. This term is also used within

CHAPTER 33 Croup and Epiglottitis

Table 33.2 Croup severity assessment

Category	Barking cough	Stridor	Recession	Distress/ agitation	Level of consciousness	Cyanosis
Mild	Occasional	None/limited at rest	None to mild	None	Normal	None
Moderate	Frequent	Audible at rest	Visible at rest	None to limited	Normal	None
Severe	Frequent	Prominent inspiratory and occasionally expiratory	Marked or severe	Substantial	Lethargic	None
Impending respiratory failure	Often not prominent due to fatigue	Audible at rest. May be quiet	May not be marked	Substantial	Lethargic, decreased level of consciousness	Present without supplemental oxygen

Source: Adapted from Bjornson, C.L. and Johnson, D.W., 2013. Croup in children. *Canadian Medical Association Journal*, 185(15), pp. 1317–1323.

some guidelines to describe patients with severe croup who have no, or a poorly sustained, response to treatment. Consequently, such patients should receive early referral to paediatric intensive care or anaesthesia for advanced clinical care,[11] In the UK, the National Institute for Health and Care Excellence guidelines on the management of croup advise that all children with evidence of moderate or severe croup, or impending respiratory failure, should be admitted.[3] A single-centre prospective study on the outcomes of 192 children attending a paediatric emergency department with a diagnosis of croup found no correlation between the initial Westley score and the length of hospitalisation.[16]

Question 3: What Are the Differential Diagnoses of this Presentation?

Although croup is a common condition with distinguishable clinical features, when evaluating a child with suspected croup, accurate and focused history taking is a key component of assessment and may alert the clinician to the presence of an alternative diagnosis. This is of particular importance when considering the initiation of inappropriate treatments, or delaying treatment, and may contribute to further clinical deterioration. In one study, 16% of patients with a final diagnosis of croup had at least one different diagnosis made prior to this, and 38% of patients with epiglottitis received alternative diagnoses before a confirmed diagnosis.[17] Croup does not present with angioedema or urticaria; therefore the patient with these signs and symptoms with stridor should be assessed for an allergic cause. Epiglottitis, peritonsillar abscess and retropharyngeal abscess should be considered in children reporting a sore throat, pain or difficulty swallowing and vocal disturbance. Causes of stridor, such as thermal injury, smoke inhalation or ingestion of caustic substances and foreign bodies, usually have a clearer precipitating event and onset without prior respiratory symptoms or viral illness. Previous trauma from the removal of foreign bodies from the airway, such as scratches caused by blind finger sweeps, may also precipitate epiglottic inflammation and infection. Congenital airway abnormalities are often reported by parents and carers during initial assessment; however, several case reports exist of croup-like symptoms as first-time presentations of airway lesions in very young infants.[18–20] The presence of a cutaneous haemangioma around the neck or face in patients with stridor should raise suspicion of subglottic haemangioma causing airway compromise.[19] COVID-19 infection may also manifest as croup in children, with severe presentations that are resistant to initial treatments[10] or biphasic, thus requiring longer periods of observation.

The list of differential diagnoses includes:[1,3,21]

- Epiglottitis
- Bacterial tracheitis
- Bacterial infection
- Retropharyngeal or peritonsillar abscess
- Neoplasm
- Congenital or acquired airway lesions
- Laryngeal diphtheria
- Foreign body ingestion
- Angioneurotic oedema
- Allergic reaction
- Toxic ingestion
- Smoke inhalation.

Epiglottitis

Epiglottitis refers to inflammation of the supraglottic structures, of which the epiglottis is a major component and commonly involved. Inflammation of this area may also affect adjacent structures, such as the aryepiglottic folds and arytenoids.[22] The epiglottis is particularly prone to swelling, as its superior surface is coated in loosely adhered epithelial tissue, which allows oedema to freely accumulate beneath it.[23] Fulminant infection within this region may also lead to the development of an epiglottic abscess.[4] Evaluation for epiglottitis is important due to the differences in treatment and clinical course of these patients, in whom there is a risk of rapid airway obstruction and clinical deterioration.

Despite often being associated with young children, epiglottitis is now more common in adults. In the US the mean age of patients admitted with epiglottitis is now 45, and patients aged 45 or older represent 68% of cases in the UK.[24] A review of death certificate information in the US found paediatric and adolescent mortality rates have substantially declined from 0.64 per 100,000 individuals in 1979 to 0.01 per 100,000 individuals in 2017.[25] Previously, it was estimated that *Haemophilus influenzae type B* (HiB) was responsible for up to 99% of cases of epiglottitis.[24] However, since the introduction of routine vaccinations for HiB the incidence of epiglottitis in children has reduced substantially. Nonetheless, previous vaccination does not exclude the possibility of epiglottitis.[26] Other causes may include *Streptococcus pneumoniae*, Group A, B, C and G beta-haemolytic *Streptococcus* and *Staphylococcus aureus*.[4,24] Cases of non-infectious epiglottitis due to thermal injury, trauma to the surface of the epiglottis or the ingestion of foreign bodies or caustic substances have also been reported.[27]

While croup and epiglottitis share similar clinical presentations, there are several key differences between these conditions. A retrospective review of 606 paediatric intensive care admissions for croup or epiglottitis was performed by Tibballs and Watson in 2011.[17] This work highlighted several differences in the presenting signs and symptoms that may assist clinicians in their assessment of a child with suspected croup or epiglottitis. The authors found that in children with a diagnosis of croup, the presence of a cough had a positive predictive value of 0.98 (0.93–0.99), and the absence of drooling had a positive predictive value of 0.83 (0.75–0.89). Whereas, in children with a diagnosis of epiglottitis, the absence of a cough and the presence of drooling had positive predictive values of 1.00 (0.96–1.00) and 0.77 (0.58–0.89) respectively. In summary, in a child with stridor, the presence of a cough and the absence of drooling make the diagnosis likely to be croup, and less likely to be epiglottitis. Alternatively, if the child has no cough and drooling is present, epiglottitis is a more likely diagnosis than croup. Other signs and symptoms suggesting epiglottitis is more likely than croup included dysphonia, dysphagia, refusing food, preferring to sit up, sore throat and vomiting (all p <0.001). A similar study was undertaken by Lee et al. and found patients with epiglottitis had a higher mean age and higher frequencies of vomiting, sore throat and dyspnoea when compared to those with croup.[28] Children and adolescents with epiglottis were up to ten times more likely to complain of a sore throat than those with croup.

Bacterial Tracheitis

Bacterial tracheitis is another rare but potentially life-threatening airway condition that may present similarly to croup with stridor, dyspnoea and a recent history suggestive of viral respiratory illness. It usually affects children aged between 6 months and 8 years[24] and has an estimated annual incidence of 0.1 cases per 100,000 children.[29] Like epiglottitis, a shift has been noted in the incidence and average age of affected patients, with mortality declining and cases occurring in older patients.[30] A case series of 36 patients reported a 69% intensive care admission rate, with 43% of patients requiring intubation.[31] A systematic review of 19 studies undertaken by Tebruegge et al. reported intubation rates of 80% to 100% of patients, and mortality ranging between 3% and 40%.[29]

Bacterial tracheitis may also be referred to as membranous croup, pseudomembranous croup or bacterial croup within the literature.[32] In bacterial tracheitis, usually as a result of a prior viral respiratory infection, bacterial invasion of the tracheal mucosa leads to the production of purulent exudate, which can lead to airway obstruction. Patients may present with stridor, hoarseness, fever and respiratory distress.[23] A cough may also be present; however, the patient may also have a reluctance to cough, due to tracheal tenderness.[32] In comparison to the mild pyrexia seen in croup, patients with bacterial tracheitis have higher temperatures and a toxic appearance. Because bacterial tracheitis often occurs following an initial viral infection, patients may present following an initial diagnosis of croup; however, this condition does not respond to the conventional croup treatments of adrenaline and corticosteroids.[32] Additionally, seasonal variance in presentations may also be seen due to its relationship with viral respiratory infections. Complications from bacterial tracheitis have been reported to include pneumothorax, pulmonary oedema, subglottic stenosis, toxic shock syndrome, hypotension, ARDS and cardiorespiratory arrest.[29]

SECTION 9 Paediatrics, Obstetrics and Gynaecology

The clinical features of croup, epiglottitis and bacterial tracheitis are compared in **Table 33.3**.

Table 33.3 Clinical features of croup, epiglottitis and bacterial tracheitis

Condition	Characteristics
Croup	'Seal-bark' cough, inspiratory stridor, hoarse voice, respiratory distress, preceding viral illness, mild upper respiratory symptoms
Epiglottitis	Absence of cough, sore throat, high fever, vomiting, 'the four Ds of epiglottis' – drooling, dysphagia, dysphonia, distress[33]
Bacterial tracheitis	High fever, tracheal tenderness, stridor, hoarse voice, poor response to croup treatment

Question 4: What Prehospital Treatments Are Available?

Epiglottitis

Epiglottitis is a life-threatening medical emergency. Extreme care should be taken during patient assessment as even minor irritation can precipitate complete airway obstruction. Stridor is a late sign and is an indicator of partial airway obstruction. Patients should be allowed to remain in an upright or 'tripod' position, as placing them in a supine position may lead to complete airway obstruction.[34,35] In the prehospital environment, when epiglottitis is suspected, a hands-off approach to minimise further distress should be undertaken, with a rapid transfer and pre-alert to the receiving hospital. Early involvement of senior clinical support is key as patients have the potential to rapidly deteriorate. Difficult airway management and ventilation should be anticipated, and the equipment for emergency tracheostomy should be readily available in any patient undergoing airway interventions.[34] Laryngoscopic view of the vocal chords is often obstructed by the enlarged epiglottis. The application of external pressure to the chest wall to force air escape through the vocal chords and create a bubble may guide endotracheal tube placement.[35]

Croup

> **PRACTICE TIP**
>
> Focus on time as the cure and everything else is temporising.

As a general principle, a hands-off approach of minimal interventions should be attempted in the majority of patients, in order to minimise further distress. Treatment strategies for croup have traditionally been based upon the assessed severity of presentation (**Table 33.4**). As croup is generally a short-lasting condition, with symptoms resolving within 7 days, management of mild cases is focused on providing supportive care. Nonetheless, patients with moderate to severe croup may require prolonged treatment with additional medications. There is a well-established consensus of treatment with oral corticosteroids and nebulised

CHAPTER 33 Croup and Epiglottitis

Table 33.4 Example croup treatment algorithm

Croup severity	Westley croup score	Treatment
Mild	0–2	• Corticosteroids • Supportive care (such as oral fluids to prevent dehydration, antipyretics if fever is causing discomfort)
Moderate	3–5	• Corticosteroids • Supportive care (such as oral fluids to prevent dehydration, antipyretics if fever is causing discomfort) • Nebulised adrenaline
Severe	6–11	• Corticosteroids • Supportive care (such as oral fluids to prevent dehydration, antipyretics if fever is causing discomfort) • Nebulised adrenaline • Supplemental oxygen
Impending respiratory failure	12–17	• Request senior clinical support • Repeat nebulised adrenaline • 15 L oxygen via non-rebreather mask • Systemic corticosteroid

Source: Adapted from BMJ Best Practice (2023) Croup [Online] Available at: https://bestpractice.bmj.com/topics/en-gb/681 and The Royal Childrens Hospital Melbourne (2020) Croup (Laryngotracheobronchitis) [Online] Available at: https://www.rch.org.au/clinicalguide/guideline_index/croup_laryngotracheobronchitis/

adrenaline, although recommendations for use, presentations and availability remain variable across prehospital services.[36]

> **PRACTICE TIP**
> Minimal handling is key: the child can be nursed in a parent's arms while being assessed.

> **PRACTICE TIP**
> Remove clothing so RR and WOB can be assessed at a distance. BP assessment is not necessary.

Nebulised Adrenaline

Nebulised adrenaline is indicated in patients with moderate to severe croup to relieve the symptoms of airway oedema. This method of administration has been widely used for many years and its efficacy has been evaluated in several randomised controlled trials. Adrenaline is thought to reduce airway oedema through stimulation of α-adrenergic receptors within the subglottic mucous membranes, which causes vasoconstriction and consequently reduces swelling.[37] A systematic review on the use of nebulised adrenaline for croup in children was undertaken by Bjornson et al.[38] who found that, when compared to a placebo, nebulised adrenaline improved croup symptoms (as defined by croup severity scores) at 30 minutes post administration. One small study that investigated longer-term effects of nebulised adrenaline versus a placebo found no significant difference in croup severity at 2 hours. Additionally, two studies compared croup scores at 6 hours following treatment and again found no difference in croup severity between those treated with nebulised adrenaline and those administered a placebo. Due to the rapid onset of action of adrenaline in comparison to glucocorticoids, adrenaline may 'buy time' and relieve symptoms while glucocorticoids take effect. Adrenaline has a plasma half-life of 2–3 minutes,[39] meaning repeat dosing may be required during this period. The use of adrenaline in children with inflammatory airway obstruction has been associated with mild side-effects, including tachycardia and pallor; therefore, cardiovascular monitoring is recommended during treatment, provided it does not cause further distress.[40]

Steroids

Steroids should be administered to all children with croup, regardless of severity, as their anti-inflammatory properties play an important role in providing a longer-term reduction in airway swelling. This treatment recommendation is based upon the findings of a Cochrane review conducted by Gates et al. This review found that, when compared to a placebo, patients treated with steroids had a lower rate of admissions, return visits or readmissions (moderate-certainty evidence).[41] No effect was seen on the requirement for additional treatments; however, this is not surprising, as steroids take longer to take effect (around 2 hours). Therefore, treatments such as adrenaline should be continued to provide relief of symptoms beforehand. In a retrospective study of 188 patients with croup, the prehospital administration of dexamethasone led to a reduced rate of in-hospital nebulised adrenaline administration.[42]

The specific type of steroid, dose and route of administration may vary depending on availability and clinical setting. Steroids are available in oral, intramuscular and inhaled presentations. Oral steroid preparations are generally well-tolerated; however, absorption may be hindered in children with vomiting or reluctance to swallow. Intramuscular administration may offer an advantage in this situation, although the use of injections may precipitate pain and anxiety in already distressed children.[43] Nebulised steroids, such as budesonide, may also offer an advantage over intramuscular administration and allow concurrent administration of oxygen to children with severe croup. Steroid administration routes have been compared in several studies, with no single method demonstrating superiority when assessed against croup severity scores, length of stay or readmission rates.[15]

> **PRACTICE TIP**
>
> Attach a sats probe under a sock if HR/oxygen saturations are critical to obtain, then retreat and observe.

CHAPTER 33 Croup and Epiglottitis

> **PRACTICE TIP**
>
> Don't be tempted to 'do something' – doing nothing other than steroids/adrenaline is safest.

> **PRACTICE TIP**
>
> If using IM steroids, always run a concurrent adrenaline nebuliser to decrease risk of acute obstruction resulting from the distress of the injection.

In the UK oral dexamethasone is the recommended steroid for the prehospital treatment of children with croup.[44] This is administered as a single dose determined by patient age, rather than the weight-based calculations utilised in other guidelines.[44] Studies have attempted to compare the efficacy of oral dexamethasone and prednisolone. Sparrow and Geelhoed investigated the rate of re-presentation in 133 children with mild to moderate croup randomised to receive single-dose oral prednisolone or dexamethasone. This study found that those treated with prednisolone were more likely to reattend medical care within the following 7 days (29% versus 7%), although no significant differences were seen in the rate of readmission, duration of symptoms or use of adrenaline.[45] When considering dosages, it has been proposed there is a 'ceiling effect', where higher doses do not offer any additional benefit.[46] Fifoot and Ting conducted a randomised, double-blinded trial comparing single oral doses of 1 mg/kg prednisolone, 0.15 mg/kg (low-dose) dexamethasone and 0.6 mg dexamethasone.[47] This study featured 99 children with a Westley Croup Score of between 2 and 7, treated within the paediatric emergency department of a tertiary care hospital. When the Westley Croup Score was reassessed at 4 hours, no significant differences were seen between all three groups. Additionally, no differences were seen in the duration of croup symptoms or rates of reattendance, readmission or adrenaline use. The authors concluded both oral prednisolone and 0.15 mg/kg dexamethasone should be considered in the treatment of mild-to-moderate croup.

More recently, the ToPDoG (Trial of Prednisolone/Dexamethasone Oral Glucocorticoid) study conducted by Parker and Cooper yielded similar results in a larger sample of 1231 patients.[48] This study investigated the impact of 1 mg/kg prednisolone, 0.15 mg/kg dexamethasone and 0.6 mg dexamethasone on Westley Croup Score at 1, 2 and 3 hours post administration and the reattendance rates of each group. No significant differences were seen in Westley Croup Score at all time intervals, and reattendance rates were 21.7% for prednisolone, 19.5% for low-dose dexamethasone and 17.8% for dexamethasone ($p = 0.59$ and 0.19). Those treated with prednisolone were found to have a higher rate of additional steroid requirement (18.9% versus 15.1% and 11.3%, respectively). The possible side-effects of short-term steroid use include restlessness and sleep disturbance, gastrointestinal disturbances and headache.[49] A systematic review of the safety of short-term corticosteroids in children with acute respiratory conditions found no evidence of an increased risk of adverse events.[50]

SECTION 9 Paediatrics, Obstetrics and Gynaecology

Question 5: Are There Any Additional Therapies That Should Be Considered?

In the prehospital environment focus should be placed on minimising distress and treating with steroids and nebulised adrenaline when required. Supplemental oxygen should be administered to all children with signs of respiratory failure. In cases of impending respiratory failure, 15 L oxygen should be delivered via a non-rebreather mask. Oral fluids should be encouraged where dehydration is suspected. Analgesic medications may be administered if associated symptoms, such as a sore throat, are causing discomfort and distress. While commonly referred to within home treatment advice, there is no evidence to support the use of inhaled hot steam or humidified air.[51] Similarly, there is no evidence to support the use of antitussive medications, decongestants or sedatives.[52,53] As croup is most often caused by viral illness, antibiotics should only be administered for suspected primary and secondary bacterial infections.[9]

Key Evidence

Bjornson, C., Russell, K.F., Vandermeer, B. et al., 2012. Cochrane review: nebulized epinephrine for croup in children. *Evidence-Based Child Health*, *7*(4), pp. 1311–1354.

Casazza, G., Graham, M.E., Nelson, D. et al., 2019. Pediatric bacterial tracheitis – a variable entity: case series with literature review. *Otolaryngology – Head and Neck Surgery*, *160*(3), pp. 546–549.

Gates, A., Gates, M., Vandermeer, B. et al., 2018. Glucocorticoids for croup in children. *Cochrane Database of Systematic Reviews*, 8.

Tibballs, J. and Watson, T., 2011. Symptoms and signs differentiating croup and epiglottitis. *Journal of Paediatrics and Child Health*, *47*(3), pp. 77–82.

Self-Reflection Questions

1. What is the value of oxygen in upper airway obstruction?
2. How might you distinguish the rare bacterial causes of upper airway obstruction from the very common viral croup?
3. Describe the characteristics of a 'croupy cough'?
4. What are the differences in location of anatomical obstruction in epiglottitis versus viral croup?
5. What urgent treatment is required in epiglottitis and bacterial tracheitis that is not required in viral croup?

References

1. Smith, D.K., McDermott, A.J. and Sullivan, J.F., 2018. Croup: diagnosis and management. *American Family Physician*, *97*(9), pp. 575–580. Available at: https://www.aafp.org/afp/2018/0501/p575.html
2. Johnson, D.W., 2014. Croup. *BMJ Clinical Evidence*. Available at: https://www.ncbi.nlm.nih.gov/pmc/articles/PMC4178284/
3. National Institute for Health and Care Excellence (2022) *Croup* [Online]. Available at: https://cks.nice.org.uk/topics/croup/
4. Kivekäs, I. and Rautiainen, M., 2018. Epiglottitis, acute laryngitis, and croup. In: Durand, M.L. and Deschler, D.G. (eds) *Infections of the Ears, Nose, Throat, and Sinuses*, Springer, Cham, pp. 247–255.
5. Hanna, J., Brauer, P.R., Morse, E. et al., 2019. Epidemiological analysis of croup in the emergency department using two national datasets. *International Journal of Pediatric Otorhinolaryngology*, *126*, p. 109641. Available at: https://pubmed.ncbi.nlm.nih.gov/31442871/

CHAPTER 33 Croup and Epiglottitis

6. Rosychuk, R.J., Klassen, T.P., Metes, D. et al., 2010. Croup presentations to emergency departments in Alberta, Canada: a large population-based study. *Pediatric Pulmonology*, *45*(1), pp. 83–91. Available at: https://pubmed.ncbi.nlm.nih.gov/19953656/
7. Rihkanen, H., Rönkkö, E., Nieminen, T. et al., 2008. Respiratory viruses in laryngeal croup of young children. *Journal of Pediatrics*, *152*(5), pp. 661–665. Available at: https://www.sciencedirect.com/science/article/pii/S0022347607010396
8. Knutson, D. and Aring, A.M., 2004. Viral croup. *American Family Physician*, *69*(3), pp. 535–540. Available at: https://www.aafp.org/pubs/afp/issues/2004/0201/p535.html
9. Sizar, O. and Carr, B., 2022. *Croup* [Online]. Available at: https://www.ncbi.nlm.nih.gov/pmc/articles/PMC4178284/
10. Almendra, M., Pereira, M.P., Gonçalves, C.S. et al., 2022. Croup and COVID-19. *Journal of Paediatrics and Child Health*. Available at: https://onlinelibrary.wiley.com/doi/10.1111/jpc.15987
11. Ortiz-Alvarez, O., 2017. Acute management of croup in the emergency department. *Paediatrics and Child Health*, *22*(3), pp. 166–169. Available at: https://academic.oup.com/pch/article/22/3/166/3852394
12. Bjornson, C.L. and Johnson, D.W., 2008. Croup. *Lancet*, *371*(9609), pp. 329–339. Available at https://www.sciencedirect.com/science/article/pii/S0140673608601701
13. Westley, C.R., Cotton, E.K. and Brooks, J.G., 1978. Nebulized racemic epinephrine by IPPB for the treatment of croup: a double-blind study. *American Journal of Diseases of Children*, *132*(5), pp. 484–487. Available at: https://pubmed.ncbi.nlm.nih.gov/347921/
14. Chan, A.K.J., Langley, J.M. and LeBlanc, J.C., 2001. Interobserver variability of croup scoring in clinical practice. *Paediatrics and Child Health*, *6*(6), pp. 347–351. Available at: https://academic.oup.com/pch/article/6/6/347/2655913
15. Bjornson, C.L. and Johnson, D.W., 2013. Croup in children. *Canadian Medical Association Journal*, *185*(15), pp. 1317–1323. Available at: https://pubmed.ncbi.nlm.nih.gov/23939212/
16. Yang, W.C., Lee, J., Chen, C.Y. et al., 2017. Westley score and clinical factors in predicting the outcome of croup in the pediatric emergency department. *Pediatric Pulmonology*, *52*(10), pp. 1329–1334. Available at: https://onlinelibrary.wiley.com/doi/10.1002/ppul.23738
17. Tibballs, J. and Watson, T., 2011. Symptoms and signs differentiating croup and epiglottitis. *Journal of Paediatrics and Child Health*, *47*(3), pp. 77–82. Available at: https://onlinelibrary.wiley.com/doi/10.1111/j.1440-1754.2010.01892.x
18. King-Schultz, L.W., Orvidas, L.J. and Mannenbach, M.S., 2015. Stridor is not always croup. *Pediatric Emergency Care*, *31*(2), pp. 140–143. Available at: https://pubmed.ncbi.nlm.nih.gov/25651384/
19. Oliveira, J.C., Azevedo, I., Gonçalves, A. et al., 2017. Stridor is not always croup: infantile haemangioma in the airway. *Case Reports*, *2017*, pp.bcr-2017. Available at: http://dx.doi.org/10.1136/bcr-2017-222449
20. Kumar, P., Kaushal, D., Garg, P.K. et al., 2019. Subglottic hemangioma masquerading as croup and treated successfully with oral propranolol. *Lung India: Official Organ of Indian Chest Society*, *36*(3), pp. 233–235. Available at: https://pubmed.ncbi.nlm.nih.gov/31031345/
21. BMJ Best Practice, 2023, *Croup* [Online]. Available at: https://bestpractice.bmj.com/topics/en-gb/681
22. Swain, S., Shajahan, N. and Debta, P., 2020. Acute epiglottitis – a life-threatening clinical entity. *Journal of Clinical and Scientific Research*, *9*(2), p. 110. Available at: https://go.gale.com/ps/i.do?id=GALE%7CA632314481&sid=googleScholar&v=2.1&it=r&linkaccess=abs&issn=22775706&p=HRCA&sw=w&userGroupName=anon%7E77ea3c5c&aty=open+web+entry
23. Davies, I. and Jenkins, I., 2017. Paediatric airway infections. *BJA Education*, *17*(10), pp. 341–345. Available at: https://www.bjaed.org/article/S2058-5349(17)30164-6/fulltext
24. Balfour-Lynn, I.M. and Wright, M., 2019. Acute infections that produce upper airway obstruction. In: Wilmott, R., Bush, A., Deterding, R. et al. (eds) *Kendig's Disorders of the Respiratory Tract in Children*, Elsevier. pp. 406–419.
25. Allen, M., Meraj, T.S., Oska, S. et al., 2021. Acute epiglottitis: analysis of US mortality trends from 1979 to 2017. *American Journal of Otolaryngology*, *42*(2), p. 102882. Available at: https://www.sciencedirect.com/science/article/abs/pii/S0196070920305767?via%3Dihub

26. BMJ Best Practice, 2023. *Epiglottitis* [Online]. Available at: https://bestpractice.bmj.com/topics/en-gb/452?q=Epiglottitis&c=suggested
27. Dowdy, R.A. and Cornelius, B.W., 2020. Medical management of epiglottitis. *Anesthesia Progress*, 67(2), pp. 90–97. Available at: https://anesthesiaprogress.kglmeridian.com/view/journals/anpr/67/2/article-p90.xml
28. Lee, D.R., Lee, C.H., Won, Y.K. et al., 2015. Clinical characteristics of children and adolescents with croup and epiglottitis who visited 146 emergency departments in Korea. *Korean Journal of Pediatrics*, 58(10), p. 380. Available at: https://www.e-cep.org/journal/view.php?doi=10.3345/kjp.2015.58.10.380
29. Tebruegge, M., Pantazidou, A., Thorburn, K. et al., 2009. Bacterial tracheitis: a multi-centre perspective. *Scandinavian Journal of Infectious Diseases*, 41(8), pp. 548–557. Available at: https://www.tandfonline.com/doi/full/10.1080/00365540902913478
30. Barengo, J.H., Redmann, A.J., Kennedy, P. et al., 2021. Demographic characteristics of children diagnosed with bacterial tracheitis. *Annals of Otology, Rhinology and Laryngology*, 130(12), pp. 1378–1382. Available at: https://journals.sagepub.com/doi/10.1177/00034894211007250
31. Casazza, G., Graham, M.E., Nelson, D. et al., 2019. Pediatric bacterial tracheitis – a variable entity: case series with literature review. *Otolaryngology – Head and Neck Surgery*, 160(3), pp. 546–549. Available at: https://aao-hnsfjournals.onlinelibrary.wiley.com/doi/10.1177/0194599818808774
32. Al-Mutairi, B. and Kirk, V., 2004. Bacterial tracheitis in children: approach to diagnosis and treatment. *Paediatrics and Child Health*, 9(1), pp. 25–30. Available at: https://academic.oup.com/pch/article/9/1/25/2648429
33. Pfleger, A. and Eber, E., 2013. Management of acute severe upper airway obstruction in children. *Paediatric Respiratory Reviews*, 14(2), pp. 70–77.
34. Abdallah, C., 2012. Acute epiglottitis: trends, diagnosis and management. *Saudi Journal of Anaesthesia*, 6(3), pp. 279–281. Available at: https://journals.lww.com/sjan/fulltext/2012/06030/acute_epiglottitis__trends,_diagnosis_and.18.aspx
35. Adil, E.A., Adil, A. and Shah, R.K., 2015. Epiglottitis. *Clinical Pediatric Emergency Medicine*, 16(3), pp. 149–153. Available at: https://www.sciencedirect.com/science/article/abs/pii/S1522840115000440?via%3Dihub
36. Cheng, T., Farah, J., Aldridge, N. et al., 2020. Pediatric respiratory distress: California out-of-hospital protocols and evidence-based recommendations. *Journal of the American College of Emergency Physicians Open*, 1(5), pp. 955–964. Available at: https://onlinelibrary.wiley.com/doi/10.1002/emp2.12103
37. Sakthivel, M., Elkashif, S., Al Ansari, K. et al., 2019. Rebound stridor in children with croup after nebulised adrenaline: does it really exist? *Breathe*, 15(1), pp. e1–e7. Available at: https://pubmed.ncbi.nlm.nih.gov/31031839/
38. Bjornson, C., Russell, K.F., Vandermeer, B. et al., 2012. Cochrane review: nebulized epinephrine for croup in children. *Evidence-Based Child Health*, 7(4), pp. 1311–1354. Available at: https://onlinelibrary.wiley.com/doi/10.1002/ebch.1856
39. Electronic Medicines Compendium, 2023. *Adrenaline (Epinephrine) Injection BP 1 in 1000* [Online]. Available at: https://www.medicines.org.uk/emc/product/6284/smpc#gref
40. Zhang, L. and Sanguebsche, L.S., 2005. The safety of nebulization with 3 to 5 ml of adrenaline (1: 1000) in children: an evidence based review. *Jornal de pediatria*, 81, pp. 193–197. Available at: https://www.jped.com.br/conteudo/Ing_resumo.asp?varArtigo=1334&cod=&idSecao=3
41. Gates, A., Gates, M., Vandermeer, B. et al., 2018. Glucocorticoids for croup in children. *Cochrane Database of Systematic Reviews*, (8). Available at: https://www.cochranelibrary.com/cdsr/doi/10.1002/14651858.CD001955.pub4/full
42. Ali, S., Moodley, A., Bhattacharjee, A. et al., 2018. Prehospital dexamethasone administration in children with croup: a medical record review. *Open Access Emergency Medicine*, 10, p. 141. Available at: https://pubmed.ncbi.nlm.nih.gov/30410413/
43. Francis, J., 2015. A critical analysis and appraisal of the management of croup in the UK out-of-hospital environment. *Journal of Paramedic Practice*, 7(6), pp. 292–298. Available at: https://www.magonlinelibrary.com/doi/abs/10.12968/jpar.2015.7.6.292

44. Joint Royal Colleges Ambulance Liaison Committee, 2019. *JRCALC Clinical Guidelines 2019*. Class Professional Publishing.
45. Sparrow, A. and Geelhoed, G., 2006. Prednisolone versus dexamethasone in croup: a randomised equivalence trial. *Archives of Disease in Childhood*, *91*(7), pp. 580–583. Available at: https://adc.bmj.com/content/91/7/580
46. Geelhoed, G.C. and Macdonald, W.B.G., 1995. Oral dexamethasone in the treatment of croup: 0.15 mg/kg versus 0.3 mg/kg versus 0.6 mg/kg. *Pediatric Pulmonology*, *20*(6), pp. 362–368. Available at: https://onlinelibrary.wiley.com/doi/10.1002/ppul.1950200605
47. Fifoot, A.A. and Ting, J.Y., 2007. Comparison between single-dose oral prednisolone and oral dexamethasone in the treatment of croup: a randomized, double-blinded clinical trial. *Emergency Medicine Australasia*, *19*(1), pp. 51–58. Available at: https://onlinelibrary.wiley.com/doi/10.1111/j.1742-6723.2006.00919.x
48. Parker, C.M. and Cooper, M.N., 2019. Prednisolone versus dexamethasone for croup: a randomized controlled trial. *Pediatrics*, *144*(3). Available at: https://publications.aap.org/pediatrics/article/144/3/e20183772/76989/Prednisolone-Versus-Dexamethasone-for-Croup-a?autologincheck=redirected
49. Great Ormond Street Hospital for Children, 2019. *Short-term steroid treatment* [Online]. Available at: https://www.gosh.nhs.uk/conditions-and-treatments/medicines-information/short-term-steroid-treatment/
50. Fernandes, R.M., Wingert, A., Vandermeer, B. et al., 2019. Safety of corticosteroids in young children with acute respiratory conditions: a systematic review and meta-analysis. *BMJ Open*, *9*(8), p. e028511. Available at: https://bmjopen.bmj.com/content/9/8/e028511
51. Moore, M. and Little, P., 2006. Humidified air inhalation for treating croup. *Cochrane Database of Systematic Reviews*, *3*. Available at: https://www.cochranelibrary.com/cdsr/doi/10.1002/14651858.CD002870.pub2/full
52. Rajapaksa, S. and Starr, M., 2010. Croup: assessment and management. *Australian Family Physician*, *39*(5), pp. 280–282. Available at: https://search.informit.org/doi/abs/10.3316/informit.143866152698583
53. Woods, C.R. and Kaplan, S.L., 2022. Patient education: croup in infants and children (beyond the basics). *UpToDate* [Online]. Available at: https://medilib.ir/uptodate/show/1201

34

Care of the Newborn: Assisting Transition, Stabilisation and Transport

Rosemarie Boland and James Yates

In this chapter you will learn:

- What changes occur during transition from intra-uterine (foetal) to extra-uterine (post-natal) life
- The importance of establishing effective breathing at birth
- Strategies for thermal control in a newborn
- Physiological benefits of delayed/deferred cord clamping
- Key principles of resuscitation of the newborn
- Stabilisation beyond resuscitation
- Considerations for transport.

Case Details

Dispatch

29-year-old female, 31 weeks pregnant, regular, strong contractions, every 3 minutes.

History

A 29-year-old female, who is 31 weeks pregnant, began experiencing strong, regular contractions at 0405. The contractions have been coming 3 minutes apart. Five minutes ago, the woman's membranes ruptured; the liquor is a straw-coloured fluid. This pregnancy has been uncomplicated to date. The woman is home alone with her 2-year-old, as her partner does shift work. This is her second child. Her first baby was born at 29 weeks.

On Arrival at the Scene

A paramedic crew arrive at the scene at 0415. The woman is in the bathroom and tells the crew she had a strong urge to push. The paramedics move the woman out of the bathroom and into the lounge. The foetal head is now visible at the perineum and with three further contractions, the baby is born. It is a male infant, with an estimated birth weight of 1.8–2 kg. The time of birth is recorded as 0424.

Decision Point

What are your clinical priorities in this case?

The priorities for care are broadly similar for all newborn babies, as are the associated interventions to reduce morbidity and mortality. The preterm newborn presents unique challenges, especially in paramedic practice, because of constraints on equipment and human resources.[1] Thermal care, establishment of effective ventilation and appropriate support for transition are three key priorities for this infant.

Question 1: What Are the Physiological, Anatomical and Biochemical Changes Involved in a Successful Transition from Foetal to Postnatal Life? What Are the Implications for Failure of Transition on the Need for Resuscitation?

The physiology of the foetus is very different from that of the newborn. In the foetus, the lungs are fluid filled, the site of gaseous exchange is the placenta, and blood is diverted away from the lungs via two shunts. At birth several key changes need to occur to allow successful transition from foetal to postnatal life. These are underpinned by the clearance of lung fluid and establishing regular effective breathing.

In the foetus, blood flow to the lungs is minimal (<8%) due to significant vasoconstriction of the pulmonary vessels, resulting in high pulmonary vascular resistance (PVR). Conversely, the systemic vascular resistance (SVR) is relatively low because resistance in the placenta is low. This results in most of the blood being shunted from right to left through the foramen ovale, an opening in the septum between the atria, and the ductus arteriosus, a small blood vessel connecting the pulmonary artery and aorta.

Following birth, an uncompromised newborn will make vigorous efforts to breathe and cry, which drive fluid out of the lungs and into the pulmonary lymphatics, establishing a functional residual capacity. Blood oxygen tension rises and SpO_2 rises from an intrapartum mean of 50–60%, to >90% within 10 minutes of birth. This leads to vasodilation of the pulmonary vasculature and a decrease in PVR, resulting in an eight- to ten-fold increase in pulmonary blood flow. The clamping of the umbilical cord and subsequent loss of the placental circulation lead to an increase in SVR. As PVR decreases and SVR increases, the pressure gradient across the ductus arteriosus reverses, resulting in shunting of blood from left to right, into the pulmonary circulation.[2] These changes cause left atrial pressure to rise, leading to closure of the foramen ovale. The rapid decrease in PVR and rise in oxygen tension, alongside withdrawal of prostaglandin E2, leads to constriction of the ductus arteriosus (DA), which then closes. Transition to extra-uterine life is then complete, with the functional closure of these foetal shunts occurring over 24–96 hours. Anatomical (permanent) closure occurs several weeks after birth.[3]

> **PRACTICE TIP**
>
> Aim to delay cord clamping by at least 60 seconds in an uncompromised newborn.

If the newborn fails to clear the foetal lung fluid and establish normal ventilatory function, the pulmonary vessels will remain constricted. Without intervention, the newborn can become rapidly hypoxic and acidotic, leading to further pulmonary vasoconstriction. This can result in the ductus arteriosus either not closing or re-opening, leading to a persistence of 'foetal-type' circulation, known as persistent pulmonary hypertension of the newborn (PPHN),

SECTION 9 Paediatrics, Obstetrics and Gynaecology

but without the placental circuit for oxygenation. This is not compatible with postnatal life. If this occurs, the newborn will require support to transition, with the primary focus being establishment of effective ventilation and oxygenation (see Question 4).

> **PRACTICE TIP**
>
> 'Resuscitation' is rarely required for newborns. Most respond to drying and stimulation alone, with only about 5% requiring help to establish effective breathing.

> **PRACTICE TIP**
>
> Effective ventilation is the key driver for transition. If the chest is not rising, check neutral head alignment, confirm mask seal, use a two-person technique or insert a supraglottic device.

Question 2: What Is the Evidence for Delayed/Deferred Cord Clamping and When Is It Indicated?

There is good evidence that delaying/deferring clamping of the umbilical cord (DCC), in uncompromised newborns, for at least 60 seconds after birth (time-based cord clamping) or after the onset or establishment of effective ventilation (physiological-based cord clamping) is beneficial.[4–6]

Establishing ventilation, either spontaneously or through positive-pressure ventilation, with the cord intact, allows pulmonary blood flow to increase before venous return from the placenta is lost. This results in a smoother transition to extra-uterine life, with increased placental transfusion, increased cardiac output, and higher and more stable neonatal blood pressure.[4,6] Longer-term benefits of DCC include increased haemoglobin levels at birth and improved iron levels. In uncomplicated preterm births <34 weeks, DCC for at least 30 seconds improves survival chances by 20%, reduces the need for inotropic support in the first 24 hours and decreases the need for blood transfusions.[7]

DCC for a minimum of 60 seconds should be undertaken for the infant born in good condition (see Question 4).[8–10]

There is less evidence and consensus about the benefits of DCC in compromised newborns[7] (see Question 4) and until there is further research to support this, initiating resuscitation interventions takes priority over delayed cord clamping. Cord milking/stripping is not recommended and can cause harm to preterm newborns.[8,9]

If undertaking DCC, thermal care must be optimised. If the paramedics arrive after the baby has been born, clamping the cord and initiating resuscitation interventions as needed are indicated.

Question 3: What Is the Evidence for Thermal Care and What Strategies Can Be Used to Maintain Normothermia?

Avoiding hypothermia and hyperthermia is essential and thermal control measures should be used to target a temperature range of 36.5–37.5 °C.[11] Newborn hypothermia is associated with a 28% increase in mortality for every 1 °C drop below 36.5 °C.[12] Multiple studies

CHAPTER 34 Care of the Newborn: Assisting Transition, Stabilisation and Transport

have demonstrated significant rates of hypothermia in infants born out of hospital,[13] likely associated with environmental stressors, lack of appropriate equipment, care priorities and education in newborn care.[14] Implementing measures to reduce hypothermia needs to be a key priority throughout the prehospital phase.

Heat is lost from the body through conduction, convection, radiation and evaporation. Newborns are particularly susceptible to heat loss as they are born wet, have less subcutaneous fat, a larger surface area to body mass ratio and a high body water content compared with older children. In addition, preterm infants <32 weeks' gestation also have immature skin, which results in greater insensible losses. There are many different interventions to prevent heat loss and a combination of approaches will be most effective.

> **PRACTICE TIP**
>
> Prevention of hypothermia is essential. Thermal care should start early and continue throughout stabilisation and transfer to hospital.

Environment

All newborns should be protected from draughts, and the temperature of the room should be increased if there is time. Alternatively, the mother or infant should be moved into a warmer environment if possible. The ambulance cabin should be preheated in case transport to hospital is required.

Term and Near-Term Infants (>32 Weeks)

Drying the newborn is an important first step immediately after birth, as this reduces evaporative losses as well as stimulating the infant. Place a hat on their head and swaddle them in a warm, clean towel. Bubble wrap, a polyethylene bag or foil blankets can be used as an external layer to surround the infant under the blanket.

If support to transition is required, an exothermic mattress should be activated, and the infant placed onto it. If no mattress is available, the newborn should be protected from any cold surfaces.

If resuscitation is not required, the infant may be placed skin-to-skin with a parent, placing a blanket over both parent and infant.

Preterm Infants (<32 Weeks' Gestation or <1800 g Birth Weight)

Due to their immature and delicate skin these infants should be placed directly into a food-grade plastic bag or wrap, without being dried.[11] This protects their skin from damage, while also reducing evaporative losses. Place them onto an activated thermal mattress, and put a hat on their head. The mattress and baby should then be wrapped in a clean, warm towel with bubble wrap or foil blankets as an outer layer.

If the infant does not need immediate resuscitation, they can be placed into the bag and then directly against the mother's chest, with a warm blanket over the top.

The temperature of the newborn should be monitored regularly after birth. Temperature is measured at the axilla as the ear canal is too narrow to facilitate accurate tympanic measurement.

SECTION 9 Paediatrics, Obstetrics and Gynaecology

Question 4: How Do We Assess Transition to Extra-Uterine Life? What Are the Key Interventions Required to Support Transition?

Initial Assessment of The Newborn

The first assessment of the newly born infant is based on three criteria: response to stimulation, breathing or crying and muscle tone. This is followed by an assessment of the heart rate.

After drying, an uncompromised newborn will cry and/or establish regular spontaneous breathing without any assistance. They will move all four limbs and adopt a flexed posture. Drying with a warmed towel provides the stimulation. Newborns should never be slapped, spanked or have their feet flicked.

The infant's heart rate is assessed via auscultation with a stethoscope after stimulating the infant to breathe. An uncompromised newborn will establish a rate >100 bpm within the first 2 minutes of postnatal age, with most achieving this within a minute of birth.

Colour does not form part of the initial assessment of the newborn because they may not have an SpO_2 >90% until up to 10 minutes of postnatal age, hence may initially appear dusky/cyanosed.[3,15]

Apgar scores are not used to guide resuscitation; these are assigned retrospectively. They are an indication of how well a newborn underwent transition unassisted or how well a newborn responded to resuscitation interventions.

The vast majority of newborns will transition successfully. Only about 6% of newborns require assistance to establish spontaneous breathing. Less than 0.7% of newborns require intubation at birth, and fewer than 0.2% require chest compressions.[11] Drugs are rarely indicated. Effective ventilation is the key to effective resuscitation of the newborn.

Signs of a Compromised Newborn Who Needs More Than Routine Care at Birth

- Flaccid, floppy, hypotonic despite stimulation.
- Apnoea or irregular, gasping respirations.
- Heart rate <100 bpm despite stimulation to breathe.
- Early onset of respiratory distress: laboured breathing, subcostal/intercostal recession.
- Severe pallor, especially in the presence of known/suspected foetal blood loss.

Immediate Care of the Uncompromised Newborn

If the newborn infant is breathing or crying, has good muscle tone and a HR >100 bpm, DCC should be undertaken and the newborn placed skin-to-skin on the mother's chest. Both mother and newborn should be covered with a warm blanket.

The infant should have regular assessment of breathing, heart rate, colour and tone, with Apgar scores being recorded at 1 and 5 minutes of age. A more detailed assessment of their condition should then be undertaken (see Question 5).

> **PRACTICE TIP**
>
> Use T(ABCDE)F to assess the newborn and identify care priorities once heart rate is >100 bpm.

CHAPTER 34 Care of the Newborn: Assisting Transition, Stabilisation and Transport

Assisting Transition of the Infant Who Needs More Than Routine Care at Birth

The first priority, after drying and stimulating the infant, is to establish effective ventilation. This takes priority over DCC in a compromised newborn. An infant who remains apnoeic or is gasping or has a heart rate that is not rising >100 bpm within a minute of birth will require positive-pressure ventilation (PPV).

A: Airway

Newborn infants have a large head with a prominent occiput, a short neck and large tongue. The trachea is shorter and narrower than that of an adult, and the larynx is higher and more anterior, positioned at C2–C3. A neutral head position, achieved with a small shoulder roll, is essential to open the airway. Flexion or hyperextension can occlude the airway.

Suctioning of the mouth and oropharynx is not routinely required. Initiating resuscitation interventions takes priority over tracheal suctioning in a compromised newborn. Only perform suctioning if a meconium plug is suspected.

B: Breathing

PPV should be provided at 40–60 inflations per minute, using a 240 mL self-inflating bag (SIB). Squeeze the bag gently, until rise and fall of the chest and upper abdomen is seen with each inflation. If a pressure manometer is available, set the peak inflation pressure to 30 cm H_2O for a term infant and 20–25 cm H_2O for a preterm infant <32 weeks. Inflation pressures of up to 50–60 cm H_2O may be needed for the first few inflations, as the lungs may still be liquid filled.[8] If a PEEP valve is available, it should be set at 5 cm H_2O. It is worth noting that some guidelines advocate the delivery of a set of sustained 'inflation breaths' before ventilations are provided.[10]

PPV should be commenced in room air. If a blender is available, then the use of supplemental oxygen should be guided by pre-ductal pulse oximetry using a neonatal sensor applied to the infant's right hand or wrist. Target SpO_2 levels in the first 10 minutes are shown in **Table 34.1**.[8]

Table 34.1 Target oxygen saturations in the first 10 minutes after birth

Time from birth	Target SpO_2
1 minute	60–70%
2 minutes	65–85%
3 minutes	70–**90%**
4 minutes	75–**90%**
5 minutes	80–**90%**
10 minutes	85–**90%**

Note: that from 3 minutes of postnatal age, the upper SpO_2 target remains **90%**

SECTION 9 Paediatrics, Obstetrics and Gynaecology

Titrating oxygen concentrations without a blender is very challenging. A flow of 6 L/min through a SIB with the reservoir bag on will deliver between 90% and 100% oxygen. Removing the reservoir bag will deliver approximately 70% oxygen and then reducing the flow to 1 L/min will deliver an oxygen concentration of 21%–70%.[16]

The effectiveness of PPV is confirmed by:

1. A rise in heart rate above 100 bpm
2. A slight rise and fall of the chest and upper abdomen with each positive-pressure inflation
3. An improvement in oxygenation.

If these are not seen:

- Check the mask seal. The mask should cover the nose and mouth but not cover the eyes.
- Ensure the head is in a neutral position.
- Increase the peak inflation pressure in 5 cm H_2O increments or squeeze the bag a bit harder.
- Consider a two-person technique – one person holding the mask seal and the other delivering inflations.
- Consider a supraglottic airway (laryngeal mask) – a size 1 is suitable for newborns >1500 g birth weight.
- Increase the oxygen according to target saturations.
- Endotracheal intubation can be considered in a compromised newborn if a person with expertise in neonatal intubation is available.

C: Circulation

After 30 seconds of *effective* PPV, if the infant's heart rate remains below 60 bpm, oxygen should be delivered at 100% and chest compressions started at ratio of 3:1. The two-thumb, hand encircling technique should be used for compressions, though the two-finger technique may be used if resources are few, such as a solo responder. Reassess the heart rate every 30 seconds. Once above 60 bpm, chest compressions can cease but PPV should continue until the heart rate is >100 bpm and the infant has established effective spontaneous breathing.

Blood loss should always be considered in an infant whose heart rate is not rising despite effective PPV, especially in the presence of suspected or known foetal blood loss. Volume replacement is indicated in this situation.[8]

D: Drugs

Drugs are rarely indicated in resuscitation of the newborn.

If the heart rate remains <60 bpm despite at least 30 seconds of chest compressions and PPV at a 3:1 ratio with 100% oxygen, adrenaline is indicated. Adrenaline 1:10,000 can be given via intraosseous (IO), intravenous (IV) or endotracheal tube (ETT), though the ETT route is the least preferable.

Volume replacement with 0.9% sodium chloride can be given via IO or IV if an infant appears shocked (pale, poor perfusion, weak pulses) or the heart rate is not rising despite effective PPV.

CHAPTER 34   Care of the Newborn: Assisting Transition, Stabilisation and Transport

Question 5: The Heart Rate Is Over 100 Bpm. How Do We Optimise the Condition of the Newborn and What Are the Considerations for Transport?

The newborn may have reached this point spontaneously after birth, or after a period of support to transition (see Question 4). It is important to now undertake a thorough assessment of the newborn using the modified T(ABCDE)F technique, which encourages ongoing thermal care and regular engagement with family members.

T: Thermal Control

- This needs to underpin all the processes of assessment, treatment and transport. Maintain existing thermal control measures but also plan ahead, for example warming up the ambulance cabin ready for departure.

A: Airway

- Wherever the newborn is positioned, either receiving skin-to-skin or lying on a surface, the head should remain in neutral alignment.
- If continued PPV is required, due to apnoea or inadequate respiratory effort, then a supraglottic airway (laryngeal mask) should be considered, if not already inserted, for newborns >32 weeks' gestation or >1500 g birth weight.[10] These can be secured with either a tie or tape.
- If the newborn is <32 weeks' gestation and/or <1500 g birth weight and requires ongoing positive-pressure ventilation, this should be delivered via an appropriately sized mask and SIB.

B: Breathing

- Assess the respiratory rate, anticipating a normal range of 40–60 breaths/min. There should be no signs of increased respiratory effort, such as subcostal recession, head bobbing or nasal flaring.
- A neonatal oxygen saturation sensor should be applied to the right hand or wrist, taking care to directly oppose the light and sensor, as well as protecting the sensor from external light. At 10 minutes, all newborns should have an SpO_2 >90% on room air, irrespective of gestational age.
- If the work of breathing is normal but oxygen saturations remain below target levels, supplemental oxygen can be delivered via a paediatric nasal cannula. The flow should be set to 1 L/min for all infants, but term newborns may have the flow titrated upwards to a maximum of 4 L/min, to reach target saturations of 90–95%.
- Face-mask CPAP, where available, set at 5–8 cm H_2O can be used for all spontaneously breathing newborns with a heart rate >100 bpm but signs of laboured breathing. Inspired oxygen concentration can be titrated to achieve target saturations.

SECTION 9 Paediatrics, Obstetrics and Gynaecology

C: Circulation

- The heart rate should be measured via auscultation over the precordial area, with an expected rate of between 140–160 bpm. A central capillary refill time should be less than 2 seconds.

D: Drugs

- A blood glucose level should be checked by a heel prick, aiming for >2.5 mmol/L.
- If blood glucose is <2.6 mmol/L:
  o Intramuscular (IM) glucagon may be administered to a compromised newborn.
  o An uncompromised infant >34 weeks' gestation can be encouraged to breast feed or be given 40% dextrose gel rubbed into the buccal membrane of the cheek.
  o A continuous intravenous (IV) or intraosseous (IO) infusion of 10% glucose may be administered at 60 ml/kg/day if appropriately skilled personnel and equipment are available and a prolonged transfer is anticipated.

E: Environment (And Everything Else)

- An axilla temperature should be measured regularly and the thermal care interventions adapted appropriately, aiming for 36.5–37.5 °C.
- Advice regarding treatment, need for onward transport and destination choice should be sought through local pathways, such as neonatal retrieval teams, receiving hospitals or remote senior clinical support.
- Plan transport with a particular focus on safety and ongoing thermal care. If possible, the newborn should not travel in a parent's arms during transport, unless in a commercially available restraint system. Travel harnesses should be used, where available, to safely restrain the newborn on the ambulance cot, with thermal control measures remaining in place, such as the thermal mattress.
- In the absence of approved restraint systems, a vacuum splint can be used to create a box shape, into which the newborn can be placed, with their thermal control packaging, and then secured to the stretcher.
- On arrival at hospital, the infant should not be carried into the department but left on, or placed into, the ambulance cot.

F: Family

- Family members should be offered the choice to be present during transitional support and ongoing care.[17]
- Regular updates and explanations to family members are essential. This will be an extremely stressful time for them.
- Conversations should be clear, with the avoidance of medical jargon, but also empathic and understanding. Open posture and body language should be adopted.

CHAPTER 34 Care of the Newborn: Assisting Transition, Stabilisation and Transport

Key Evidence

Knol, R., Brouwer, E., van den Akker, T. et al. (2020) 'Physiological-based cord clamping in very preterm infants – Randomised controlled trial on effectiveness of stabilisation', *Resuscitation*, 147, pp. 26–33.

Wyckoff, M. H., Wyllie, J., Aziz, K et al. (2020) 'Neonatal life support: 2020 International Consensus on Cardiopulmonary Resuscitation and Emergency Cardiovascular Care Science with Treatment Recommendations', *Circulation,* 142(16 suppl 1), pp. S185–S221.

Dainty, K. N., Atkins, D. L., Breckwoldt, J. et al. (2021) 'Family presence during resuscitation in paediatric and neonatal cardiac arrest: A systematic review', *Resuscitation*, 162, pp. 20–34.

Self-Reflection Questions

1. What maternal, foetal and intrapartum risk factors increase the likelihood of a newborn needing more than routine care at birth?
2. How would you manage failure to achieve chest rise after initial attempts via a self-inflating bag and mask?
3. How would you keep a preterm newborn <32 weeks' gestation warm, and how would you safely transport them to hospital?
4. What are the indications for advanced life support (advanced airway management, chest compressions, adrenaline) in newborn infants?
5. What differential diagnosis should be considered in a newborn who is not responding to effective positive pressure ventilation?

References

1. Boland, R. A., Davis, P. G., Dawson, J. A. et al. (2018) 'Very preterm birth before arrival at hospital', *Australia and New Zealand Journal of Obstetrics and Gynaecology*, 58(2), pp. 197–203.
2. Crossley, K. J., Allison, B. J., Polglase, G. R. et al. (2009) 'Dynamic changes in the direction of blood flow through the ductus arteriosus at birth', *Journal of Physiology*, 587(19), pp. 4695–4704.
3. van Vonderen, J. J., Roest, A. A. W., Siew, M. L. et al. (2014) 'Measuring physiological changes during the transition to life after birth', *Neonatology*, 105(3), pp. 230–242.
4. Polglase, G. R., Dawson, J. A., Kluckow, M. et al. (2015) 'Ventilation onset prior to umbilical cord clamping (physiological-based cord clamping) improves systemic and cerebral oxygenation in preterm lambs', *PLoS One*, 10(2), p. e0117504.
5. Knol, R., Brouwer, E., van den Akker, T. et al. (2020) 'Physiological-based cord clamping in very preterm infants – Randomised controlled trial on effectiveness of stabilisation', *Resuscitation*, 147, pp. 26–33.
6. Bhatt, S., Alison, B. J., Wallace, E. M. et al. (2013) 'Delaying cord clamping until ventilation onset improves cardiovascular function at birth in preterm lambs', *Journal of Physiology*, 591(8), pp. 2113–2126.
7. Katheria, A., Hosono, S. and El-Naggar, W. (2018) 'A new wrinkle: Umbilical cord management (how, when, who)', *Seminars in Foetal and Neonatal Medicine*, 23(5), pp. 321–326.
8. Australian and New Zealand Committee on Resuscitation (2021) *Section 13: Neonatal Guidelines*. Available at: https://www.anzcor.org/home/neonatal-resuscitation/
9. Wyckoff, M. H., Singletary, E. M., Soar, J. et al. (2021) '2021 international consensus on cardiopulmonary resuscitation and emergency cardiovascular care science with treatment recommendations: Summary from the Basic Life Support; Advanced Life Support; Neonatal Life Support; Education, Implementation, and Teams; First Aid Task Forces; and the COVID-19 Working Group', *Resuscitation,* 169, pp. 229–311.
10. Madar, J., Roehr, C. C., Ainsworth, S. et al. (2021) 'European Resuscitation Council Guidelines 2021: Newborn resuscitation and support of transition of infants at birth', *Resuscitation,* 161, pp. 291–326.

11. Wyckoff, M. H., Wyllie, J., Aziz, K et al. (2020) 'Neonatal life support: 2020 International Consensus on Cardiopulmonary Resuscitation and Emergency Cardiovascular Care Science with Treatment Recommendations', *Circulation,* 142(16 suppl 1), pp. S185–S221.
12. Laptook, A. R., Salhab, W. and Bhaskar, B. (2007) 'Admission temperature of low birth weight infants: predictors and associated morbidities', *Pediatrics,* 119(3), pp. e643–e649.
13. Goodwin, L., Voss, S., McClelland, G. et al. (2022) 'Temperature measurement of babies born in the pre-hospital setting: Analysis of ambulance service data and qualitative interviews with paramedics', *Emergency Medicine Journal*, 39(11), pp. 826–832.
14. McLelland, G. E., Morgans, A. E. and McKenna, L. G. (2014) 'Involvement of emergency medical services at unplanned births before arrival to hospital: A structured review', *Emergency Medicine Journal*, 31(4), pp. 345–350.
15. Dawson, J. A., Kamlin, C. O. F., Vento, M. et al. (2010) 'Defining the reference range for oxygen saturation for infants after birth', *Pediatrics*, 125, pp. 1340–1347.
16. Thió, M., Bhatia, R., Dawson, J. A. et al. (2010) 'Oxygen delivery using neonatal self-inflating resuscitation bags without a reservoir', *Archives of Disease in Childhood. Foetal and Neonatal Edition*, 95(5), pp. F315–319.
17. Dainty, K. N., Atkins, D. L., Breckwoldt, J. et al (2021) 'Family presence during resuscitation in paediatric and neonatal cardiac arrest: A systematic review', *Resuscitation*, 162, pp. 20–34.

Maternal Bleeding: Postpartum Haemorrhage and Active Management of the Third Stage of Labour

35

Mark Durham and Dawn Kerslake

> **In this chapter you will learn:**
> - The definition(s) of postpartum haemorrhage (PPH)
> - The different pathologies behind PPH
> - Management options and priorities.

Case Details

Dispatch
30-year-old female, bleeding after delivery.

History
A 30-year-old woman has just given birth to her fourth child (fifth pregnancy). The caller advises that this was an unexpected delivery at 37 weeks. The woman had suffered sudden abdominal cramps, then birthed and is losing 'a lot of blood' now. Two double-crewed ambulances and a critical care paramedic were dispatched.

On Arrival of the First Crew
The scene is safe, and the patient is sitting on the bathroom floor upstairs in a two-storey house. Her primary survey findings and initial vital signs are:

Airway	Patent
Breathing	RR 20, SpO$_2$ 99% on room air
Circulation	Peripheral pulses present, HR 118, BP 140/96, warm peripheries
Disability	GCS E4, V5, M6 (15), BGL 7.1 mmol/L
Environmental	Temp 37.6 °C

The first crew arrive on scene and pass an update that the patient is losing blood rapidly. They cut the cord and dry the baby, noting him to be healthy and vigorous. They pass him to his mother and apply oxygen to her. The crew begin massaging the uterus to slow bleeding.

They ask whether there have been any concerns during the pregnancy and the patient's partner advises there have not, but that she also bled last time she gave birth.

SECTION 9 Paediatrics, Obstetrics and Gynaecology

On Your Arrival as the Critical Care Paramedic

The patient is becoming pale and drowsy, and the blood loss is likely more than a litre and continuing rapidly. The crew tell you that the uterus still feels 'boggy' despite uterine massage.

AMPLE

The patient was normally fit and well prior to pregnancy, working as a delivery driver and generally active. Non-smoker. During her second trimester she developed gestational hypertension.

Allergies	NKDA
Medications	Pregnancy vitamin supplements Nifedipine
Past history	Gravid 5, Para 4 (now) Previous postpartum haemorrhage
Last ins and outs	Normal; passed faeces during birth
Events prior	Unexpected delivery at 37 weeks Problem-free pregnancy until now, aside from essential hypertension

Decision Point

What are your clinical priorities in this situation?

What are your options regarding management? How should you prioritise them?

Question 1: What Are Primary and Secondary Postpartum Haemorrhage?

Postpartum haemorrhage (PPH) is generally defined by volume, though details vary across the world (**Table 35.1**). Broadly speaking, primary PPH is held to be significant blood loss soon after

Table 35.1 Example definitions of postpartum haemorrhage

Issuing body	Definition (primary PPH)	Comments
World Health Organization[1]	>500 ml blood loss (regardless of route of delivery)	Probably the widest accepted definition; also, the simplest.
Royal College of Obstetricians and Gynaecologists[2]	Mild PPH = 500–1,000 ml Moderate PPH = 1,000–2,000 ml Severe PPH = 2,000+ ml	Allows for a more targeted response but relies more heavily on accurate estimation of blood loss.
American College of Obstetrics and Gynecology[3]	>1,000 ml (regardless of route of delivery) Any bleeding that causes haemodynamic instability	This allows for inaccuracy on estimating blood loss; however, clinical signs of haemodynamic instability are known to present late in third trimester pregnancy.

CHAPTER 35 Maternal Bleeding: Postpartum Haemorrhage and Active Management

the second stage of labour (within 24 hours) and is often associated with very rapid blood loss. Secondary PPH on the other hand is generally considered significant bleeding over the days/weeks following birth (usually up to six weeks) and can be associated with a more insidious loss.

There is nonetheless strong consensus that PPH is a leading (and often preventable) cause of maternal death.[4,5] Depending on the country, and on the definition used, PPH can occur in 5–20% of all births taking place in higher-income countries.[6,7] The fact that 94% of deaths due to PPH occur in lower- and middle-income countries[8] therefore illustrates how preventable these deaths can be if the right interventions can be brought to bear in a timely fashion, and within a co-ordinated healthcare system. Indeed, a confidential enquiry into UK maternal deaths has consistently shown that these deaths can be avoidable.[9]

One of the key factors in preventing death from PPH is early recognition.[9] If recognition depends on the blood volume lost, one must also bear in mind how consistently inaccurate healthcare staff are at estimating this. For instance, an American case review report identified inaccuracy in estimation of loss to be a major cause of delay in implementing PPH protocols,[10] while an older in vitro study of 92 EMS providers showed that across a range of scenarios, 24% of estimates failed to be within 50% of the actual volume, with just 8% managing to be within 20%.[11] Evidence suggests that clinicians will tend to overestimate in cases of lower blood loss, or when blood is on clothing, and underestimate blood on carpet or in cases of more significant blood loss.[12,13] **Figure 35.1** shows two different volumes of 'blood'.

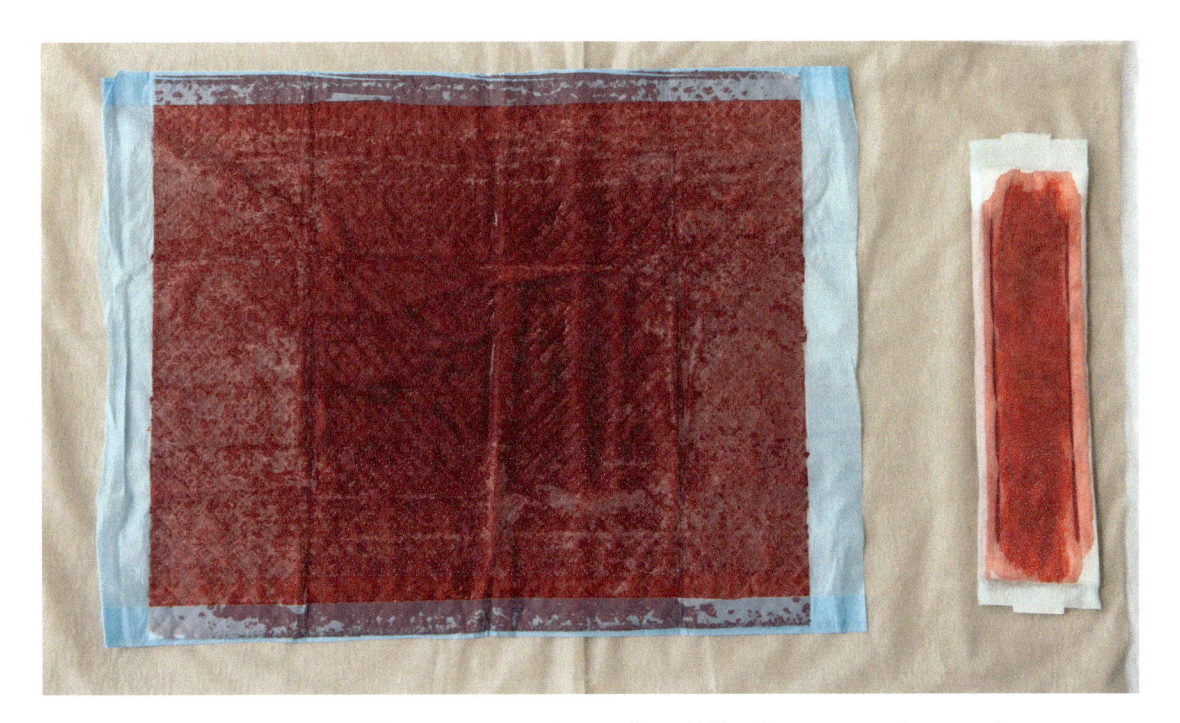

Figure 35.1 500 mL blood loss on maternity pad and 50 mL on maternity towel.
Source: Joint Royal Colleges Ambulance Liaison Committee, Association of Ambulance Chief Executives (2022). *JRCALC Clinical Guidelines*. Bridgwater: Class Publishing Ltd.

SECTION 9　Paediatrics, Obstetrics and Gynaecology

Estimate the amount of blood yourself, then read the caption for the answer. In practice, estimates can be further refined/contextualised by including other factors, such as rate of loss and clinical presentation.

Question 2: What Is the Physiology/Pathophysiology Behind Postpartum Haemorrhage?

Of the many maternal changes of the third trimester, the most relevant in the context of PPH includes a slight increase in red blood cell count, but a greater (40%) increase in plasma volume. This leads not just to a relative anaemia, but also to a dilutional reduction in clotting factors. Not only does this impact on someone's ability to clot, but it also means that they will show signs of shock much later than might be expected.

As the organ for blood exchange between a foetus and its mother, the placenta is a crucial organ to consider in postpartum haemorrhage. It functions as lungs, liver and kidneys for the baby in utero; it is highly vascular, perfused by something in the order of 120 spiral arteries.[14] Elsewhere in this book, one will consider that bleeding from an artery is a medical emergency. Here, one must consider bleeding from 120 arteries, simultaneously.

During pregnancy, the spiral arteries perfusing the placenta lose their own muscle layer (to increase flow capacity). During the third stage of labour, therefore, these arteries are entirely dependent on myometrial contraction to 'tie off', control bleeding and facilitate endometrial separation for the third stage of labour.

The most common causes of postpartum haemorrhage can be broadly categorised into 'four Ts':

- Tone (lack of effective myometrial contraction)
- Tissue (retained tissue in the uterus)
- Tears/trauma
- Thrombin (clotting disorders).

These have been listed in order of commonality, with uterine atony making up 60–80%.[15,16] These can occur concomitantly, especially tissue retention and uterine atony. Before going into these causes in greater detail, it is important to observe evidence from a large case-control study from Norway:[16] the single greatest risk factor for severe PPH is previous history of the same. Some of the more common other risk factors include over-distension of the uterine muscle (such as may occur with twins or very large infants), very rapid or very prolonged births, placenta praevia and pregnancy-induced hypertension. Predicting the possibility of PPH before it begins can save vital minutes in implementing care in time.

> **PRACTICE TIP**
>
> The single biggest risk factor to look for with severe PPH is previous history of the same. Predicting a PPH before it happens can save time – and life!

Tone

If the arteries of the placenta are dependent upon myometrial contractions, it is perhaps unsurprising that uterine atony is a significant majority cause of PPH. Accordingly, many of

CHAPTER 35 Maternal Bleeding: Postpartum Haemorrhage and Active Management

the approaches to managing primary PPH seek primarily to achieve uterine tone. Risk factors for uterine atony include prolonged labour, precipitate labour (as in the case study above), uterine distension (such as multi-foetal gestation, polyhydramnios or foetal macrosomia), prolonged use of oxytocin (inducing labour) or magnesium sulphate infusions (for example, for eclampsia), since it is a smooth muscle relaxant.

Tissue

The myometrium will not contract effectively and fully close the spiral arteries if the placenta is still in situ. Retained placenta is therefore closely associated with uterine atony and can be a cause of primary PPH. Over the longer term, retained placental tissue will become necrotic, and the resulting endometritis (not to be confused with endometriosis) can cause sepsis, thrombotic disorders and secondary PPH.

Tears

It is not just the placenta that can bleed postpartum. The genital and peri-genital areas are also extremely vascular and can bleed profusely if torn during the second stage of labour. The most common sites are the cervix or tissues of the vagina, perineum or bleeding into a haematoma, for example, in the pelvic space. Bleeding from such causes is slightly distinct from others in that it may be compressible.

Thrombin

Unsurprisingly, disorders of the body's ability to clot play a significant role in PPH. This is especially the case given the dilutional reduction in clotting factors mentioned previously. If, during pregnancy, a person needs to be put on anticoagulants (for example, for a pulmonary embolus, itself predisposed by pregnancy), this can be a delicate balance.

Disseminated intravascular coagulopathy (DIC) further impacts upon risk/severity of haemorrhage. This can be a direct consequence of haemorrhage, especially in severe primary PPH. It is worth noting, however, that DIC can also be caused/further disposed by conditions such as eclampsia, HELLP syndrome (closely related to eclampsia – a syndrome characterised by haemolysis, elevated liver enzymes and low platelet count) and placental abruption. A retrospective case control study from a tertiary centre in Seoul suggested that DIC was implicated in 22.4% of the 255 patients with primary PPH that it looked at.[17] DIC can be associated with more subacute conditions as well, such as sepsis arising from retained tissue, leading to secondary PPH.

Question 3: What Are the Common Treatment Options?

Fundal Massage

In cases of haemorrhage, massage will form the initial mainstay of most prehospital treatment regimes. It is quick to implement, simple to teach and retain, and effective. The fundus (top of the uterus) will be roughly the same number of centimetres above the pubic bone as the gestational age. At term therefore, it will be roughly halfway between the umbilicus and the sternum (40 cm above the pubic bone).

With the side of the hand, press into the abdomen just above the fundus and press downwards, massaging in circles. An atonic uterus will feel boggy. As the massage stimulates myometrial contraction, it will feel more like a cricket ball/baseball under the skin. In cases of haemorrhage (distinct from active management of the third stage), massage will have to be maintained, otherwise the muscles may relax again and bleeding will recommence.

Uterotonic drugs

Uterotonic drugs include oxytocin, ergot alkaloids and prostaglandins. **Table 35.2** shows some of the typical agents used. These agents can be given in combination and are often supplied as combination drugs themselves (such as Syntometrine – an oxytocin/ergot alkaloid combination).

Tranexamic Acid

Tranexamic acid is an antifibrinolytic agent which stabilises clots and has been shown by an international, double-blinded, randomised controlled trial to reduce deaths by up to a third if administered within three hours of childbirth, but with no evidenced benefit thereafter.[20,22]

Table 35.2 Typical uterotonic drugs in use today

Type of agent	Example (trade name)	Pharmacokinetic overview[18–21]	Pharmacodynamic overview[18,19]	Notes
Oxytocin/ oxytocin analogue	Syntocinon	IV or IM use. Half-life = 1-6 mins.	Binds directly to myometrial smooth muscle, inducing rhythmic contraction of upper uterus. Almost immediate IV effect, peak concentration ~30 mins; IM onset 3–7 minutes; clinical effect ~1 hour.	Preparations usually light- and temperature-sensitive (requires refrigeration).
Long-lasting oxytocin analogue	Duratocin	IV or IM use. Half-life = 40 mins.	Binds directly to myometrial smooth muscle, inducing rhythmic contraction of upper uterus. Takes effect over a few minutes IV, and lasts up to an hour. IM injection will take effect over around 10 minutes, clinical effect ~2 hours.	Available as heat-stable preparation.

CHAPTER 35 Maternal Bleeding: Postpartum Haemorrhage and Active Management

Type of agent	Example (trade name)	Pharmacokinetic overview[18–21]	Pharmacodynamic overview[18,19]	Notes
Prostaglandins	Carboprost, misoprostol (synthetic analogue)	Depending on the presentation, can be administered IM (carboprost) or sublingually/rectally/vaginally (misoprostol). Half-life (injection) = 8 minutes. Half-life (sublingual/PR administration) = 20–40 minutes.	Enhance generalised uterine contractility, by promoting the expression of oxytocin receptors. Also promote vasoconstriction by direct action. Injectable preparations peak plasma concentrations = 15 minutes or more. Sublingual/rectal onset of action ~9–15 minutes.	Carboprost requires refrigeration but can tolerate being removed for short periods. Misoprostol tablets are heat stable.
Ergot alkaloids	Ergometrine	IM or IV use. Half-life = 30–120 minutes.	Induce tetanic smooth muscle contraction of upper and lower uterus. IV onset almost immediate (<1 minute), clinical effect ~45 minutes. IM onset 2–3 minutes, clinical effect up to 3 hours.	Will raise blood pressure, which can be problematic if hypertension is already pathologically present.

N.B. Before giving any uterotonic drug you **must** be sure there is no other foetus in utero.

It can be given IV, but a currently small and preliminary pool of research (currently restricted to the trauma setting) suggests that intramuscular administration may be a viable option also.[21–24]

Volume Replacement

There is currently a degree of controversy surrounding optimal strategy for fluid resuscitation in PPH. Traditional wisdom supports the use of large volumes of fluid replacement (for example, up to 3.5 litres of crystalloid).[23,25] There is a growing movement, however, to investigate use of more controlled volumes[24–27] to minimise dilutional coagulopathy, chloraemic acidosis and (in services without ambulance-borne fluid warmers) hypothermia – in line with thinking from trauma research.[26,28] Regardless of what locally approved strategy dictates, volume replacement in uncontrolled PPH will require wide-bore IV access, possibly in multiple sites.

Non-Pneumatic Anti-Shock Trousers

Pneumatic anti-shock trousers work by applying pressure to the lower body, reducing blood flow there and reducing bleeding, while increasing preload and perfusion to the vital organs. They were developed by NASA for high-G flying and adopted into prehospital trauma care in the late twentieth century. They fell out of use in trauma because of the risks of over-inflation, causing problems such as kidney injury and compartment syndrome, as well as a blood pressure crash upon removal, which was difficult to deal with in the ED.[18,27]

In more recent years, non-pneumatic variants have received attention for treatment of PPH (**Figure 35.2**), especially in lower- and middle-income countries.[19,28] Evidence suggests that in this context they are safer and provide significant benefits in terms of mortality and extreme adverse incidents. For instance, a large (n = 142) before/after study compared mortality and adverse events rates in Nigeria and Egypt,[28] while a more recent study was non-comparative, but looked at a case series in Colombia.[18] To date there has been no study looking at their use in any prehospital system that fields advanced prehospital care; in fact, evidence of their use in higher-income systems generally is currently lacking.

Bi-Manual Compression

Bi-manual compression is a recognised and accepted method for providing direct pressure to an otherwise incompressible bleed, to slow blood loss pending definitive control.[1] It is an aggressive manoeuvre to be used only in extremis and should only be considered when both uterotonics and fundal massage have already been attempted (and have proven insufficient). It is a uniquely invasive and socially sensitive manoeuvre, and the importance of maternal consent and clear communication with all those on scene cannot be overstated – regardless of time criticality.

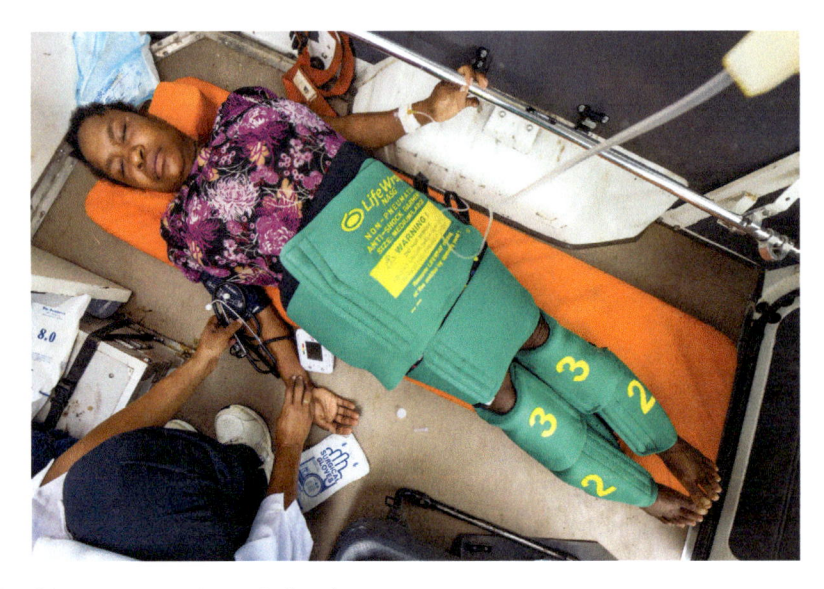

Figure 35.2 Non-pneumatic anti-shock trousers.
Source: UNICEF/UNI328410/Dozier. Reproduced with permission.

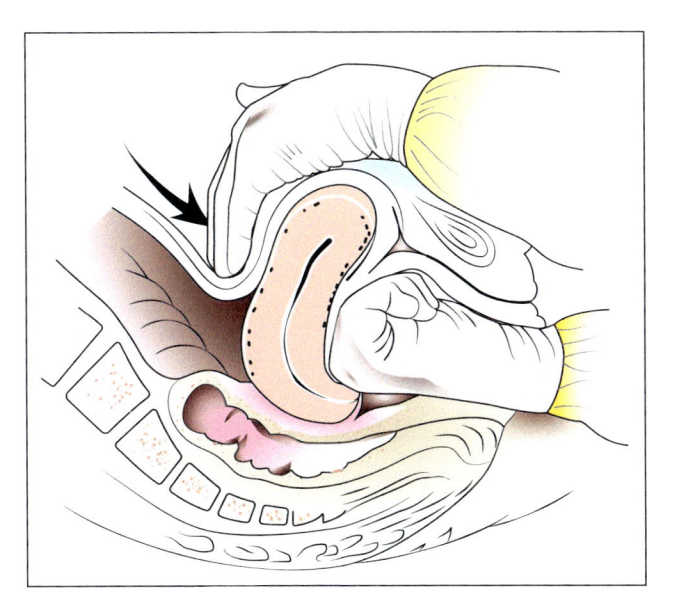

CHAPTER 35 Maternal Bleeding: Postpartum Haemorrhage and Active Management

Figure 35.3 Bi-manual compression.

As per **Figure 35.3**, one hand is inserted into the lower vagina with fingers curled, and then clenched into a fist (as best as possible). The other hand then presses from the fundus down onto this hand.

> **PRACTICE TIP**
>
> Bi-manual compression is an aggressive and invasive manoeuvre that requires both hands and effectively ties up one team member for the duration of the incident. While it may be the senior clinician who decides upon the need for bi-manual compression, a good strategy would be to find the team member with the smallest hands and talk them through performing the procedure.

> **PRACTICE TIP**
>
> Suckling stimulates the release of oxytocin and, in turn, uterine contractions. While it has many benefits in the management of an uncomplicated third stage, there is insufficient evidence to recommend its use in PPH under any definitions given in this chapter.

Question 4: What Is the Order of Priorities in the Management of This Patient With PPH?

In light of the discussion of treatment options, the case study above might look like this (**Figure 35.4**):

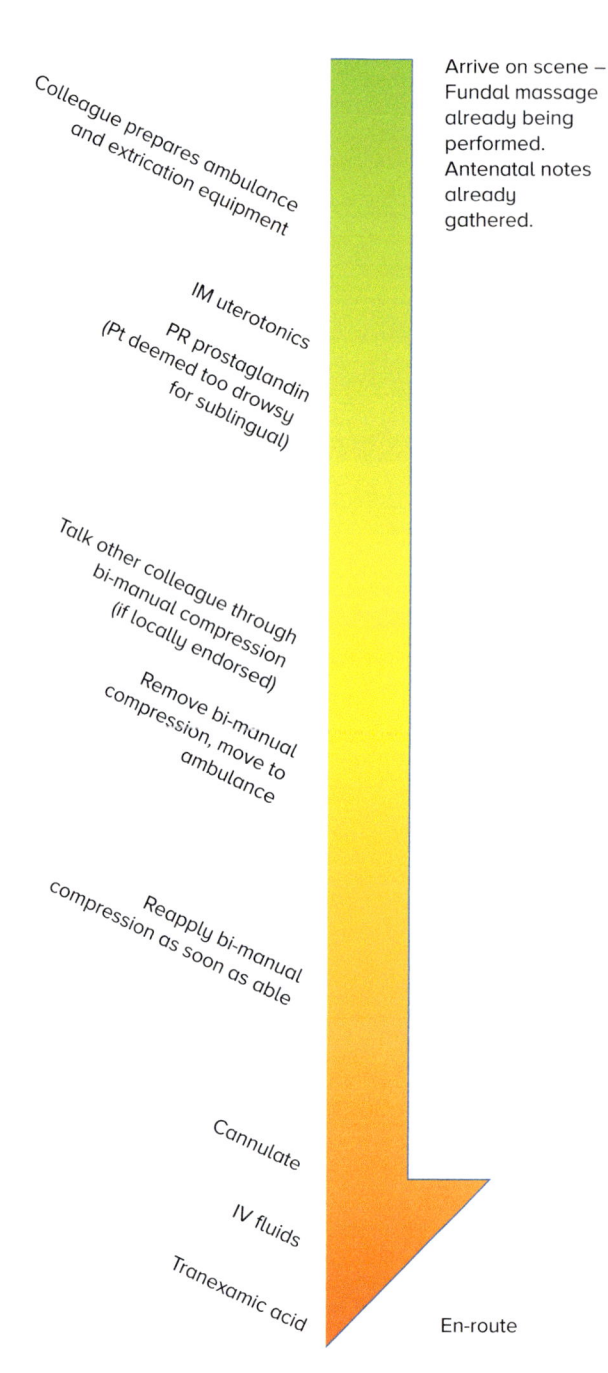

SECTION 9 Paediatrics, Obstetrics and Gynaecology

Figure 35.4 Illustrative timeline for the case study.
Source: Image by Dawn Kerslake and Mark Durham

CHAPTER 35 Maternal Bleeding: Postpartum Haemorrhage and Active Management

- You send a colleague out to prepare for extrication (ambulance facing in the right direction with the heating running, and extrication equipment brought in); meanwhile, you gather the mother's antenatal records.
- You draw and administer an intramuscular uterotonic (such as Syntometrine).
- By this stage, you consider the patient too drowsy for oral misoprostol, so you elect to give it per rectum.
- Your crewmate is not yet back from the ambulance, so you gather specific consent and talk a second colleague through the process of bi-manual compression (depending on regional guidance). Your colleague applies bi-manual compression, pending extrication.
- The first crew member returns from the ambulance with the trolley bed at the bottom of the stairs. Unfortunately, bi-manual pressure must be removed while you assist the patient onto a carry sheet/lifting chair and get her down the stairs (you would have preferred to walk her for the sake of speed, but she is too drowsy by this stage).
- You load the patient into the ambulance and bi-manual compression is recommenced.
- You transport to the nearest consultant-led obstetric unit (somewhere with an obstetric theatre attached).
- You attach monitoring, reassess the patient as the vehicle is pulling away, and pass a pre-alert to the receiving centre, indicating the need for blood.
- You gain IV access en route and give tranexamic acid and fluids, as per local guidance.

> **PRACTICE TIP**
>
> If secondary PPH presents in the first couple of days after labour, it is likely to be a similar cause to primary PPH – uterine atony or retained tissue (note: when considering tranexamic acid, this is still over three hours after presentation).
>
> If secondary PPH presents later than this, and especially if accompanied with dysmenorrhoea, consider necrotic retained tissue, endometritis and sepsis.

Key Evidence

This is some of the current pool of evidence and international guidance significantly shaping management of postpartum haemorrhage in the world today.

Systematic Review/Meta-Analyses

Begley C.M., Gyte G.M.L., Devane D. et al. 2014. Active versus expectant management for women in the third stage of labour. *Cochrane Database of Systematic Reviews*, (11):1–161.

Randomised Controlled Trials

Mavrides E., Allard S., Chandraharan E. et al. on behalf of the Royal College of Obstetricians and Gynaecologists. 2016. Prevention and management of postpartum haemorrhage (Green-top Guideline No. 52). *British Journal of Obstetrics and Gynaecology*, 124(5):e106–e149.

Shakur H., Roverts I., Fawole B. et al. 2017. Effect of early tranexamic acid administration on mortality, hysterectomy, and other morbidities in women with post-partum haemorrhage (WOMAN): an international, randomised, double-blind, placebo-controlled trial. *Lancet*, 389(10084):2105–2116.

SECTION 9 Paediatrics, Obstetrics and Gynaecology

Van der Nelson H., O'Brien S., Burnard S. et al. 2020. Intramuscular oxytocin versus Syntometrine® versus carbetocin for prevention of primary postpartum haemorrhage after vaginal birth: a randomised double-blinded clinical trial of effectiveness, side effects and quality of life. *British Journal of Obstetrics and Gynaecology*, 128(7):1236–1246.

National/International Guidelines

Escobar M.F., Nassar A,H., Therno G. et al. 2022. FIGO recommendations on the management of postpartum hemorrhage 2022. *International Journal of Gynecology and Obstetrics,* 1557(Suppl.1):3–50.

Self-Reflection Questions

1. What do you think is the best fluid resuscitation strategy for PPH in the prehospital setting?
2. How is the pathophysiology of bleeding different between PPH and trauma in terms of tissue damage and cell mediators? To what extent do you think this difference holds in the presence of decompensating shock and global hypoperfusion?
3. If the baby requires clinical attention as well, how will you split your attention/resources between them? How might this change your priorities/actions?
4. When might you walk the patient out of the house for speed, and at what stage would you resort to extricating them?
5. Depending on local systems, these patients are unlikely to go to the emergency department for handover, but rather directly to obstetric theatres. How might this affect your handover process?

References

1. World Health Organization. 2012. *WHO recommendations for the prevention and treatment of postpartum haemorrhage.* Geneva: WHO Press.
2. Mavrides E., Allard S., Chandraharan E. et al. on behalf of the Royal College of Obstetricians and Gynaecologists. 2016. Prevention and management of postpartum haemorrhage (Green-top Guideline No. 52). *British Journal of Obstetrics and Gynaecology*, 124(5):e106–e149.
3. Shields L.E., Goffman D. and Caughey A.B. on behalf of the American College of Obstetricians and Gynecologists. Postpartum hemorrhage (practice bulletin No.183). *Obstetrics and Gynecology*, 130(4): e168–e186.
4. Say L., Chou D., Gemmill A., et al. 2014. Global causes of maternal death: a WHO systematic analysis. *Lancet*, 2(6):e323–e333.
5. Aukes A.M., Arion K., Bone J.N. et al. 2021. Causes and circumstances of maternal death: a secondary analysis of the Community-Level Interventions for Pre-eclampsia (CLIP) trials cohort. *Lancet Global Health*, 9(9):e1242–e1251.
6. Knight M., Callaghan W.M., Berg C. et al. 2009. Trends in postpartum hemorrhage in high resource countries: a review and recommendations from the International Postpartum Hemorrhage Collaborative Group. *Biomed Central Pregnancy and Childbirth*, 27(9):55.
7. Flood M., McDonald S.J., Pollock W. et al. 2019. Incidence, trends and severity of primary postpartum haemorrhage in Australia: a population-based study using Victorian Perinatal Data Collection data for 764 244 births. *Australian and New Zealand Journal of Obstetrics and Gynaecology*, 59(2):228–234.
8. World Health Organization. 2019. *Maternal Mortality.* [online] Available at: https://www.who.int/news-room/fact-sheets/detail/maternal-mortality#:~:text=94%25%20of%20all%20maternal%20deaths,lives%20of%20women%20and%20newborns.
9. Knight M., Bunch K., Patel R. et al. (eds), on behalf of MBRRACE-UK. 2022. *Saving Lives, Improving Mothers' Care Core Report – Lessons learned to inform maternity care from the UK and Ireland Confidential Enquiries into Maternal Deaths and Morbidity 2018–20.* Oxford: National Perinatal Epidemiology Unit, University of Oxford.

CHAPTER 35 Maternal Bleeding: Postpartum Haemorrhage and Active Management

10. Seacrist M.J., VanOtterloo L.R., Morton C.H. et al. 2019. Quality improvement opportunities identified through case review of pregnancy-related deaths from obstetric hemorrhage. *Journal of Obstetrics, Gynecologic and Neonatal Nursing*, 48(3):288–299.
11. Patton K.R., Funk D.L., McErlean M. et al. 2001. Accuracy of estimation of external blood loss by EMS personnel. *Journal of Trauma*, 50(5):914–916.
12. Tall G., Wise D., Grove P. et al. 2003. The accuracy of external blood loss estimation by ambulance and hospital personnel. *Trauma and Emergency Medicine*, 15(4):318–321.
13. Natrella M., Di Naro E., Loverro M. et al. 2018. The more you lose the more you miss: accuracy of postpartum blood loss visual estimation. A systematic review of the literature. *Journal of Maternal–Fetal and Neonatal Medicine*, 31(1):106–115.
14. Brosens I.A. (1988). The utero-placental vessels at term – the distribution and extent of physiological changes. In: Kaufmann P., Miller R.K. (eds), *Placental Vascularization and Blood Flow. Trophoblast Research, vol 3*. Boston: Springer.
15. Solanki S., Bijarniya R. and Mittal D. 2021. Study of risk factors of post-partum hemorrhage and its outcome at tertiary care. *International Journal of Science and Research,* 10(2):1367–1369.
16. Nyfløt L.T., Sandven, I., Stray-Pedersen B. et al. 2017. Risk factors for severe postpartum hemorrhage: a case-control study. *BMC Pregnancy and Childbirth*, 17(1):17–26.
17. Sohn C.H., Kim S.R., Kim Y-J. et al. 2017. Disseminated intravascular coagulation in emergency department patients with primary postpartum hemorrhage. *Shock*, 48(3):329–332.
18. World Health Organization. 2018. *WHO Recommendations: Uterotonics for the Prevention of Postpartum Haemorrhage*. Geneva: World Health Organization.
19. Joint Formulary Committee. 2022. *British National Formulary September 2022–March 2023*. 84th edn. London: BMJ Group and the Royal Pharmaceutical Society of Great Britain.
20. Shakur H., Roverts I., Fawole B. et al. 2017. Effect of early tranexamic acid administration on mortality, hysterectomy, and other morbidities in women with post-partum haemorrhage (WOMAN): an international, randomised, double-blind, placebo-controlled trial. *Lancet,* 389(10084):2105–2116.
21. Grassin-Delyle S., Shakur-Still H., Picetti R. 2021. Pharmacokinetics of intramuscular tranexamic acid in bleeding trauma patients: a clinical trial. *British Journal of Anaesthesia*, 126(1):201–209.
22. Vu E.N., Wan W.C.Y, Yeung T.C. et al. 2018. Intramuscular tranexamic acid in tactical and combat settings. *Journal of Special Operations Medicine*, 18(1):62–68.
23. Mavrides E., Allard S., Chandraharan E. et al. on behalf of the Royal College of Obstetricians and Gynaecologists. 2016. Prevention and management of postpartum haemorrhage. *British Journal of Obstetrics and Gynaecology*, 124:e106–e149.
24. Schol P.B.B., de Lange N.M., Woiski M.D. et al. 2021. Restrictive versus liberal fluid resuscitation strategy, influence on blood loss and hemostatic parameters in mild obstetric hemorrhage: an open label randomized controlled trial. (REFILL study). *PLoS ONE*, 16(6): e0253765.
25. Gillissen A., van den Akker T., Caram-Deelder C. 2018. Association between fluid management and dilutional coagulopathy in severe postpartum haemorrhage: a nationwide retrospective cohort study. *BMC Pregnancy and Childbirth*, 18(1):398–407.
26. Chang R., Holcomb J.B. 2017. Optimal fluid therapy for traumatic hemorrhagic shock. *Critical Care Clinics*, 33(1):15–36.
27. Roberts I., Blackhall K., Dickinson K.J. 1999. Medical anti-shock trousers (pneumatic anti-shock garments) for circulatory support in patients with trauma. *Cochrane Database of Systematic Reviews*, (4):1–11.
28. UNICEF. 2019. *Non-pneumatic Anti-shock Garment (NASG)* [Online]. Available at: https://www.unicef.org/innovation/non-pneumatic-anti-shock-garment-nasg#:~:text=The%20Non%2Dpneumatic%20Anti%2DShock,and%20Space%20Administration%20(NASA).

SECTION 10

Special Circumstances

The Older Patient

36

David Anderson and Tegwyn McManamny

In this chapter you will learn:
- Why older people form an increasing proportion of ambulance service call-outs
- How the physiological changes of ageing influence the response to illness and injury
- The role of the critical care paramedic (CCP) in the assessment and care of older people
- The role of advanced care directives (ACD) in CCP practice.

Case Details

Dispatch
83-year-old male, fallen, possible altered level of consciousness.

History
An 83-year-old man has fallen down a step at a residential aged care (RAC) home, landing on concrete. An aged-care worker calls for an ambulance and advises that the patient may have hit his head, and that one of his legs appears shortened and externally rotated. A double-crewed ambulance is dispatched.

On Arrival of the First Crew
The patient is lying supine in an outdoor patio area, with several concerned staff members in attendance. His primary survey findings and initial vital signs are:

Airway	Patent
Breathing	RR 8, SpO$_2$ 90% on air
Circulation	Peripheral pulses present, HR 120, irregular, BP 110/70, warm peripheries
Disability	GCS E2, V3, M5 (10), pupils 5 mm and sluggish, BGL 5.5 mmol/L
Environmental	Temp 36.1 °C

The first paramedic crew apply high-flow oxygen via a non-rebreather mask. Their secondary survey reveals a significant haematoma in the right parietal region and a shortened and externally rotated right leg with urinary incontinence evident. Due to the patient's reduced

SECTION 10 Special Circumstances

conscious state and need for ongoing ventilatory support, a critical care paramedic is requested to assist.

On Your Arrival as the Critical Care Paramedic

The initial paramedic team have placed a cervical collar on the patient and are providing intermittent positive pressure ventilation with a bag-valve-mask (BVM) and supplementary oxygen to achieve a rate of 12 breaths/minute. They are having some difficulty maintaining this as the patient is making intermittent voluntary movements towards them, trying to move the mask off his face. He is moaning and appears very uncomfortable.

AMPLE

The patient has a significant past medical history, which is provided to you on a printed summary by a RAC staff member. His past medical history includes hypertension, atrial fibrillation, congestive cardiac failure, osteoarthritis, hearing loss and prostate cancer. His medications include rivaroxaban, atenolol, amlodipine, perindopril, digoxin, frusemide and Panadol Osteo. He is allergic to penicillin (anaphylaxis). He is in the RAC home for respite as his wife of 60 years has recently died. He walks with a four-wheeled walker and does a lap of the RAC home garden every day.

Allergies	Penicillin (anaphylaxis)
Medications	Rivaroxaban, atenolol, amlodipine, perindopril, digoxin, frusemide and paracetamol
Past history	Hypertension, atrial fibrillation, congestive cardiac failure, osteoarthritis, hearing loss and prostate cancer
Last ins and outs	Normal
Events	Fall down a single step while navigating with his four-wheeled walker to the patio – presumed mechanical fall

Decision Point

What are your clinical priorities in this situation?

You are faced with a patient with an altered conscious state, who requires assisted positive pressure ventilation. He has a closed head injury, and appears to be in significant pain.

Question 1: Why Do Older People Form an Increasing Proportion of Ambulance Service Call-Outs?

In the UK, US, Canada, Australia and New Zealand (and most developed countries) 'old age' is defined as being 65 years and over, and typically aged 50 years and over for those from an indigenous background, such as Aboriginal and Torres Strait Islanders and Māori. This population continues to grow in number and as a proportion of the population – older people made up 16% of the total Australian population in 2020, and it is projected that by 2066 older people in Australia will make up between 21% and 23% of the total population.[1] In the UK,

CHAPTER 36   The Older Patient

18.6% of the total population of England and Wales are aged 65 years and over.[2] Globally, the number of persons aged 80 years or over is projected to increase from 137 million in 2017 to 425 million in 2050, with two thirds of older people living in developing countries.[3] The number of people entering old age is growing and older people are representing an increasing share of the total population.[4]

With demographics including a large cohort born between 1946 and 1964 (the 'baby boomers') now entering old age, there are several key reasons for this population ageing, including increasing life expectancy, declining fertility and improved healthcare quality. Older people form an increasing proportion of ambulance service call-outs, with ambulance service utilisation rates increasing with age. Ambulance transportation to emergency departments also increases with increasing age.

This is not just because of the size of the older population, but also due to injuries and illnesses associated with the biological impacts of ageing, as well as natural age-related changes. As people age, they are increasingly likely to experience more than one condition at the same time, with chronic obstructive pulmonary disease, ischaemic heart disease, infections, diabetes, depression and dementia common reasons for ambulance requests. In addition, falls become more common and can result in serious injury.

PRACTICE TIP

Older people are often assumed to be frail or dependent and a burden to society. However, paramedics must be aware of this potential for bias and base their assessment and care of older people on an individually tailored approach.

Question 2: How Do the Physiological Changes of Ageing Influence the Response to Illness and Injury?

The physiological changes of ageing influence the response of older people to illness and injury, with alterations in normal homeostatic mechanisms resulting in changes in baseline physiological characteristics that CCPs are likely to rely on for clinical decision-making, such as blood pressure, heart rate and oxygen saturation levels. In addition, seemingly innocuous illnesses and injuries can have life-altering outcomes for older people. Ageing is a natural process, but it is also associated with various age-related illnesses, including chronic medical conditions and both physical and cognitive dysfunction, which influence the response of older people to illness and injury.

It is useful to understand the differences between normal age-related changes and the geriatric syndromes that CCPs might commonly encounter while caring for unwell older people in the community. Age-related changes affect nearly every body system, but this should not be automatically interpreted as pathology, and instead, CCP assessment and management should be tailored to address the needs of the older person. There is great variability in the manner in which people age; however, **Table 36.1** highlights some predictable age-related changes and their potential implications.

The physiological changes of ageing also have implications for CCPs in terms of pharmacological management of older people who are ill or injured. This group of patients is prone to challenges due to drug interactions and adverse effects, not just due to the physiological

Table 36.1 Predictable age-related changes and their potential implications

Body system	Change	Implications
Integumentary	• Epidermal thinning. • Loss of elasticity and subcutaneous fat. • Loss of sensory receptors. • Decrease in skin cell turnover rate. • Reduced dermal blood vessels.	• Older people have higher risk of skin tears. • Skin repair is protracted – prolonged wound healing time means higher infection risk.
Musculoskeletal	• Relative decline in lean body mass and progressive reduction in total body water with relative increase in adipose tissue. • Loss and atrophy of muscle cells. • Increased bone loss with reduction in bone mass. • Reduced strength of muscular contraction, leading to changes in strength and movement. • Cartilaginous degeneration, impaired remodelling, leading to joint instability and disease.	• Movement restriction (speed and strength), which may require adjustments to patient extrications undertaken by CCPs. • Increased risk of fracture from relatively benign injuries. • Prolonged healing time.
Cardiovascular	• Decreased cardiac output, reduced cardiac contractility. • Increased myocardial stiffness. • Increasing stiffness of arteries (including thoracic aorta) resulting in increased cardiac afterload. • Increased amyloid deposits in myocardium. • Increased arteriosclerosis. • Increased peripheral vascular resistance.	• Decreased inotropic response to catecholamines (both endogenous and exogenous) – reduced ability of older people to increase cardiac output in response to stress. • Higher baseline blood pressure (may not respond predictably to stress/illness, may be hypotensive despite a relatively 'normal' systolic blood pressure).
Respiratory	• Reduced vital capacity. • Decrease in arterial oxygen pressure. • V/Q mismatch with reduced lung elastic recoil, reduced lung compliance and diffusion capacity. • Reduced chemoreceptor response to hypercapnia and hypoxia. • Slowed mucociliary function.	• Reduced ability to compensate for increased respiratory demands (stress/illness/exertion). • Decreased ability to generate normal expiratory pressures, increased risk of early airway collapse. • Older people experience increase in pneumonia and other infections.

CHAPTER 36 The Older Patient

Body system	Change	Implications
Neurological	• Brain size decreases. • White and grey matter volume loss. • Neuronal loss, structural changes to neurons, synaptic loss. • Increased permeability of blood–brain barrier. • Decreased cerebral blood flow. • Changes in hypothalamic function lead to diminished thermoregulation capabilities.	• Slowing of some key functional processes and cognitive tasks, for example, speed of processing and working memory. CCPs should be aware of slowed processing speed and attentional function and allow for this during patient assessment.
Genitourinary	• Decrease in kidney volume and weight and reduction in tubular function and in the number of glomeruli per kidney, leading to deterioration in renal function. • Reduction in renal clearance. • The concentrating and diluting abilities of the kidneys slow, resulting in higher potential for dehydration and hyponatraemia.	• Prolonged half-life of some medications due to delayed clearance. CCPs must be aware of the consequences of reduced renal function when considering medication regimes and doses. • Always assess for signs of dehydration and manage accordingly.
Gastrointestinal	• Oesophageal function deteriorates, with a decrease in peristalsis and potential delay in transit time, leading to dysphagia. • Decrease in intestinal motility, hypotonic colon leading to stool dehydration and increased risk of constipation. • Liver function changes; reduction in liver blood flow, leading to delay in the metabolisation of some medications (for example, diazepam).	• May influence ability of older people to self-administer oral medications or participate in oral rehydration.
Endocrine	• Deterioration in number and function of beta cells, leading to insulin insufficiency and hyperglycaemia. Insulin resistance develops with age. • Combination of decreased renal function with decrease in maximal reabsorption of glucose may cause hyperglycaemic hyperosmolar non-ketotic coma (HONK).	• Increased glucose intolerance may manifest in older people with no prior diagnosis of diabetes. • Mild hyperglycaemia in the setting of an infection (such as urinary tract) may lead to osmotic diuresis and rapid progression to severe illness.

(Continued)

Table 36.1 (*Continued*)

Body system	Change	Implications
Senses	• Diminished olfactory function, motor tone, power, co-ordination and reflexes. • Decreased sensitivity to temperature. • Decreased sensitivity to proprioception. • Changes in visual acuity and field, and depth and motor perception. • Decreased hearing perception and vestibular function.	• CCPs should be aware of changes in the visual system, hearing and balance of older people, and allow for this in patient assessment (particularly in history-taking and interviews with older people).
Immune	• Reduced T and B cell production, diminished lymphocyte function leads to increases in vulnerability to certain infections. • Increase in immunosenescence. • Increase in low-grade inflammation in the absence of an overt infection.	• Older people are at increased risk of infection, including iatrogenic infections from healthcare providers or facilities.

changes listed in Table 36.1, but also due to polypharmacotherapy and multimorbidity.[5] CCPs will be familiar with the Webster Packs of medications that many older people are on, and an awareness of common pharmacological interactions in older people (as well as altered pharmacokinetics and pharmacodynamics) is essential to ensure that prehospital care involves safe and effective pharmacological management. Key concepts include the following.

- **Bioavailability** – a reduction in first-pass metabolism occurs with advancing age, with a resultant increased bioavailability in some medications (including those commonly administered by CCPs, such as metoclopramide and opioids). CCPs should therefore consider a smaller initial dose of these medications, watch for effect, and titrate subsequent doses accordingly.
- **Distribution** – due to the changes outlined in Table 36.1 around body composition, volume of distribution changes with age. For example, hydrophilic medications (such as gentamicin, digoxin, lithium and theophylline) are inclined to have a smaller volume of distribution leading to higher serum levels in older people, potentially requiring smaller loading doses. However, this is balanced to some extent by the delayed renal clearance experienced by older people. Lipophilic medications, such as amiodarone, morphine and benzodiazepines, have a higher volume of distribution and a resultant prolongation of their half-life. CCPs should be aware of this and titrate medication doses according to close observation.
- **Clearance** – age-related changes in the speed of clearance of metabolised medications are linked to reduced liver blood flow and liver volume, a reduction in glomerular

CHAPTER 36   The Older Patient

filtration rate and a reduction in CYP enzymes. The most clinically relevant point is that accumulation of medications with a narrow therapeutic index can have significant implications for older people (some antibiotics, lithium and digoxin are examples) with potentially serious adverse effects.

- **Polypharmacy** – this is common in older people. In Australia, approximately 40% of people aged 75 years and older are dispensed five or more medications,[6] with higher rates in metropolitan areas and increasing with socioeconomic disadvantage. CCPs should recognise the potential for medication interactions and include a focused medication analysis as part of patient assessment.

The physiological changes of ageing also have implications for CCPs in terms of patient assessment in the context of 'normal' vital signs and symptoms of illness and injury. The changes outlined in Table 36.1 underpin alterations to baseline characteristics, such as blood pressure, heart rate and oxygen saturations. An increase in peripheral vascular resistance, for example, may lead to older people experiencing a higher baseline blood pressure. For example, a systolic reading that sits within a 'normal' range (for example, 100–120 mmHg systolic) may actually represent hypotension for that person, and the presence of acute physiological derangement requiring CCP intervention. Similarly, common medications that an older person may be prescribed may mask the ability of the individual to respond to injury or illness in a predictable manner. One example of this is beta-blockers (such as metoprolol and atenolol), which may impair the ability of older people to mount a tachycardia in response to injury, illness or stress. CCPs should be mindful that the vital signs of older adults may differ from 'normal' values, and take into account individual variability when assessing pain, stress, injury and illness. This should include a focused history-taking, with attention paid to the normal vital signs parameters *for that individual*.

Question 3: What Is the Role of the CCP in the Assessment and Care of Older People?

As the CCP attending this scene you have an important role in the assessment and care of this older person. Your understanding of ageing's physiologically mediated changes on baseline characteristics, such as a patient's vital signs, is essential to recognising the clinical status of the patient and their potential for deterioration. In addition, your awareness of pharmacological considerations, including the implications of prescribed medications, as well as the pharmacokinetic changes associated with ageing and how that may influence your chosen drug regimens, equips you with enhanced decision support tools. The opportunity to advocate for the wishes of older people during their assessment and care is extremely important, and your role should be led by any expressed wishes or the presence of an advanced care directive (ACD) if a patient is unable to express their own thoughts or wishes around a particular treatment, resuscitation or end-of-life care.

The patient described in this chapter has experienced a low-level fall with resultant head strike and multiple injuries. His outcome is dependent on a range of factors, including his own individual physiological reserves, the prehospital care provided and the ability for him to be triaged swiftly to a major trauma service. Older people are commonly under-triaged, with an under-estimation of the burden of their injuries leading to delays in reaching a major trauma service and resultant prolonged hospital admissions. Older people experience

SECTION 10 Special Circumstances

significant morbidity and mortality due to traumatic injuries, with their physiological changes, co-morbidities and potential for polypharmacy all combining to make prehospital trauma care more challenging.

Older People, Trauma Systems and Prehospital Triage

We are gradually understanding that prehospital triage decisions can have a significant impact on the outcomes of older people experiencing traumatic injuries. However, there are few empirical studies assessing how well prehospital triage systems perform with older people, with experts noting that traditional triage measures, such as blood pressure and age, poorly identify older patients at risk of adverse outcome, and that better prognostic measures for older trauma patients are required.[7] Trauma tools should be sensitive enough to identify major trauma patients so they can benefit from access to major trauma services, while still being sensitive enough to predict patients whose injuries are not classified as major trauma, so they can be treated at non-major trauma services (such as local hospitals). Older people with traumatic injuries are more likely to be under-triaged, and instead be transported by ambulance to non-major trauma services, where their definitive care may be delayed while secondary transfer to a more appropriate service is organised. Prehospital decision making around the triage of this patient group may be affected by the following.

- **Physiological responses to trauma** – as previously discussed, the physiological changes of ageing, as well as levels of co-morbidity, can result in the vital signs of older people differing from commonly accepted 'normal' values, and medications may mask responses to severe injury. Multimorbidity and frailty also complicate the physiological reserve of older people and the manner in which they respond to trauma.
- **Poor recognition of 'minor' injury mechanisms and the major implications they can have** – low-level falls is a key example here, with falls <2 m often perceived to be insignificant mechanism, despite clear evidence that even standing-height falls in the older person can result in severe injuries and are the most common reason for injury and death in older adults.[8,9]
- **Clinician bias** – age bias in medicine (including in paramedicine) can have a significant impact on older people. Misconceptions about ageing and the physical and mental capacity of older adults can result in poorer access to healthcare and medical treatments,[10] and it is paramount that healthcare providers (including CCPs) work to acknowledge and challenge both implicit and explicit bias in their emergency care of older people.

Assessment

Following a structured approach to assessment is essential to any form of patient care. This can be achieved by applying a systematic method of assessment, that takes into account the specific needs of individual older people. It is important to consider the likely physiological changes that occur with ageing, and ensure that assessment is adapted to account for them. For example:

- CCPs should ideally position themselves in front of the conscious patient when asking questions and should speak clearly and with adequate volume throughout conversation.

CHAPTER 36 The Older Patient

- If a patient has been previously diagnosed with a cognitive impairment, attempt to ascertain what their baseline level of functioning is, and whether there are new deficits today.
- Reduce interruptions and background noise as much as possible, with one person (ideally the same person) asking questions at a time.
- Do not rush questions and history taking – allow appropriate time for the older person to answer the question. Repeat the question if needed.
- Obtain data from other sources if the older person does not recall information such as medications, hospitalisations and past illnesses. Family members, carers, a phone call to the local GP, and historical medical records may all assist.
- Give **examples** to check for changes in function, such as mobility. Questions such as 'How long have you been unable to walk to your mailbox?' and 'Can you normally do your own shopping?' can give a more helpful picture of symptoms, activity and potential functional decline.
- The **physical assessment** of the older person should include a full vital signs survey, secondary survey, relevant adjuncts (such as temperature, blood glucose level, oxygen saturations) and careful visual observation of the older person in the environment they are being assessed within. Observation of their movements (sitting and standing, walking with frame, for example), as well as general appearance (restless, anxious, comfortable, pale, dyspnoeic), is important and can add critical information to the CCP's assessment. An observation of the physical environment itself (clean/tidy, unclean, no food in the refrigerator, very hot/cold room temperature) can also yield important data to add to a holistic patient assessment.
- The assessment of the older person in pain is just as important as that of other age groups. Evidence suggests that older people are often untreated or under-treated for pain,[11] potentially due to older people under-reporting their pain, but also due to challenges with pain assessment and misconceptions about pain that are likely linked to ageism. Pain in older people may manifest as agitation, inactivity, decreased function without a reliable explanation, fatigue and sleeplessness. Untreated pain is associated with worse outcomes, with both physical and psychological consequences. A patient self-report should underpin any pain assessment; however, if an older person is unable to provide this, validated observational pain scales can be used to assess management and guide treatment. These may include the Pain Assessment in Advanced Dementia (PAINAD) tool, the Pain Assessment Checklist for Seniors with Limited Ability to Communicate (PACSLAC) and the Abbey Pain Scale. Take care to assess pain both when the patient is at rest and when they are active (for example, being transferred or moving). Consideration should be given to treating the underlying causes of pain and a multi-modal approach to pain management should include both pharmacological and non-pharmacological means (such as a splint, limb elevation and analgesia for a limb fracture).
- An assessment of frailty is essential, as it can aid decision making with regard to prehospital interventions, by identifying patients who are at increased risk of adverse health outcomes, including mortality, disability, worsening mobility, falls, hospitalisation and death.[12] Frailty is defined as a condition of decreased physiological reserve that leads to a vulnerable state. For older adults, being frail increases the risk of adverse

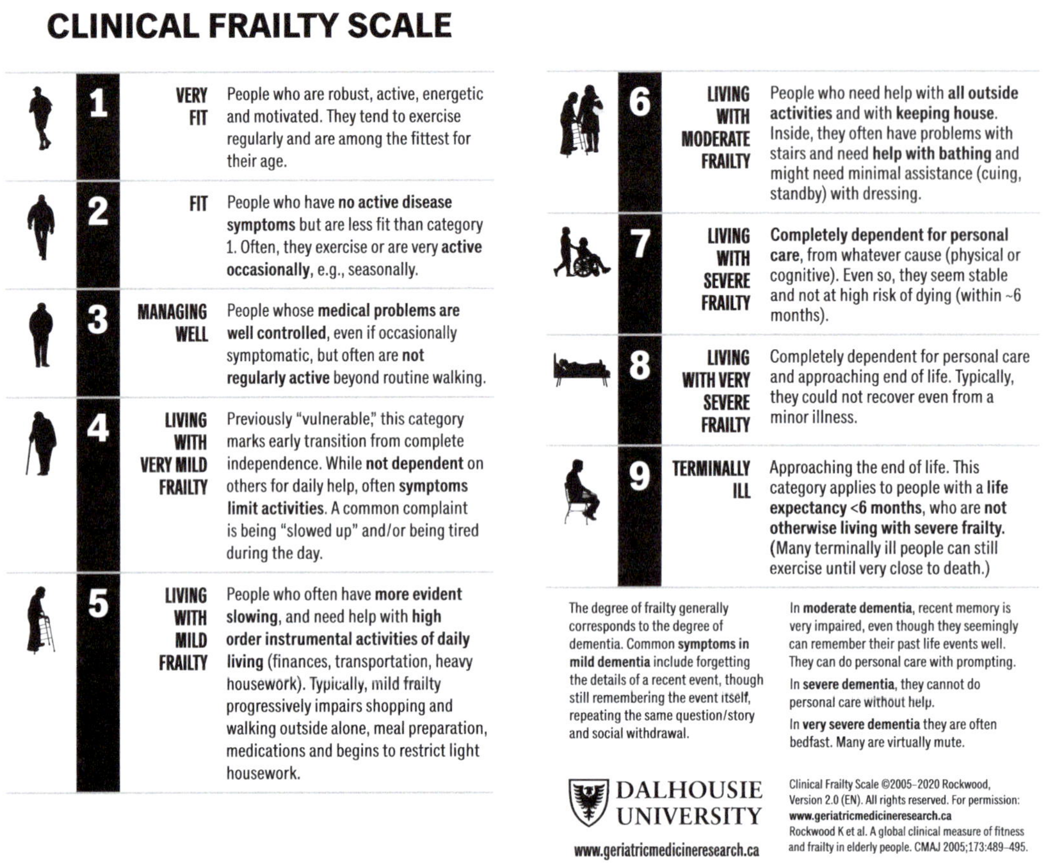

SECTION 10　Special Circumstances

CLINICAL FRAILTY SCALE

1	**VERY FIT**	People who are robust, active, energetic and motivated. They tend to exercise regularly and are among the fittest for their age.
2	**FIT**	People who have **no active disease symptoms** but are less fit than category 1. Often, they exercise or are very **active occasionally**, e.g., seasonally.
3	**MANAGING WELL**	People whose **medical problems are well controlled**, even if occasionally symptomatic, but often are **not regularly active** beyond routine walking.
4	**LIVING WITH VERY MILD FRAILTY**	Previously "vulnerable," this category marks early transition from complete independence. While **not dependent** on others for daily help, often **symptoms limit activities**. A common complaint is being "slowed up" and/or being tired during the day.
5	**LIVING WITH MILD FRAILTY**	People who often have **more evident slowing**, and need help with **high order instrumental activities of daily living** (finances, transportation, heavy housework). Typically, mild frailty progressively impairs shopping and walking outside alone, meal preparation, medications and begins to restrict light housework.
6	**LIVING WITH MODERATE FRAILTY**	People who need help with **all outside activities** and with **keeping house**. Inside, they often have problems with stairs and need **help with bathing** and might need minimal assistance (cuing, standby) with dressing.
7	**LIVING WITH SEVERE FRAILTY**	**Completely dependent for personal care**, from whatever cause (physical or cognitive). Even so, they seem stable and not at high risk of dying (within ~6 months).
8	**LIVING WITH VERY SEVERE FRAILTY**	Completely dependent for personal care and approaching end of life. Typically, they could not recover even from a minor illness.
9	**TERMINALLY ILL**	Approaching the end of life. This category applies to people with a **life expectancy <6 months**, who are **not otherwise living with severe frailty**. (Many terminally ill people can still exercise until very close to death.)

The degree of frailty generally corresponds to the degree of dementia. Common **symptoms in mild dementia** include forgetting the details of a recent event, though still remembering the event itself, repeating the same question/story and social withdrawal.

In **moderate dementia**, recent memory is very impaired, even though they seemingly can remember their past life events well. They can do personal care with prompting.

In **severe dementia**, they cannot do personal care without help.

In **very severe dementia** they are often bedfast. Many are virtually mute.

DALHOUSIE UNIVERSITY
www.geriatricmedicineresearch.ca

Clinical Frailty Scale ©2005–2020 Rockwood, Version 2.0 (EN). All rights reserved. For permission: www.geriatricmedicineresearch.ca
Rockwood K et al. A global clinical measure of fitness and frailty in elderly people. CMAJ 2005;173:489–495.

Figure 36.1 Clinical Frailty Scale.
Source: Dalhousie University, Halifax, Nova Scotia, Canada (https://www.dal.ca/sites/gmr.html). Reproduced with permission.

- health outcomes when exposed to a stressor,[13] such as illness or an injury. There is a range of frailty assessment tools, and many ambulance services worldwide use some form of scale to aid prehospital assessment of frailty and help inform decision making around interventions, referral options and requirements for critical care support. One such example is the Clinical Frailty Scale (CFS) (**Figure 36.1**).
- There is a higher prevalence of frailty in females than males, and prevalence increases with age,[14] with 43.7% of adults aged ≥65 years and 69% of adults aged ≥85 years being assessed as frail.[15] A frailty assessment should be used in conjunction with other prehospital assessments to help form a holistic approach to patient care that considers the overall health status of the patient and their goals of care, and opportunities for frailty-informed care management.
- In the older patient with time-critical injuries and illnesses, history may need to be obtained from bystanders, carers or family rather than the patient themselves. However, a structured approach to assessment should underpin every episode of patient care, and the observational skills of the CCP should be utilised at every opportunity.

CHAPTER 36 The Older Patient

Question 4: What Is the Role of Advance Care Directives in CCP Practice?

An advance care directive (ACD) is a document that allows a competent adult to outline their values and treatment wishes so that these can be adhered to should they lose decision-making capacity. In some jurisdictions ACDs are legally binding documents. There are two broad types of ACD: instructional and values based. An instructional directive contains definitive instructions for treatments that the patient does not wish to receive. Note that, while a patient can refuse treatment, patients cannot demand treatments that are not indicated. The most common statements in instructional ACDs include 'I do not wish to receive CPR' or 'I do not wish to be intubated'. Values directives can be more helpful, as they give an indication of the patient's values and allow the clinician to make a decision based on this. For example, a values directive may state: 'I value independence and being able to drive'. If a patient has a serious illness that, even with successful treatment, would not result in them retaining this degree of independence, then treatment would not be in keeping with the patient's values and should not be offered.

If an ACD is available, it should be adhered to, even if this results in the patient not receiving potentially life-saving treatment. In settings where it is likely that an ACD will be present (for example, in an RAC), CCPs should ask the facility staff if there is an ACD.

Surrogate decision makers (typically close family members) may also request that treatments be withheld if they do not believe these to be in keeping with the patient's values. Less experienced paramedics or other prehospital providers, such as EMTs or firefighters, often find such requests difficult to comply with and may insist on continuing treatment against the wishes of surrogate decision makers. Critical care paramedics will typically be senior and experienced enough to consider the instructions of a surrogate decision maker in the context of the patient's clinical condition and trajectory, as well as their co-morbidities.

Very occasionally, the views of a surrogate decision maker will contradict those in an ACD. In these cases, the ACD should be adhered to unless there is very good reason to suspect that the patient has recently changed their mind. However, these situations can be quite challenging, and it would be appropriate to consult with a senior ambulance service doctor (or perhaps the patient's GP – if they are contactable) or senior paramedic leader, and in some cases to transport the patient to hospital while still providing the minimum treatment required to stabilise the patient so that a more considered decision can be made by a multidisciplinary team.

In most cases, however, patients' families are relieved to know that an ACD exists and will support the CCP to act in accordance with the patient's values. In most cases this will involve providing treatment aimed at maintaining comfort and dignity, rather than providing advanced critical care.

> **PRACTICE TIP**
>
> Advance care directives can help guide treatment. Ensure you provide symptom relief and comfort, and involve next of kin, family and loved ones where possible.

> **PRACTICE TIP**
>
> Older people living in residential aged care are generally older and more frail than those living independently in the community.

SECTION 10 Special Circumstances

Key Evidence

Alshibani A., Banerjee J, Lecky F. et al., 2021. New horizons in understanding appropriate prehospital identification and trauma triage for older adults. *Open Access Emergency Medicine*, *13*, 117–135.

Dwyer R.A., Gabbe B.J., Tran T. et al., 2021. Residential aged care homes: Why do they call '000'? A study of the emergency prehospital care of older people living in residential aged care homes. *Emergency Medicine Australasia*, *33*, 447–456.

Lum H.D., Sudore R.L., Bekelman D.B., 2015. Advance care planning in the elderly. *Medical Clinics*, *99*(2), 391–403.

Preston J., Biddell B., 2021. The physiology of ageing and how these changes affect older people. *Medicine*, *49*(1), 1–5.

Self-Reflection Questions

1. What changes might you make to your clinical practice when caring for older people?
2. How might the physiological changes that occur through ageing affect the response of an older person to a traumatic insult (for example, motor vehicle collision)?
3. Why are falls the leading cause of trauma-related mortality in older people?
4. What fluid resuscitation and analgesic regime might you consider for a hypotensive older person in pain, and why?
5. How might you approach an older person with a potentially life-threatening illness, who has an advance care directive stating that they should not receive CPR or intubation?

References

1. Australian Bureau of Statistics (ABS), 2018. *Population Projections, Australia*. ABS cat. no. 3222.0 [Online]. Canberra, ACT: Australian Bureau of Statistics. Available at: https://www.abs.gov.au/statistics/people/population/population-projections-australia/2017-base-2066
2. Office for National Statistics, 2022. *Voices of our ageing population: Living longer lives* [Online]. Available at: https://www.ons.gov.uk/peoplepopulationandcommunity/birthsdeathsandmarriages/ageing/articles/voicesofourageingpopulation/livinglongerlives#:~:text=The%20population%20of%20England%20and,the%20previous%20census%20in%202011
3. United Nations, Department of Economic and Social Affairs, Population Division, 2017. *World Population Ageing 2017 – Highlights* [Online]. Available at: https://www.un.org/en/development/desa/population/publications/pdf/ageing/WPA2017_Highlights.pdf (ST/ESA/SER.A/397)
4. Australian Research Council Centre of Excellence in Population Ageing Research (CEPAR), 2021. *CEPAR Population Ageing Futures Data Archive* [Online]. Sydney, NSW: CEPAR. Available at: https://cepar.edu.au/cepar-population-ageing-projections
5. Błeszyńska, E., Wierucki, Ł., Zdrojewski, T. et al., 2020. Pharmacological interactions in the elderly. *Medicina (Kaunas, Lithuania)*, *56*(7), 320. Available at: https://www.mdpi.com/1648-9144/56/7/320
6. Australian Commission on Quality and Safety in Healthcare, 2021. *Medicines use in older people. The Fourth Australian Atlas of Healthcare Variation* [Online]. Available at: https://www.safetyandquality.gov.au/our-work/healthcare-variation/fourth-atlas-2021/medicines-use-older-people
7. Cubitt, M., Downie, E., Shakerian, R. et al., 2019. Timing and methods of frailty assessments in geriatric trauma patients: A systematic review. *Injury*, *50*(11), 1795–1808. Available at: https://www.injuryjournal.com/article/S0020-1383(19)30425-5/abstract
8. Rau, C.-S., Lin, T.-S., Wu, S.-C. et al., 2014. Geriatric hospitalizations in fall-related injuries. *Scandinavian Journal of Trauma, Resuscitation and Emergency Medicine*, *22*(1), 63. Available at: https://www.ncbi.nlm.nih.gov/pmc/articles/PMC4232632/

9. Wu, M.Y., Chen, Y.L., Yiang, G.T. et al., 2018. Clinical outcome and management for geriatric traumatic injury: Analysis of 2688 cases in the emergency department of a teaching hospital in Taiwan. *Journal of Clinical Medicine*, *7*(9). Available at: https://www.mdpi.com/2077-0383/7/9/255
10. Chang, E.-S., Kannoth, S., Levy, S. et al., 2020. Global reach of ageism on older persons' health: A systematic review. *PLoS ONE*, *15*(1), e0220857. Available at: https://journals.plos.org/plosone/article?id=10.1371/journal.pone.0220857
11. Cavalieri, T.A., 2005. Management of pain in older adults. *Journal of the American Osteopathic Association*, *105*(3 Suppl 1), S12–17. Available at: https://pubmed.ncbi.nlm.nih.gov/18154193/
12. Bandeen-Roche, K., Seplaki, C.L., Huang, J. et al., 2015. Frailty in older adults: A nationally representative profile in the United States. *Journals of Gerontology, Series A. Biological Sciences and Medical Sciences*, *70*(11), 1427–1434. Available at: https://pubmed.ncbi.nlm.nih.gov/26297656/
13. Won, C.W., 2019. Frailty: Its scope and implications for geriatricians. *Annals of Geriatric Medicine and Research*, *23*(3), 95–97. Available at: https://pubmed.ncbi.nlm.nih.gov/32743296/
14. O'Caoimh, R., Sezgin, D., O'Donovan, MR. et al., 2020. Prevalence of frailty in 62 countries across the world: A systematic review and meta-analysis of population-level studies. *Age and Ageing*, *50*(1), 96–104. Available at: https://pubmed.ncbi.nlm.nih.gov/33068107/
15. Fogg, C., Fraser, S.D.S., Roderick, P. et al., 2022. The dynamics of frailty development and progression in older adults in primary care in England (2006–2017): A retrospective cohort profile. *BMC Geriatrics*, *22*(1), 30. Available at: https://pubmed.ncbi.nlm.nih.gov/34991479/

37 Providing Paramedic Care in Resource-Limited Settings

Matt Cannon and Felix Ho

> **In this chapter you will learn:**
> - What the considerations are for paramedics providing prolonged field care in the out-of-hospital environment
> - The fluid balance
> - The potential complications of medication administrations
> - The environment and improvisation of resources.

Case Details

You are a critical care paramedic working in Port Moresby, Papua New Guinea (PNG).

Dispatch

28-year-old-male, post fall from tree, fractured tib/fib.

History

A 28-year-old man was climbing down from a coconut tree on a farm when he fell awkwardly onto the ground. He has fallen approximately 1 metre. He was found by family, who were unable to move him due to pain. The patient is four hours' drive from Port Moresby, the nearest hospital with an emergency department. A double-crewed ambulance is dispatched.

On Arrival of the First Crew

The scene is safe, and the patient is in a semi-recumbent position. There is an obvious open lower limb fracture, onto which the family has placed mud in the hopes of protecting the wound while waiting for the ambulance. The patient's primary survey findings and initial vital signs are:

Airway	Patent
Breathing	RR 20, SpO$_2$ 98% on air
Circulation	Peripheral pulses present, HR 124, regular, BP 148/92, warm peripheries
Disability	GCS E4, V5, M6 (15), BGL 6.3 mmol/L
Environmental	Temp 36.8 °C

CHAPTER 37 Providing Paramedic Care in Resource-Limited Settings

The first paramedic crew to arrive provides analgesia and an improvised splint to the open right lower tibia/fibula fracture. Secondary survey reveals tenderness, deformity and ecchymosis to the right ankle, right knee and right hip. There are superficial grazes to bilateral hands and forearms. Other examinations appear unremarkable.

On Your Arrival as the Critical Care Paramedic

Weather conditions prohibit helicopter operations, so you have responded by road, and it is dusk by the time you arrive at the scene. The initial paramedic crew are struggling to extricate the patient due to extreme pain and inability to bear weight on the right ankle. IV access is obtained but the patient does not tolerate morphine, with associated nausea and vomiting. An improvised splint has been applied and appears to provide some pain relief while at rest. The open compound wound has mud in situ and there are flies and mosquitoes lingering around it.

AMPLE

The patient has a past medical history of anxiety and depression. His only medication is sertraline (Zoloft) 50 mg daily and he has no known allergies. He works as a school teacher and is of average fitness level. He is a smoker of 15 pack years (1 packet per day for 15 years).

Allergies	NKDA
Medications	Sertraline (Zoloft) 50 mg PO daily
Past history	Anxiety/depression
Last ins and outs	Last oral intake
Events prior	Was climbing down from a coconut tree when he lost his footing and fell approximately 1 m onto hard ground

Decision Point

What are your clinical priorities in this situation?

With the difficulty in access and egress, long transport distance, inability to weight bear, pain management, potential source of wound infection with mud and foreign debris, and it now being nighttime, prolonged field care in a resource-limited setting is paramount.

Question 1: What Are the Priorities of Prolonged Field Care in Resource-Limited Settings?

A structured, systematic approach should occur within the prehospital environment, regardless of the setting. A primary survey to detect and correct any immediately life-threatening conditions is essential to ensure prioritisation of care. Recognition and correction of these life threats are vital, ensuring a time-critical approach and transport of these patients.

Prolonged field care occurs on completion of the primary survey until arrival at the hospital. Within this case study, there are considerable logistical and transport challenges, complicated by nightfall, which may result in delayed stabilisation, extrication and transport times. A systematic approach during the prolonged field care phase ensures patient safety

SECTION 10 Special Circumstances

and delays a therapeutic vacuum. The prolonged field care algorithm devised by Smith et al.[1] provides a useful summary of considerations and priorities for prolonged field care. A brief summary of these considerations includes the following.

- Preparing for prolonged field care, which includes logistical considerations, ensuring sufficient supplies, optimising the field environment, optimising the available resources and being in the right frame of mind for a prolonged period of care.
- Monitor and resuscitate, ensuring the patient maintains homeostasis with baseline monitoring, observing trends and reducing overall therapeutic vacuum.
- Pain relief and medications are vital for patient comfort, reducing cardiac output, decreasing metabolic demands, increasing compliance and increasing paramedic credibility for the treatment regime. (Analgesia selection will be discussed later in this chapter.)
- Wound care and infection control are vital to prevent localised and systemic infections, reducing forensic contamination and decreasing length of hospital stay. (Antibiotic selection will be discussed later in this chapter.)
- Patient care should be vital to the work of any paramedic. The principles of beneficence (to promote the wellbeing of the patient) and non-maleficence (to avoid or prevent further harm) are core to overall patient care. Medical-legal responsibility and a health care code of ethics and practice must be complied with regardless of the prolonged field care, environment or situation.
- Documentation is important to maintain continuity of care, reduce harm through prevention of medication errors and ensure that the patient condition and trends are reflected for long-term care.
- Preparing for evacuation includes determining the most appropriate, accessible and reliable form of transport to remove the patient to the most appropriate facility. This may be the closest facility or could be a larger tertiary centre further away. The availability of surgical expertise, an airstrip for aeromedical evacuation or further resources are factors that need to be considered. Consultation with the receiving facility or a centralised co-ordination centre may reduce this overall burden on the paramedic while in the prolonged field care phase of treatment.
- Kit management is vital in knowing what resources are available immediately, and what additional resources are required during the prolonged field phase. It is impossible to stock every conceivable piece of equipment or consumable within a prehospital setting (or even a hospital setting). Knowledge of the limitations and flexibility of different pieces of equipment and consumables will improve overall patient care within a resource-limited environment. For example, a triangular bandage can be used as a sling, a pad or a gallows for a fracture; it can be turned into an improvised short rope or paracord, a tourniquet or a cloth face mask; it can be used for pre-filtering water and as a fire starter. A rough itemisation of consumables utilised during the case will also reduce time during restocking after the case has been completed.
- Team and self-management ensure that you are able to assist the patient. Consider the use of the IMSAFE checklist, which is widely used within the aviation sector to assist with crew resource management. This checklist, courtesy of the FAA,[2] comprises the following items.

CHAPTER 37   Providing Paramedic Care in Resource-Limited Settings

- o   Illness: Do I have any symptoms of illnesses?
- o   Medication: Have I taken my required prescription or over-the-counter medications? Do these affect my work performance?
- o   Stress: Am I under psychological pressure from this case? Am I worried about other matters, such as family, post-shift commitments, personal safety, financial matters, health problems or family discord?
- o   Alcohol: Am I under the effects of alcohol? Am I withdrawing from alcohol?
- o   Fatigue: Am I tired and not adequately rested?
- o   Emotion: Am I emotionally affected or upset?

There are multiple priorities encountered during the prolonged field care phase of treatment, which occur following the completion of the primary survey and last until arrival at the hospital. The use of algorithms and checklists will ensure a systematic and reproducible pattern to ensure that priorities of care are achieved.

Question 2: What Are the Considerations For Analgesia Management?

Pain management is vital for patient comfort, reducing cardiac output, decreasing metabolic demands, increasing compliance and increasing paramedic credibility for the treatment regime and patient. The consideration for analgesia within a resource-limited environment during prolonged field care includes the effectiveness, duration and availability of the analgesic agents. In this case study, the patient does not appear to have adequate analgesia, and past attempts at using morphine resulted in side-effects.

Assessment of pain should be performed to ascertain the location, type and characteristics of the pain, which aids in diagnosing the underlying cause. The standard assessment of pain through a numerical system is traditionally favoured, with an alternative being the Wong-Baker Faces scale or the Alder Hey Triage Pain Score.

The World Health Organization[3] three-step analgesic ladder, while originally produced for cancer pain, can be adapted for use within a resource-limited, prehospital environment. The ladder consists of three steps (**Figure 37.1**).

1. For patients in mild pain, non-opioid analgesics, such as paracetamol, aspirin (in some cases) and NSAIDS (non-steroidal anti-inflammatory drugs), +/- adjuvants should be considered. These have relatively long half-lives and are generally well tolerated. Paracetamol inhibits central prostaglandin synthesis, but not peripheral prostaglandin production. NSAID inhibits the cyclo-oxygenase enzymes (COX), which results in prostaglandin synthesis; non-selective NSAIDs affect the COX-1 (constitutive expression and regulates physiological function in the gut and kidney) and COX-2 (induced by cytokines and is induced in inflammation and repair) isoforms, whereas COX-2 selective NSAIDs affect COX-2 only. Different NSAIDs have different COX-2 selectivity (**Figure 37.2**).
2. For patients in moderately severe pain, where non-opioid analgesics are ineffective, a weak opioid should be considered. These include codeine, tramadol or similar. Remember to include a non-opioid and/or an adjuvant, which works in conjunction with the weak opioid.

SECTION 10 Special Circumstances

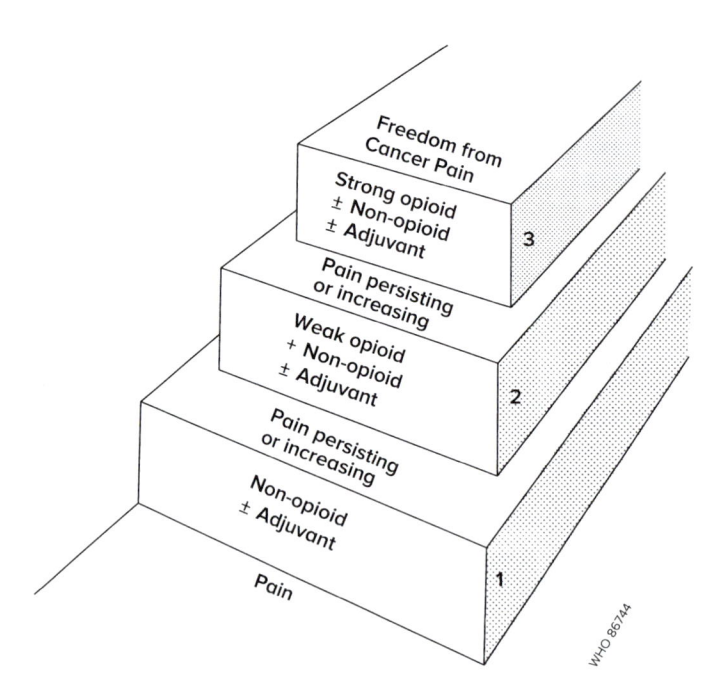

Figure 37.1 The three-step analgesic ladder.
Source: World Health Organization, 1986. Reproduced with permission.

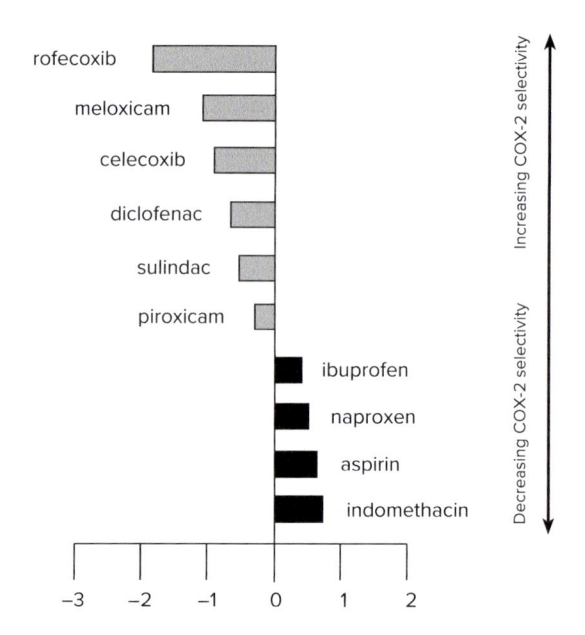

Figure 37.2 COX selectivity of NSAIDs.
Source: Brooks, 2000. Therapeutic Guidelines Ltd. https://australianprescriber.tg.org.au/articles/cox-2-inhibitors.html. Reproduced with permission.

CHAPTER 37 Providing Paramedic Care in Resource-Limited Settings

3. For patients in severe pain, a strong opioid should be administered, such as morphine, fentanyl, pethidine, hydromorphone and buprenorphine. Pharmacological effects are relatively linear; therefore, titration can be used to manage analgesia. Remember to include a non-opioid and/or an adjuvant, which works in conjunction with the weak opioid.

Non-pharmacological adjuvant therapies provide a synergic effect and can be used in conjunction along all steps of the analgesic ladder. Examples that could be considered, depending on environment or equipment available, include, but are not limited to, splintage and immobilisation of fractures; use of temperature such as cold (for burns, sprains or musculoskeletal injury) or heat (for sprains and strains); elevation; local anaesthesia infiltration; and psychosocial reassurance (providing reduction of anxiety and comfort from friends or family).

Consider the use of antiemetics, which is a common side-effect of opioid use. Within the case, the patient was found to experience nausea and vomiting after morphine administration.

Local anaesthesia infiltration, such as the use of lidocaine (lignocaine), bupivacaine and prilocaine, is common within the hospital environment and could be considered should the clinician be trained and within their scope of practice. Ensure that prior to administration of local anaesthetics, there is adequate venous access and availability of resources. The use of surface anatomy is usually sufficient, but ideally the use of ultrasound will improve success. Contraindications to consider include allergy to local anaesthetics, infection at the proposed site, and bleeding disorders (anticoagulant therapy and thrombocytopenia in the event of an arterial puncture). Recognition of local anaesthetic toxicity and a knowledge of where and how to access lipid emulsion (Intralipid) are important considerations when using large volumes of local anaesthetics.

Peripheral nerve blocks can be a very useful option in remote or resource-limited settings. The use of POCUS in paramedic practice is increasing, and along with it the options available to paramedics for nerve blocks. However, even in the absence of POCUS, landmark-guided nerve blocks of the femoral nerve or fascia iliaca compartment can be valuable.

In a resource-limited environment, consideration of the availability of analgesia is important. The half-life elimination of a medication can be helpful in titration of analgesic administration, but this should be taken as a guide to assist with dosage titration (**Table 37.1**).

Table 37.1 Half-life for various analgesics

Analgesic	Half-life (hours)
Paracetamol	2–4
Aspirin	2–4
Ibuprofen	3–4
Codeine	2–3
Oxycodone (PO)	2–3
Hydrocodone (PO)	2–4
Morphine	2–3
Fentanyl	20–30 minutes

Source: Based on Hameed, M., Hameed, H. and Erdek, M., 2010. Pain management in pancreatic cancer. *Cancers*, 3(1), pp. 43–60.

SECTION 10   Special Circumstances

A stepwise, multi-regime analgesic selection, taking into consideration half-life elimination, should be considered for patient management within a resource-limited environment.

Question 3: What Are the Considerations for Fluid Balance?

Fluid balance is important in the prolonged field care phase in a resource-limited setting. The case study presents the distance to the patient as a four-hour drive; therefore, it could be safely assumed that the injury has occurred more than hours ago. In tropical environments like PNG, dehydration is a major factor with loss of body fluids through sweating and urination. Brearley et al.[4] conducted studies of physiological responses of heat-acclimatised health care workers in tropical conditions (mean ambient temperatures of 29.3 °C and relative humidity of 50.3%, apparent temperature of 27.9 °C) for 150 minutes (3.5 hours), which resulted in average sweating of 0.54 L per hour, consumption of 0.36 L of fluid per hour with a net loss of 0.7% of body mass. This would be different based on the workload intensity, fitness, environmental factors and the type of clothing the patient was wearing; however, a 0.5 L per hour rate of loss could be presumed for this patient.

Dehydration predisposes individuals to heat illnesses and electrolyte changes. In addition, dehydration compromises wound healing due to compromised perfusion, increases length of hospital stay and increases morbidity. Sweating is a means for thermoregulation and results in incidental losses of electrolytes. Mao et al.[5] found that mean losses of various electrolytes among teenage soccer players compared with sedentary students amounted to electrolyte loss of 1800 mg sodium, 240 mg potassium and 20 mg calcium per hour in sweat. Normal urine output for a healthy adult male patient should be in the range of 0.5 mL/kg/hour.

Monitoring for dehydration is important. Some common physical signs of dehydration include (in an average 70 kg male patient = 40 L circulating volume):[6]

- **Mild (<5%) = 2.5 L deficit**
    o   Mild thirst
    o   Dry mucous membranes
    o   Concentrated urine
- **Moderate (5%–8%) = 4 L deficit**
    o   Moderate thirst
    o   Reduced skin turgor (elasticity), especially arms, forehead, chest and abdomen
    o   Tachycardia
- **Severe (9%–12%) = 6 L deficit**
    o   Great thirst
    o   Reduced skin turgor and decreased intraocular pressure (eyeball)
    o   Collapsed veins, sunken eyes, 'gaunt' face
    o   Postural hypotension
    o   Oliguria (<400 mL urine/24 hours)
- **Very severe (>12%) >6 L deficit**
    o   Signs of shock.

In a remote, resource-limited setting, replacement of fluids and electrolytes is challenging. An accurate method of assessment for fluid status can be achieved in a critical care

CHAPTER 37 Providing Paramedic Care in Resource-Limited Settings

setting through documenting fluid intake, fluid output and daily weights. This will be challenging in resource-limited settings. Physical assessment of fluid hydration status can be performed to provide the prehospital clinician with clues to the amount of net fluid deficit. End-organ perfusion is the ultimate goal and to prevent hypovolaemic shock from occurring.

In a resource-limited setting, the availability of intravenous fluids is challenging. Crystalloids are normally carried within a prehospital setting; generally, a combination of normal saline, Hartmann's solution or compound sodium lactate, and 5% or 10% dextrose in water. None of these are normal in any respect and do not replace all incidental losses. Even in small amounts, hypotonic intravenous fluids may cause dilutional hyponatraemia. There are also the secondary issues of carriage to remote conditions; a severe dehydration could indicate approximately 6 L deficits and most carriage of 6 kg of intravenous fluids is impractical.

Oral fluid replacement should therefore be encouraged to maintain end-organ perfusion in prolonged field care in resource-limited settings. Fluid should be consumed in approximately 200 mL aliquots to promote gastric emptying. Oral rehydration solution should be considered if there is excess sweating or exercise. Be aware of formulations and concentration if using oral rehydration solution; excess glucose will delay gastric emptying and promote osmotic diarrhoea; excess sodium can cause nausea. Direct consumption of salt tablets without dilution could cause gastric irritation and vomiting. The Wilderness Medical Society guidelines suggest 250 mL of oral rehydration solution intake every 30 minutes for the first four to six hours to make up for incidental losses in moderate dehydration.[7]

End-organ perfusion is the ultimate goal, and in prolonged field care and in resource-limited settings, urine output measurement is a good surrogate for critical care monitoring and is a sensitive marker for volume status and end-organ (renal) perfusion through adequate renal blood flow. Urine output of approximately 0.5 mL/kg/hour in adults, 1 mL/kg/hour in paediatric patients and 2 mL/kg/hour in infants aged less than one year should be aimed for.[8] Urine should appear clear or straw coloured on visual inspection; dark or cola coloured is a serious sign of dehydration and lack of end-organ perfusion.

Question 4: What Wound Management Should You Consider in Prolonged Field Care?

Wound management of the open fracture should be considered within this patient. In this case study, it appears there have been several hours between the initial injury and paramedic arrival. The wound has also been grossly contaminated by local improvised health care by placing mud onto the wound. Flies and mosquitoes are another source of zoonotic infection. Irrigation of the wound in prolonged field care in resource-limited settings is important.

Saline Irrigation

Saline irrigation, be it in the form of 30 mL containers or 1000 mL saline bags, is cumbersome to carry and administer in resource-limited settings. The traditional use of an intravenous giving set to irrigate a wound will only suffice where access to such equipment is available.

If there are clean sources of water, then tap water has been shown to be as effective in wound irrigation as saline in non-contaminated wounds.[9] The use of cooled boiled water could be considered to irrigate a wound. Pressure irrigation with an adequate pressure is required to ensure its effectiveness; the ideal is 5 to 8 psi, which is approximately the same pressure as that achieved from an 18-gauge needle or catheter attached to a syringe. An alternate source could also be achieved from a plastic bag filled with water and a hole the size of a toothpick.[6] Gross contamination should be removed (such as mud or other foreign debris), and once irrigated with at least 500 mL, the wound should ideally be covered with a moist, sterile dressing. In resource-limited settings, the use of clean clothes or even plastic cling wrap should be considered as an alternative. The wound should be left open and should **NOT** be closed or sutured.

Antibiotics

Administration of antibiotics, if available, should be considered in heavily contaminated compound fractures or other open wounds where there is a significant distance to hospital. An open fracture allows for communication of the bone and/or joint to the external environment, potentially increasing the risk for bacterial infection, which in turn increases the potential for osteomyelitis, necrotising fasciitis and delays in wound healing. A rule of thumb is that if an open wound is located near a joint, it is assumed to be connected with the joint. Prehospital probing of a wound does not change any management and increases the risk of osteomyelitis; therefore it should not be performed. Time duration is another significant factor; delays of more than three hours to operative washout increase the risk of infection. Ideally, intravenous antibiotics should be considered. The most common would be a first-generation cephalosporin for gram-positive coverage, or clindamycin if allergies exist for penicillin. Consider gram-negative coverage if in contact with contaminated water. Schmitt et al.[10] provide a good guide for antibiotic choice for open fractures (**Table 37.2**). Oral amoxicillin-clavulanic acid could also be considered in resource-limited settings.

Tetanus

Tetanus should also be considered in those requiring prolonged field care. Tetanus is a potentially fatal disease caused by the tetanospasmin toxin from the *Clostridium tetani* spore-forming gram-positive bacillus. The spores are hardy and are commonly found in soil and faeces of humans and animals. These spores are generally resistant to heat and antiseptics, and once they have accessed the body through wounds or open fractures, they tend to grow under anaerobic conditions with low oxygen. Incubation occurs in one to two days, but can be as long as 21 days. The tetanospasmin toxin causes the clinical condition of tetanus through blocking of the inhibitory pathways (gamma-aminobutyric acid), resulting in sustained excitatory nervous impulses and the tetany observed from sustained muscular contractions. Clinically, initial contractions are observed in the wounded area before becoming generalised. Pain, headache, muscle rigidity and trismus (lock-jaw) from severe contraction of the masseter muscle are seen in 80% of cases of generalised tetanus. Laryngeal obstruction and chest wall rigidity lead to respiratory failure which is the most common cause of direct death from tetanus. Autonomic dysfunction including arrhythmias, hypermetabolism, hypertension, diaphoresis and fever can also result, and these, along with spasms, can be observed for weeks to months.

CHAPTER 37 Providing Paramedic Care in Resource-Limited Settings

Table 37.2 Antibiotic choices for contaminated open fractures in prolonged field care

Type of injury and level of contamination	First-generation cephalosporin (gram +ve coverage) Cefazolin / Cephazolin	If anaphylactic to penicillin Clindamycin	Aminoglycocide (gram −ve coverage) Gentamicin	Broad spectrum (gram +ve and gram −ve coverage) Piperacillin / Tazobactam (Tazocin)
Wound <1 cm; minimal contamination or soft tissue damage	<50 kg: 1 g Q 8 hr 50–100 kg: 2 g Q 8 hr >100 kg: 3 g Q 8 hr	<80 kg: 600 mg Q 8 hr >80 kg: 900 mg Q 8 hr		
Wound 1–10 cm; moderate soft tissue damage; comminution of fracture	<50 kg: 1 g Q 8 hr 50–100 kg: 2 g Q 8 hr >100 kg: 3 g Q 8 hr	<80 kg: 600 mg Q 8 hr >80 kg: 900 mg Q 8 hr		
Severe soft tissue damage and substantial contamination with associated vascular injury	<50 kg: 1 g Q 8 hr 50–100 kg: 2 g Q 8 hr >100 kg: 3 g Q 8 hr	<80 kg: 600 mg Q 8 hr >80 kg: 900 mg Q 8 hr	Loading dose: Child or <50 kg: 2.5 mg/kg Adult: 5 mg/kg	
Farmyard, soil or standing water, irrespective of wound size or severity				<100 kg: 3.375 g Q 6 hr >100 kg: 4.5 g Q 6 hr

Source: Adapted from Alam, N., Oskam, E., Stassen, P.M et al., 2018. Prehospital antibiotics in the ambulance for sepsis: a multicentre, open label, randomised trial. *Lancet Respiratory Medicine*, 6(1), pp. 40–50 and Schmitt, S.K., Sexton, D.J. and Baron, E.L., 2014. Treatment and Prevention of Osteomyelitis Following Trauma in Adults [Online]. UpToDate. http://www.uptodate.com/contents/treatment-and-prevention-of-osteomyelitis-following-trauma-in-adults

Treatment of tetanus is through wound debridement in a medical facility to remove devitalised tissue and foreign bodies. It is for this reason that open wounds should not be closed in the field and should not be sutured. Passive immunisation with tetanus immunoglobulin should be considered if available. Typical dosages are:

- 250 units human tetanus immunoglobulin (IM) for adults
- 500 units if the wound is >12 hours old, heavily contaminated or the patient's weight is >90kg.

SECTION 10 Special Circumstances

Adverse reactions from tetanus immunisations include pain, a palpable lump around the injection site, swelling and erythema within two to eight hours of injection (20%) and anaphylaxis (0.6 to 3 per million doses).

Key Evidence

Reviews

- Brearley, M.B., Heaney, M.F. and Norton, I.N., 2013. Physiological responses of medical team members to a simulated emergency in tropical field conditions. *Prehospital and Disaster Medicine*, 28(2), pp. 139–144.
- Moscati, R.M., Mayrose, J., Reardon, R.F. et al., 2007. A multicenter comparison of tap water versus sterile saline for wound irrigation. *Academic Emergency Medicine*, 14(5), pp. 404–409.
- O'Brien CL, Menon M, Jomha NM., 2014. Controversies in the management of open fractures. *Open Orthopaedics Journal*, 8, pp. 178–184.
- Tobias, J.D., 2014. Acute pain management in infants and children – part 2: intravenous opioids, intravenous nonsteroidal anti-inflammatory drugs, and managing adverse effects. *Pediatric Annals*, 43(7), pp. e169–e175.

Randomised Controlled Trials

- Alam, N., Oskam, E., Stassen, P.M et al., 2018. Prehospital antibiotics in the ambulance for sepsis: a multicentre, open label, randomised trial. *Lancet Respiratory Medicine*, 6(1), pp. 40–50.
- Rickard, C., O'Meara, P., McGrail, M. et al., 2007. A randomized controlled trial of intranasal fentanyl vs intravenous morphine for analgesia in the prehospital setting. *American Journal of Emergency Medicine*, 25(8), pp. 911–917.

Self-Reflection Questions

1. What do you think the role of a paramedic is in prolonged field care?
2. What role do you think long-acting analgesics have in prolonged field care?
3. What is the role of antibiotics?
4. What alternatives for equipment do you have in your practice?
5. These complex patients require a detailed handover when you arrive at the hospital. Using the table below, prepare a handover of the patient described using the IMIST AMBO format.

Introduction
Mechanism
Injuries
Symptoms
Treatment
Allergies
Medications
Background history
Other information

References

1. Smith, M., Johnston, K. and Withnall, R., 2021. Systematic approach to delivering prolonged field care in a prehospital care environment. *BMJ Military Health*, 167(2), pp. 93–98.
2. Federal Aviation Authority, 2015. *Single-pilot crew resource management* [Online]. Available at: https://www.faa.gov/sites/faa.gov/files/2022-01/Single%20Pilot%20Crew%20Resource%20Management.pdf
3. World Health Organization, 1986. *Cancer Pain Relief*. Geneva: World Health Organization.
4. Brearley, M.B., Heaney, M.F. and Norton, I.N., 2013. Physiological responses of medical team members to a simulated emergency in tropical field conditions. *Prehospital and Disaster Medicine*, 28(2), pp. 139–144.
5. Mao, I., Chen, M.L. and Ko, Y.C., 2001. Electrolyte loss in sweat and iodine deficiency in a hot environment. *Archives of Environmental Health: An International Journal*, 56(3), pp. 271–277.
6. Talley, N.J. and O'Connor, S., 2010. *Clinical Examination: A Systematic Guide to Physical Diagnosis*, 6th edn. Chatswood: Elsevier Health Sciences.
7. Wilderness Medical Society, 2006. *Practice Guidelines for Wilderness Emergency Care*, 5th edn. Austin: Wilderness Medical Society.
8. American College of Surgeons, 2018. *Advanced Trauma Life Support*, 10th edn. Chicago: American College of Surgeons.
9. Moscati, R.M., Mayrose, J., Reardon, R.F. et al., 2007. A multicenter comparison of tap water versus sterile saline for wound irrigation. *Academic Emergency Medicine*, 14(5), pp. 404–409.
10. Schmitt, S.K., Sexton, D.J. and Baron, E.L., 2014. Treatment and prevention of osteomyelitis following trauma in adults [Online]. UpToDate. Available at: http://www.uptodate.com/contents/treatment-and-prevention-of-osteomyelitis-following-trauma-in-adults.

Index

NOTE: Page numbers followed by *f* denote figures; those followed by *t* denote tables.

A

ABD. *See* Acute behavioural disturbance
Acid-suppressive therapies, 129
ACS. *See* Altered conscious state
ACT-FAST stroke algorithm, 171, 171*f*
Acute behavioural disturbance (ABD)
    adverse events, 314–315, 314*t*
    case history, 307–308
    causes of, 308–309
    definition of, 308
    IM medication, 312–313
    indications, 311–312
    patient assessment, 309
    sedation assessment tool, 309, 310*t*
    verbal and non-verbal techniques, 310–311
Acute chest pain, 116–122
    case history, 116–117
    causes of, 84
Acute coronary syndromes (ACS), 119
Acute ischaemic stroke
    assessment and management of, 168–179
    case history, 168–170
    clinical diagnosis, 172–174
    general stroke screening tools, 170
    prehospital management responsibilities, 178–179
    treatment, 175–178
Acute pulmonary oedema
    case history, 133–134
    clinical features, 135*t*
    contraindications of CPAP for, 139, 139*t*
    diagnosis, 134–136
    NIV role of, 136–137
    paramedic management of, 136–137
    risks, complications and, 139, 139*t*
    treatment, 139–142
Acute respiratory failure (ARF), 51
Acute trauma coagulopathy (ATC), 279–280
    haemostatic therapy, 279
    management of, 279
Adenosine, 104
Adrenaline, 78, 78*t*, 122*t*
Advance care directive (ACD), 379
Airway protection, 5
Altered conscious state (ACS), 5–6, 57, 103, 204
Altered level of consciousness
    AEIOU-TIPS, 149*f*
    assessment, 149–151
    case history, 147–148
    clinical syndromes, 153–154
    hazards, 148
    management strategies, 151–153
Altered mental status (AMS), 298–299
Aminophylline, 64–65
Anaesthesia drugs, 7–8, 8*t*–9*t*
Analgesia, multimodal, 183–186, 185*t*
    administration, 186–188, 187*t*
    analgesic ladder, 385, 386*f*
    plan for, 189
    procedural sedation, 188, 188*t*
    purposes of, 189–190
Anatomically difficult airway, 24–33
    case history, 24–25
    defined, 26
Anticipated clinical course, 5, 6, 57
Apnoeic oxygenation, hypoxia, 18
ARF. *See* Acute respiratory failure

395

Index

Asthma. *See* Severe asthma
ATC. *See* Acute trauma coagulopathy
Atrioventricular nodal re-entrant tachycardia (AVNRT), 102
Atrioventricular re-entrant tachycardia (AVRT), 102

B
Bacterial tracheitis, 333–334, 334t
Basic life support
    high-performance CPR, 213, 214f
Bi-level positive airway pressure (BiPAP), 56
Bradycardia, 94
Brain injury, 163
    brain imaging, 172–174
    Brainstem stroke, 173
Breath, shortness of, 116–122
Broad complex tachycardia
    case history, 108–110
    defined, 110
    ECG characteristics of, 110–112, 111t
    intervention in, 113
    management strategies, 113–114
    requirement for sedation, 114
    treatment of, 112–113

C
Calcium channel blockers, 104
Canadian Airway Focus Group (CAFG), 26
Capture beat, 111, 111t
Cardiac arrest, 7
    case history, 239–240
    causes of, 240–241
    diagnosing hyperkalaemia, 241
    ECG signs of, hyperkalaemia, 241–242
    in pregnancy, 243
        algorithm, 244–245, 244f
        manually displacing uterus, 244, 244f
        obstetric and non-obstetric causes, 243, 244t
    steps of, hyperkalaemic, 242–243
Cardiogenic shock (CS), 73, 85
    causes, 119
    defined, 117–118
Cardiopulmonary resuscitation (CPR), 211

Cardiovascular toxicity, 303
    alkalinisation of serum, 303
    serum sodium load, 303
Cerebellar stroke, 173
Choreography role, CPR, 215
Cincinnati Prehospital Stroke Scale (CPSS), 170, 171t
Clinical frailty scale (CFS), 378f
C-Mac hyperangulated video laryngoscope, 9, 10f
Compensated shock, 75
Compound sodium lactate (CSL), 77
Congestion
    features of, 119t
    initial assessment for, 119–120
Continuous pulmonary airway pressure (CPAP), 136–137, 136f
    use of, 137–139, 138f
Conventional cardiopulmonary resuscitation (CCPR), 220
COVID-19 pandemic, 332
    respiratory failure, 6, 56
Cricothyroid membrane (CTM), 30, 31f
Cricothyroidotomy, 30–33
Critical care paramedic (CCP), 189, 229, 291
Critically ill patients, complications of, 6–7
Croup
    additional therapies, 338
    bacterial tracheitis, 333–334, 334t
    case history, 327–328
    clinical features, 329, 331t, 334t
    definition of, 328–329
    differential diagnosis, 331–332
    vs. epiglottitis, 332–333, 334
    nebulised adrenaline, 335–336
    steroids, 336–337
    symptoms, 329
    treatments algorithm, 334, 335t
    Westley croup severity score, 329, 330t
Crystalloids, 77
c-spine injuries (CSIs), 259

D
Damage control resuscitation (DCR), 279
DCC. *See* Delaying/deferring clamping of the umbilical cord

Index

Decompensated shock, 75, 270
Delayed-sequence intubation (DSI), 18
Delaying/deferring clamping of the umbilical cord (DCC), 344
Difficult airway, 26
Difficult face-mask ventilation, 29, 29t
Difficult tracheal intubation
    HEAVEN criteria for, 28t
    history and anatomical features, 26–28
    LEMON mnemonic for, 27t, 28f
Distributive shock, 74
Dobutamine, 78t, 79, 122t
Dopamine, vasoactive agent, 78t, 79
Drug therapies, evidence for, 64–65

E

ECMO. *See* Extracorporeal membrane oxygenation
ECPR. *See* Extracorporeal cardiopulmonary resuscitation
Endovascular thrombectomy, 175–176, 176f
Epiglottitis, 332–333
    vs. croup, 334
    treatments algorithm, 334, 335t
European Society of Cardiology (ERC), 139
Extracorporeal cardiopulmonary resuscitation (ECPR)
    case history, 218–219
    complications and challenges, 224–225
    CPR survival curves, 222, 223f
    definition of, 220
    ECMO, 220–221
    eCPR *vs.* mechanical CPR, 220f
    equipment set up, 224, 225f
    hospital *vs.* prehospital, 223
    OOHCA to ECPR, 222f
    phases of, 224
    V-A ECMO, 221f
Extracorporeal membrane oxygenation (ECMO), 220–221
Extra-uterine life, newborn, 346–348

F

Face-mask ventilation (FMV), 29
Fentanyl, 7–9, 184, 187–9, 285

Finger thoracostomy, technique for, 290
Fluid administration, 121
Foetus, physiology of, 343–344
Fusion beat, 111, 111t

G

General stroke screening tools, 170, 171t
GINA. *See* Global Initiative for Asthma
Glasgow coma score (GCS), 159, 159t, 171–172
Global Initiative for Asthma (GINA), 65

H

Haemorrhagic loss, 74
Haemorrhagic shock, 277–278
Head or neurological injury, 20–21
Head-up positioning, hypoxia, 18
Heart failure, 19, 79, 94, 134–140
High-performance CPR
    basic life support, 213, 214f
    case history, 211–212
    communication and team leadership, 215–216
    definition of, 212–213
    education and training, 215
    elements of, 213
    feedback and performance monitoring, 215
    role of choreography, 215
Humanitarian, 5, 6, 57
Hyperkalaemia, cardiac arrest
    causes of, 241
    ECG signs, 241–242
Hyperthermia
    case history, 195–196
    heat loss, 196–197
    stages of, 197–198
    treatment, 198
Hypoglycaemia, 177
Hypoperfusion
    features of, 119t
    initial assessment for, 119–120
Hypotension, 6–7, 18–19, 94
Hypothermia
    case history, 195–196
    heat loss, 196–197
    stages of, 196
    treatment for, 197

Index

Hypovolaemia, cardiac arrest, 231–232
Hypovolaemic shock, 74
Hypoxaemia, 6, 7
Hypoxia, 18
    cardiac arrest, 233

I
Inodilators, 121
Inotropy, 73, 121, 122*t*
Intubation
    considerations for, 57
    indications and, 57
    physiological goals of, 21
Irreversible shock, 75

K
Ketamine, 7, 7*t*, 184, 185, 187
King vision channelled videolaryngoscope, 9, 10*f*

L
Left hemispheric stroke, 173
Levosimendan, 122*t*

M
Macintosh-style videolaryngoscope, 9, 10
Magnesium, 64–65
Mechanical ventilation
    benefits of, 41–42
    case history, 39–40
    considerations for, 57
    high pressure alarms, paramedic response to, 44
    indications, 57
    patient with life-threatening asthma, principles in, 66
    problems associated with, 45–46
    settings guide, 42, 43*f*
    sources of, 44–45
Metaraminol, 8
Methoxyflurane, 186
Mid-arm point (MAP), 291
Milrinone, 122*t*
Minnesota tube, UGIB, 130
Mobile Stroke Unit (MSU), 174

Multimodal analgesia, 183–186, 185*t*
Myocardial infarction
    case history, 82–84
    complications of, 84–85
    contemporary outcomes for, 88–89
    features in, 84
    in-hospital trajectory of, 88
    thrombolysis, 85–86
Myocardial ischaemia, 94

N
NACA. *See* National Asthma Council Australia
Narrow complex tachycardia
    case history, 100–101
    defined, 101
    diagnosis for, 101, 101*f*
    management options for, 103–105
    paramedic management of, 106
National Asthma Council Australia (NACA), 63–64
Nebulised adrenaline, 335–336
Needle thoracocentesis (NT), 286, 287*f*
Neurological toxicity, 304
Neurosurgery, 176–177
Newborn, care of
    apnoeic, 347–348
    case history, 342–343
    DCC, 344
    environment, 345
    extra-uterine life, 346–348
    heart rate, 349–350
    immediate care, 346
    initial assessment, 346
    physiology of, 342–343
    preterm infants, 345
    signs of, 346
    term and near-term infants, 345
NIV. *See* Non-invasive ventilation
Non-haemorrhagic loss, 74
Non-invasive ventilation (NIV), 6, 18, 20, 56
    in APO, role of, 136–137
    in asthma, role of, 65
    prehospital application of, 57
    use of, 6

Index

Non-ST-elevation myocardial infarction (NSTEMI), 119
Noradrenaline, 122t
    vasoactive agent, 78, 78t

O

Obstructive lung pathology, 44, 44t, 46
Obstructive shock, 73–74, 277
Occasional intubators, 5
Older patient
    advance care directive, 379
    ambulance requests, 370–371
    bioavailability, 374
    case history, 369–370
    CCP role, 375
    clearance, 374–375
    clinician bias, 376
    distribution, 374
    'minor/major' injury mechanisms, 376
    physical assessment, 377
    physiological changes, 371, 372t–374t
    polypharmacy, 375
    trauma physiological responses, 376
Out-of-hospital cardiac arrest (OHCA), 222, 230
Oxygen therapy, 56, 84

P

Packed red blood cells (PRBC), 128, 279
Patient with life-threatening asthma
    intubation and ventilation in, risks of, 66
mechanical ventilation principles in, 66
    PEEP. See Positive end-expiratory pressure
Penetrating trauma
    acute trauma coagulopathy, 279–280
    case history, 275–277
    haemorrhagic shock, 277–278
    management hierarchy, 280–281
    obstructive shock, 277–278
    tranexamic acid, 282
Perfusion, 72
    prehospital therapies, 119, 120, 120f
Permissive hypotension, 279–281
Phenylephrine, 8, 78t, 79
Physiologically difficult airway, 13–22
    case history, 13–15
    concept of, 16
    definition of, 15
    prediction factors, 17
    strategies, 17–21
    types of, 15, 16f
    VAPOUR mnemonic, 17
Point-of-care ultrasound (POCUS), 31, 52, 286
Positive end-expiratory pressure (PEEP), 18
Positive-pressure ventilation (PPV)
    airway, 347
    breathing, 347–348
    circulation, 348
    drugs, 348
Post-intubation phase
    strategies in, 22
Postpartum haemorrhage (PPH)
    blood volume lost, 354–355
    case history, 353–354
    definitions of, 354t
    management of, 361–363
    physiology/pathophysiology
        causes of, 356
        tears, 357
        thrombin, 357
        tissue, 357
        tone, 356–357
    treatment for
        bi-manual compression, 360, 361f
        fundal massage, 357–358
        non-pneumatic anti-shock trousers, 360f
        tranexamic acid, 358–359
        uterotonic drugs, 358t–359t
        volume replacement, 359
PPH. See Postpartum haemorrhage
PPV. See Positive-pressure ventilation
Pregnancy, cardiac arrest, 243
    algorithm, 244–245, 244f
    manually displacing uterus, 244, 244f
    obstetric and non-obstetric causes, 243, 244t
Prehospital airway management, 31
    cricothyroidotomy, 33
    development of, 32–33, 33f
    rescue techniques, 32–33
    risk-benefit analysis, 31–32
    tracheal intubation, 32

Index

Prehospital point-of-care blood lactate assessment (POCBLA), 205–206
Prehospital rapid sequence intubation (RSI)
   case history, 3–4
   complications of, 6–7
   drugs, 7–8, 8t–9t
   evidence based for, 4–5
   indications for, 5–6, 57
   video laryngoscopes used in, 9, 10f
Prehospital sepsis management
   aetiologies, 201–202
   benefits and challenges, 203–205
   case history, 200–201
   definition of, 202
   incidence and impact, 201–202
   management of, 203
   POCBLA, 205–206
Pre-oxygenation, hypoxia, 18
Prolonged field care, 383–385
Pulseless electrical activity (PEA), 229

R

Rapid sequence intubation (RSI), prehospital
   case history, 3–4
   complications of, 6–7
   drugs, 7–8, 8t–9t
   evidence based for, 4–5
   indications for, 5–6
   video laryngoscopes used in, 9, 10f
REBOA. See Resuscitative endovascular balloon occlusion of the aorta
Refractory cardiac arrest
   case history, 218–219
   complications and challenges, 224–225
   CPR survival curves, 222, 223f
   definition of, 220
   ECMO, 220–221
   eCPR vs. mechanical CPR, 220f
   equipment set up, 224, 225f
   hospital vs. prehospital, 223
   OOHCA to ECPR, 222f
   phases of, 224
   V-A ECMO, 221f
Resource-limited settings, paramedic care
   antibiotic choices, 390, 391t
   case history, 382–383

COX-2 selective NSAIDs, 385, 386f
fluid balance, 388–389
half-life analgesics, 387t
IMSAFE checklist, 384–385
prolonged field care, 383–384
saline irrigation, 389–390
tetanus, 390
three-step analgesic ladder, 385, 386f
typical dosages, 391–392
Respiratory failure, 5, 6
   ABCDE approach, 52, 53f–55f, 55
   aetiologies and prevalence of, 51
   BLUE protocol, 55f
   case history, 49–50
   management of, 55–56
   type 1 vs. type 2, 57–58
Restrictive lung pathology, 44, 44t, 46–47
Resuscitative endovascular balloon occlusion of the aorta (REBOA), 271, 281
Right heart failure, 19–20
   diagnosis and assessment of, 19
   fluid and vasopressor resuscitation, 19
   principles of intubation, 20
Right hemispheric stroke, 173 Rocuronium, 7, 8t
RSI. See Rapid sequence intubation

S

Sedation assessment tool (SAT), 309, 310t
Sedation-facilitated pre-oxygenation, 18
Sengstaken-Blakemore tube, 128, 130f
Sepsis. See Prehospital sepsis management
Severe asthma
   beta-2 agonist role, 63–64
   classification of, 61–62, 62t, 63t
   intubation and ventilation, risks of, 66
   role of NIV in, 65
Severe metabolic acidosis
   bicarbonate role, 321–322
   blood gas measurement, 320
   case history, 317–318
   clinical assessment, 319
   diabetic ketoacidosis, 319
   end-tidal carbon dioxide ($EtCO_2$), 320
   hyperchloraemic metabolic acidosis, 319
   identification and assessment, 20

Index

lactic acidosis, 318–319
loss of bicarbonate, 319
management of, 320–321
non-invasive ventilation, 20
principles of intubation, 20
Severe/uncontrolled pain
administration risks, 186–188, 187t
case history, 182–183
methoxyflurane role, 186
multimodal analgesia, 183–186, 185t
plan for, 189
procedural sedation, 188, 188t
purposes of, 189–190
Severity-based triage tools, 170–171
Shock
cardiogenic, 73
case history, 71–72
definition of, 72–73
distributive, 74
fluid administration in, 75–77
hypovolaemic, 74
obstructive, 73–74
progress, 75
stabilising patient in, 75
types of, 73–74, 74f
vasoactive medications, 77–79, 78t
Shocked blunt trauma
'CABc' approach, 267
case history, 266–267
devices, 268f
fluids and medications, 270
permissive hypotension, 269–270
prehospital blood transfusion, 270–271
prehospital intervention, 272
REBOA, 271
role of tourniquets, 269
thoracic injury, 272
treatable causes, 268t
Short-acting beta agonists (SABA), 63–64
Society for Cardiovascular Angiography and Interventions (SCAI), 117, 118t
Somatostatin analogues, 129
ST-elevation myocardial infarction (STEMI), 119
Steroids, 336–337
Supraglottic airway devices (SADs), 29–30
Supraventricular tachycardia (SVT), 102, 103–105

paramedic management of, 106
post-reversion management of, 105
Survival curves, ECPR, 222, 223f
Synchronised cardioversion, 104–105
Synchronised intermittent mandatory ventilation (SIMV), 45
Syncope, 94

T

Targeted treatment, 5–6
TCA. *See* Traumatic cardiac arrest
Tension pneumothorax, cardiac arrest, 233
anatomical locations, 288f
case history, 284–285
diagnosis of, 290
finger thoracostomy, 289–291
lung ultrasound, 286
mid-arm point, 291
mid-clavicular line, 289f
needle thoracocentesis, 286, 287f
POCUS, 286
Termination of resuscitation
algorithms and decision-making, 252
bystander support, 251
case history, 247–248
clinical evidence, 248
ethical justification, 248–249
family needs, 251
patient death, 250t
review of, family, 249
Thrombolysis, 175
complications of, 87
contraindications for, 86–87, 86t
evidence for, 85–86
indications for, 87
Tranexamic acid (TXA), 282
Transcutaneous pacing, 97–98, 97f
Trapped patient
case history, 257–258
definition of, 258
extrication methods, 261, 262t
medical management, 263
morbidity and mortality rates, 258–259
predict pattern of injury, 260–261, 261t
rescue teams, 261
treatment of, 262–263

Index

Traumatic brain injury (TBI)
    assessment, 159–160
    case history, 157–158
    epidemiology of, 160–161
    management strategies, 162–163
    'red flags,' 161, 162t
    signs of, 164–165
Traumatic cardiac arrest (TCA)
    algorithm, 232f
    case history, 228–230
    causes of, 230–233
    factors of, 234t
    hypovolaemia, 231–232
    hypoxia, 233
    out-of-hospital cardiac arrest, 230
    tension pneumothorax, 233
    treatment for, 233–234
Treatment for, PPH
    bi-manual compression, 360, 361f
    fundal massage, 357–358
    non-pneumatic anti-shock trousers, 360t
    tranexamic acid, 358–359
    uterotonic drugs, 358t–359t
    volume replacement, 359
Tricyclic antidepressant toxicity
    aetiologies of, 300f
    altered mental status, 298–299
    cardiovascular toxicity, 303
    case history, 297–298
    clinical effects/toxidromes, 300–301
    ECG, 302
    neurological toxicity, 304
    summary of, 305f
Types 1 and 2 respiratory failure, 57–58

U

Undifferentiated shock. *See* Shock
Unstable bradycardia, management of
    algorithm for, 96f
    case history, 92–93
    categories, 94
    causes, 94–95
    management of, 95–96
    methods and challenges in, 97–98
Upper gastrointestinal bleed (UGIB)
    blood administration in, 128
    case history, 124–125
    causes of, 127f
    defined, 126
    early management priorities in, 126–128
    endoscopic view of, 129f
    management, 129–130

V

VA-ECMO. *See* Veno-arterial extracorporeal membrane oxygenation
Valsalva manoeuvres, 103–104
Vasoactive agents, 121–122, 122t
Vasopressin, 78t, 79
Vasopressors, 19, 121, 122t
Veno-arterial extracorporeal membrane oxygenation (VA-ECMO), 221f
Ventilator-patient asynchrony, 45
Ventricular tachycardia (VT), 110, 111t
Video laryngoscopes (VL), 9, 10f

W

Westley Croup Severity Score, 329, 330t
Wolff-Parkinson-White (WPW) syndrome, 102